Introduction to PHYSICAL THERAPY

THIRD EDITION

Introduction to PHYSICAL THERAPY

THIRD EDITION

Michael A. Pagliarulo, PT, EdD
Professor
Department of Physical Therapy
Ithaca College
Ithaca, New York

MOSBY

ELSEVIER

MOSBY
ELSEVIER

11830 Westline Industrial Drive
St. Louis, Missouri 63146

INTRODUCTION TO PHYSICAL THERAPY, THIRD EDITION

ISBN-13: 978-0-323-03284-1
ISBN-10: 0-323-03284-2

Notice

Neither the Publisher nor the Authors assume any responsibility for any loss or injury and/or damage to persons or property arising out of or related to any use of the material contained in this book. It is the responsibility of the treating practitioner, relying on independent expertise and knowledge of the patient, to determine the best treatment and method of application for the patient.

The Publisher

ISBN-13: 978-0-323-03284-1
ISBN-10: 0-323-03284-2

Publishing Director: Linda Duncan
Senior Editor: Kathy Falk
Senior Developmental Editor: Christie M. Hart
Publishing Services Manager: Patricia Tannian
Design Direction: Bill Drone

Printed in the United States of America

Last digit is the print number: 9 8 7 6 5 4 3 2 1

Contributors

BARBARA C. BELYEA, PT, MS, CSCS

Clinical Associate Professor
Department of Physical Therapy
Ithaca College
Ithaca, New York

SUSAN E. BENNETT, PT, EdD, NCS, MSCS

Clinical Associate Professor
Departments of Rehabilitation Sciences and
    Neurology
State University of New York at Buffalo
Buffalo, New York

RAY A. BOONE, PT, MEd

Adjunct Associate Professor
Department of Physical Therapy
Ithaca College, Rochester Campus
Rochester, New York

CHERYL A. CARPENTER-DAVIS, PTA, EdD

Associate Dean and Articulation Coordinator
The Metropolitan Community Colleges
Independence, Missouri

JENNIFER E. COLLINS, PT, MPA, EdD

Chair and Associate Professor of Physical
    Therapy
Physical Therapy Department
Nazareth College
Rochester, New York

STACEY C. DUSING, PT, PhD

Assistant Professor
Department of Physical Therapy
Medical College of Virginia
Virginia Commonwealth University
Richmond, Virginia

HILARY B. GREENBERGER, PT, PhD, OCS

Associate Professor of Physical Therapy
Department of Physical Therapy
Ithaca College
Ithaca, New York

HELEN L. MASIN, PT, PhD

Associate Professor
Department of Physical Therapy
University of Miami
Miami, Florida

MICHAEL A. PAGLIARULO, PT, EdD

Professor
Department of Physical Therapy
Ithaca College
Ithaca, New York

SHREE PANDYA, PT, MS

Assistant Professor of Neurology and of
    Physical Medicine and Rehabilitation
School of Medicine and Dentistry
University of Rochester
Rochester, New York

v

ANGELA EASLEY ROSENBERG, DPH, PT

Assistant Professor
Division of Physical Therapy
Director of Training
Clinical Center for the Study of Development
    and Learning
University of North Carolina
Chapel Hill, North Carolina

LAURIE A. WALSH, PT, JD

Associate Professor of Physical Therapy
Physical Therapy Department
Daemen College
Amherst, New York

R. SCOTT WARD, PT, PhD

Professor and Chair
Division of Physical Therapy
University of Utah
Salt Lake City, Utah

JENNIFER WILSON, PT, MBA

Manager of Clinical Operations
Department of Physical Therapy
Nazareth College
Rochester, New York

Dedication

This book is dedicated to the communities and (former) residents who were so dramatically affected by the brutal force of Hurricane Katrina, which hit the Gulf Coast on August 29, 2005. While at this writing the region celebrates Mardi Gras to demonstrate its will to survive, this area will need years to recover from the massive destruction and personal upheaval. To that end, I am pledging 10% of my annual royalties from this edition to the community of Pearlington, Mississippi. Let me explain the connection with this edition.

My wife Tricia (who is also a physical therapist) and I enjoyed the sights and culinary delights of New Orleans while attending the Combined Sections Meeting of the American Physical Therapy Association in February 2005. We agreed to revisit the city during our travel from Ithaca, New York, to Portland, Oregon, where I planned to be on sabbatical for the spring of 2006. Completion of this edition was a primary purpose for the sabbatical. As we watched the disaster of Katrina unfold on CNN, we decided that during our southern journey across the United States we would offer assistance to Habitat for Humanity rather than travel as tourists. Opportunities at the time were limited, however, because the focus was on cleanup of the massive destruction rather than rebuilding. As we approached the area from Florida, we heard about a small organization, Hands On USA (now Hands On Network), that was providing relief services in Biloxi, Mississippi. After learning more about the agency, we decided to volunteer for a week. It was enlightening to see the extensive results and long-term impact that an agency with little or no bureaucracy could produce.

When we continued west through Mississippi, Tricia wanted to stop in Pearlington, a town she had seen featured in a CNN segment. This small community in Katrina's path had experienced the full force of the hurricane, but because of its size was not receiving the attention of major cities such as New Orleans. As we drove through town, the destruction caused by the combination of high winds and flooding was apparent. The elementary school gym (where the floodwater mark could be seen on the regulation-height basketball backboard) had been converted into a center for relief goods and services. As we chatted with the coordinator, we were impressed by the resiliency of those who remained (700 of the 1500 residents) and their determination to resurrect the town. The effort, however, will take years.

This dedication and my pledge are minuscule relative to the ongoing needs of the region. I am happy to offer assistance and encourage others to continue their support for this area in the years to come.

Michael A. Pagliarulo
Tuesday, February 28, 2006
Mardi Gras

Preface

The content and organization of this text continue to evolve, as do the profession and practice of physical therapy. Each chapter has been updated to reflect current data, clinical practice, changes within the American Physical Therapy Association (APTA), influence of Vision 2020, and attention to professionalism. Several photos have been replaced, and new ones have been added. Two new chapters address the issues of communication and reimbursement, which are so essential in our profession.

Before the revisions are described in more detail, readers should be assured that the fundamental intent and approach of the text have not changed. This text continues to provide a comprehensive description of the profession (Part I) and practice (Part II) of physical therapy. The book is not intended to teach the skills of practice, but rather to provide a description of the major areas of practice following the *Guide to Physical Therapist Practice*. The role of the physical therapist using the patient/client management model shows the broad scope of practice. The role of the physical therapist assistant is addressed in a separate chapter but is also incorporated throughout the text to demonstrate the critical partnership between this position and the physical therapist. The text continues to serve the primary population of students in physical therapist and physical therapist assistant education programs, as well as others who desire to learn about this profession.

The major changes to this edition are two additional chapters in Part I. Chapter 4, Communication in Physical Therapy in the 21st Century, reflects the importance of communication in our profession and describes current approaches as they relate to health care. This includes communicating with individuals who have different abilities or attitudes, are of different ages, and come from different cultures. The chapter is written in a more personal tone than the rest of the text and encourages readers to reflect on and practice the techniques presented. Chapter 6, Financing and Reimbursing Health Care in Physical Therapy, provides a logical and organized description of an area that causes great frustration among health care providers in general and among physical therapists and physical therapist assistants specifically. The chapter describes major factors, such as managed care and Medicare, and their impact on physical therapy.

Other content revisions in Part I include a full description of the language and influence of Vision 2020, the organizational change within APTA as it pertains to the governance opportunities of the physical therapist assistant, and the significance of the document Professionalism in Physical Therapy: Core Values. The former chapter on current issues has been retitled Current Issues: Physical Therapy in Evolution to reflect the ongoing changes in the profession, and some of the former chapter's content was moved to the two new chapters. Part I (Profession) now concludes with the chapter on the APTA to present this organization as the foremost body representing the profession of physical therapy.

As in previous editions, I encourage feedback from readers of this text, particularly those who use it in their educational programs. I am pleased by the success of the first two editions and look forward to suggestions for future enhancements.

ACKNOWLEDGMENTS   As I consider all the assistance and support I received while writing and editing this edition, I must begin with my wife and three adult children. The latter continue to marvel that their father ever wrote a book!

Certainly, the personnel at Elsevier have been essential in bringing this into fruition. With any project that spans years to complete, personnel changes are not uncommon and such was the case with this edition. These individuals include Marj Fraser and Marion Waldman, who were instrumental in the early phase, and Meghan Ziegler, who began the manuscript reviews. Christie Hart and Patricia (Trish) Tannian were involved in the last phase of this production. Trish provided excellent assistance in the final editing, which is always so tedious and critical. It is fascinating how this project required extensive and ongoing communication with these individuals, yet I rarely, if ever, met many of them.

These acknowledgments would be incomplete if I did not recognize the outstanding chapters from the contributors. Each submitted updates to this edition in his or her respective area of expertise. Their clinical or academic (or both) knowledge of the material was evident as they submitted their manuscripts. In addition, two new contributors, Helen Masin and Jennifer Wilson, provided excellent material in the new chapters on communication and financing/reimbursement, respectively. These content areas are essential for the practice and management of physical therapy services and broaden the scope of this text. The continued success of this text is largely due to the work of all these individuals, and I am deeply gratified.

Michael A. Pagliarulo

Contents

Part I

Profession

Physical therapy is knowledge. Physical therapy is clinical science. Physical therapy is the reasoned application of science to warm and needing human beings. Or it is nothing.[1]

Helen J. Hislop, PT, FAPTA

1

Profession of Physical Therapy: Definition and Development

Michael A. Pagliarulo

CHAPTER OUTLINE

KEY TERMS

American Physiotherapy Association (APA)
American Women's Physical Therapeutic Association
autonomous practice
client
disability
disablement model
functional limitation
impairment
National Foundation For Infantile Paralysis ("the Foundation")
pathology/pathophysiology
patient
physiatrist
physical therapist
physical therapy
physiotherapist
physiotherapy
profession
reconstruction aide
Vision 2020

OBJECTIVES

After reading this chapter, the reader will be able to:
■ Define physical therapy
■ Describe the components of the model of disablement
■ Describe the characteristics of a profession
■ Describe a brief history of the profession of physical therapy in the United States and the major factors that influenced its growth and development

The profession of physical therapy has evolved and grown significantly in the past three decades. Although it has received substantial publicity, confusion remains regarding its unique characteristics. For example, how does physical therapy differ from occupational or chiropractic therapy? This chapter's first purpose, then, must be to present and define this profession.

To define physical therapy thoroughly, we must present a brief history of its development. A review of the past will demonstrate how the profession has responded to societal needs and gained respect as an essential component of the rehabilitation team. It will also link some current trends and practices with past events.

DEFINITION

Part of the confusion regarding the definition of **physical therapy** results from the variety of legal definitions seen from state to state. Each state has the right to define the profession of physical therapy and regulate its practice. Such definitions are commonly included in legislation known as "practice acts," which pertain to specific professions (practice acts are further described in Chapter 5).

To limit the variety of definitions, the Board of Directors of the American Physical Therapy Association (APTA) created the Physical Therapist Scope of Practice (Box 1-1), which was originally titled Model Definition of Physical Therapy for State Practice Acts.[2] This definition identifies several activities

BOX 1-1   *Guidelines:* **Physical Therapist Scope of Practice**

Physical therapy, which is limited to the care and services provided by or under the direction and supervision of a physical therapist, includes:
1. Examining (history, systems review and test and measures) individuals with impairments, functional limitations, and disability or other health-related conditions in order to determine a diagnosis, prognosis, and intervention. Tests and measures may include the following:
   - Aerobic capacity and endurance
   - Anthropometric characteristics
   - Arousal, attention, and cognition
   - Assistive and adaptive devices
   - Circulation (arterial, venous, lymphatic)
   - Cranial and peripheral nerve integrity
   - Environmental, home, and work (job/school/play) barriers
   - Ergonomics and body mechanics
   - Gait, locomotion, and balance
   - Integumentary integrity
   - Joint integrity and mobility
   - Motor function (motor control and motor learning)
   - Muscle performance (including strength, power, and endurance)

Continued

BOX 1-1   *Guidelines: Physical Therapist Scope of Practice—cont'd*

- Neuromotor development and sensory integration
- Orthotic, protective, and supportive devices
- Pain
- Posture
- Prosthetic requirements
- Range of motion (including muscle length)
- Reflex integrity
- Self-care and home management (including activities of daily living and instrumental activities of daily living)
- Sensory integrity
- Ventilation, and respiration/gas exchange
- Work (job/school/play), community, leisure integration or reintegration (including instrumental activities of daily living)

2. Alleviating impairment and functional limitation by designing, implementing, and modifying therapeutic interventions that include, but are not limited to:
   - Coordination, communication and documentation
   - Patient/client-related instruction
   - Therapeutic exercise
   - Functional training in self-care and home management (including activities of daily living and instrumental activities of daily living)
   - Functional training in work (job/school/play) and community and leisure integration or reintegration activities (including instrumental activities of daily living, work hardening, and work conditioning)
   - Manual therapy techniques (including mobilization/manipulation)
   - Prescription, application, and, as appropriate, fabrication of devices and equipment (assistive, adaptive, orthotic, protective, supportive, and prosthetic)
   - Airway clearance techniques
   - Integumentary repair and protection techniques
   - Electrotherapeutic modalities
   - Physical agents and mechanical modalities

3. Preventing injury, impairment, functional limitation, and disability, including the promotion and maintenance of health, wellness, fitness, and quality of life in all age populations.

4. Engaging in consultation, education, and research.

From Guidelines: Physical Therapist Scope of Practice, BOD G03-01-09-29. Board of Directors Standards, Positions, Guidelines, Policies, and Procedures. Alexandria, VA, American Physical Therapy Association, 2005.

inherent in the practice of physical therapy. It uses language and terminology based on the Guide to Physical Therapist Practice,[3] a pivotal document describing the physical therapist's approach to patient care. One of the three fundamental concepts of the Guide is the five elements of the patient/client management model, and these are incorporated into the definition. First and foremost, physical therapy begins with an *examination* to determine the nature and status of the condition. An *evaluation* is then conducted to interpret the findings and establish a *diagnosis* and *prognosis* that includes a plan of care. *Interventions* are then administered and modified in accordance with the patient's responses. Interventions focus on musculoskeletal, neuromuscular, cardiopulmonary, and integumentary disorders. Other important activities in the role of the physical therapist (PT) include consultation, education, and research. These may be separate from, but ultimately contribute to, effective practice.

In addition to identifying the activities of a PT, the definition states that physical therapy is "provided by or under the direction and supervision of a physical therapist." This qualification is further stipulated in a section of another policy (adopted by the House of Delegates, the highest policymaking body of the APTA) specifying that PTs and physical therapist assistants (PTAs) working under the direction of a PT are the *only* individuals who provide physical therapy (Box 1-2).[4]

Another link between the definition of physical therapy and the Guide is that the definition anchors examination and intervention to the concept of disablement, a second key concept of the Guide. The **disablement model** focuses on functional abilities that result from a medical condition, unlike the medical model, which focuses on treating the ailment. Several versions of the disablement model exist and were well described by Jette[5] (see the model of enablement and disablement developed by the World Health Organization and described in Chapter 13), although the Guide is based on the scheme presented by Nagi.[6,7] As described in the Guide, the process of disablement includes pathology/pathophysiology, impairment, functional limitations, and disability. **Pathology/pathophysiology** is an interruption of normal processes, usually at the

---

BOX 1-2   *Provision of Physical Therapy Interventions and Related Tasks*

Physical therapists are the only professionals who provide physical therapy interventions. Physical therapist assistants are the only individuals who provide selected physical therapy interventions under the direction and at least general supervision of the physical therapist.

From Provision of Physical Therapy Interventions and Related Tasks, HOD P06-00-17-28. House of Delegates Standards, Policies, Positions, and Guidelines. Alexandria, VA, American Physical Therapy Association, 2005.

cellular level, is exhibited as abnormal signs or symptoms, and is generally reflected in the medical diagnosis. A disease is an example of a pathology/ pathophysiology. **Impairment** is an abnormality of a body function or structure at the tissue, organ, or system level. An example of an impairment is decreased muscle strength or range of motion at a joint. Impairment causes **functional limitation**, which is a decreased ability of a *person* to perform a task without regard to the context or environment. Decreased strength in the upper limbs might result in a functional limitation, such as problems with feeding. A **disability** occurs if the functional limitation restricts activity in a particular context or environment. Feeding could be a disability if the individual with decreased upper limb strength has no assistive devices but the use of assistive devices could reduce or eliminate this disability. A disability, then, becomes situation dependent. Through the examination the PT determines the presence and extent of impairment, functional limitation, and disability before establishing a plan of care.

The definition of physical therapy also reflects the areas of prevention; health promotion, wellness, and fitness; and consultation, all of which occur across the life span. This is the third and last key concept in the Guide. Traditionally, PTs have provided care to **patients**—individuals who have disorders that require interventions to improve their function. **Client** is the term used to refer to an individual who seeks the services of a PT to maintain health or a business that hires a PT for consultation.[3] These areas of involvement have become more significant in the recent development of the profession.

PHYSICAL THERAPY AS A PROFESSION

The definition of physical therapy provides a broad description of the *scope of practice* of physical therapy. A companion document addresses physical therapy

---

BOX 1-3   *Position on Physical Therapy as a Health Profession*

> Physical therapy is a health profession whose primary purpose is the promotion of optimal health and function. This purpose is accomplished through the application of scientific principles to the processes of examination, evaluation, diagnosis, prognosis, and intervention to prevent or remediate impairments, functional limitations and disabilities as related to movement and health.
>
> Physical therapy encompasses areas of specialized competence and includes the development of new principles and applications to meet existing and emerging health needs. Other professional activities that serve the purpose of physical therapy are research, education, consultation and administration.

From Physical Therapy as a Health Profession, HOD P06-99-19-23. House of Delegates Standards, Policies, Positions, and Guidelines. Alexandria, VA, American Physical Therapy Association, 2005.

as a *profession* (Box 1-3).[8] This position was adopted by the House of Delegates of the APTA in 1983 and was subsequently revised to incorporate Guide language. Although the position states, "Physical therapy is a health profession…," it does not offer a spectrum of characteristic evidence to support this statement. Perhaps one reason is the difficulty in conclusively defining a profession.

Swisher and Page[9] presented a comprehensive review of the variety of descriptions of a profession. They addressed definitions based on a description of characteristics, stages of evolution, or power, but they focused on three qualities commonly held in high regard: autonomy, ethical standards, and accountability. Distinct applications of these qualities were made to physical therapy.

Moore[10] also included autonomy in a description of a **profession** and positioned it at the peak of a hierarchy of characteristics (Figure 1-1). This description is particularly applicable to physical therapy. The first characteristic, a lifetime commitment requiring an individual's dedication to the profession, is formidable yet admirable. PTs and PTAs do not commonly leave this profession. The second characteristic, a representative organization, provides standards, regulations, structure, and a vehicle for communication. In physical therapy this characteristic is fulfilled by the APTA. The third characteristic, specialized education, ensures competency to practice. For example, evaluative criteria for accreditation stipulate that the degree for professional level physical therapist education programs must be at the postbaccalaureate level and that

Figure 1-1 ■ Hierarchy of the criteria to define a profession.

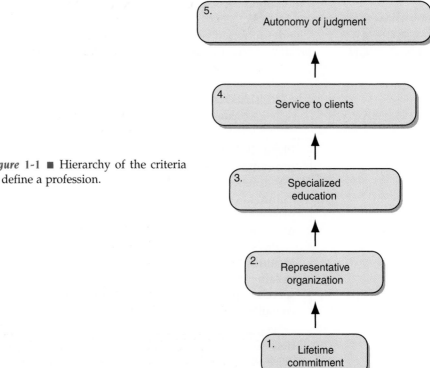

5. Autonomy of judgment

4. Service to clients

3. Specialized education

2. Representative organization

1. Lifetime commitment

the degree for physical therapist assistant education programs is the associate degree.[11,12] The fourth characteristic, service to clients, is obvious in physical therapy and provides a direct benefit to society. In this context the term "patients" would also apply. The final feature, autonomy of judgment, applies regardless of whether the therapist practices in a jurisdiction where a physician's referral is required by law.

Independent and accurate judgment is inherent in every evaluation, plan of care, and discharge plan conducted by the PT. This last criterion is frequently used to distinguish a professional from a technician (an individual who requires supervision).

In the past two decades the concept of autonomy has received a great deal of attention, not only in the description of physical therapy as a profession, but also as a driving force in the recognition of a PT as an autonomous practitioner. **Autonomous practice** is one of the six key components of the APTA Vision Statement for Physical Therapy 2020 (see Box 1-7).[13] The APTA Board of

---

BOX 1-4   *Autonomous Physical Therapist Practice: Definitions and Privileges*

Autonomous physical therapist practice is characterized by independent, self-determined professional judgment and action. Physical therapists have the capability, ability and responsibility to exercise professional judgment within their scope of practice, and to professionally act on that judgment.

Privileges of Autonomous Practice in 2020
Each of these elements includes two over-arching concepts: recognition of and respect for physical therapists as the practitioners of choice, and recognition of and respect of the education, experience, and expertise of physical therapists in their professional scope of practice.

1. Direct and unrestricted access:
   The physical therapist has the professional capability and ability to provide to all individuals the physical therapy services they choose without legal, regulatory, or payer restrictions.
2. Professional ability to refer to other health care providers:
   The physical therapist has the professional capability and ability to refer to others in the health care system for identified to possible medical needs beyond the scope of physical therapist practice.
3. Professional ability to refer to other professionals:
   The physical therapist has the professional capability and ability to refer to other professionals for identified patient/client needs beyond the scope of physical therapist practice.
4. Professional ability to refer for diagnostic tests:
   The physical therapist has the professional capability and ability to refer for diagnostic tests that would clarify the patient/client situation and enhance the provision of physical therapy services.

From Autonomous Physical Therapist Practice: Definitions and Privileges, BOD P03-03-12-28. Board of Directors Standards, Positions, Guidelines, Policies, and Procedures. Alexandria, VA, American Physical Therapy Association, 2005.

Directors has issued a position listing and describing the elements of autonomous practice (Box 1-4).[14] This position indicates that PTs have the capability to exercise professional judgment to practice under direct access within their scope of practice and refer patients and clients to other health care professionals when necessary. These attributes reiterate the importance of autonomy of judgment as one of the highest, if not the highest, characteristics of a profession.

The second common quality of a profession identified by Swisher and Page, ethical standards, is also related to the second highest level in Moore's hierarchy, service to clients. Should the individuals providing physical therapy aspire to some standards? Six of the seven APTA Core Documents (documents that identify or describe standards and principles of practice and behavior) either specifically focus on ethical conduct or include a section that refers to ethical standards (Table 1-1)[15]:

1. Standards of Practice for Physical Therapy (see Figure 2-1)
2. Code of Ethics (see Box 5-1)
3. Guide for Professional Conduct
4. Standards of Ethical Conduct for the Physical Therapist Assistant (see Box 5-2)
5. Guide for Conduct of the Physical Therapist Assistant
6. Professionalism in Physical Therapy: Core Values

Moreover, all members of the APTA have agreed in writing to either comply with (PTs or PTAs) or be guided by (students) the respective Code of Ethics (PTs and students) or Standards of Ethical Conduct for the Physical Therapist Assistant (PTAs and students).

Graduates of professional programs commonly recite an oath that they will uphold high standards of practice and behavior as they take up their profession. Although a formal oath does not exist in physical therapy, the Education Section of the APTA has adopted a model oath (Box 1-5).[16] As a model, this permits physical therapist students and PTs freedom to use it, modify it, use another one entirely, or not use anything at all. The important feature of this oath, however, is its relationship to the APTA Code of Ethics (compare Boxes 1-5 and 5-1). Anchored to the Code, the model oath provides a verbal commitment to this standard of conduct.

A strategy recently adopted by the APTA to promote physical therapy as a profession was to define and describe the professionalism component of the Vision Statement. In 2003 the Board of Directors approved the document "Professionalism in Physical Therapy: Core Values," developed by a consensus conference method (Table 1-1).[17] The purpose of the document was to assist the transition to a doctoring profession by articulating what a physical therapist practitioner would do in her or his daily practice to demonstrate professional behavior. This document has focused greater attention on professional behaviors and how to teach and emulate them.

As a profession, physical therapy is guided by the criteria listed in Figure 1-1. Such was not always the case, and evolution of the profession has entailed significant change and varying degrees of recognition from other professions. The next section provides a brief overview of the history of physical therapy.

Table 1-1
Core Values of Professionalism in Physical Therapy

Core Value	Definition
Accountability	Accountability is active acceptance of the responsibility for diverse roles, obligations, and actions of the physical therapist, including self-regulation and other behaviors that positively influence patient/client outcomes, the profession, and health needs of society.
Altruism	Altruism is the primary regard for or devotion to the interest of patients/clients, thus assuming the fiduciary responsibility of placing the needs of the patient/client ahead of the physical therapist's self-interest.
Compassion/ caring	Compassion is the desire to identify with or sense something of another's experience; a precursor of caring. Caring is the concern, empathy, and consideration for the needs and values of others.
Excellence	Excellence is physical therapy practice that consistently uses current knowledge and theory while understanding personal limits, integrates judgment and the patient/client perspective, embraces advancement, challenges mediocrity, and works toward development of new knowledge.
Integrity	Integrity is steadfast adherence to high ethical principles or professional standards.
Professional duty	Professional duty is the commitment to meeting one's obligations to provide effective physical therapy services to individual patients/clients, to serve the profession, and to positively influence the health of society.
Social responsibility	Social responsibility is the promotion of a mutual trust between the profession and the large public that necessitates responding to societal needs for health and wellness.

From Professionalism in Physical Therapy: Core Values, BOD 05-04-02-03. House of Delegates Standards, Policies, Positions, and Guidelines. Alexandria, VA, American Physical Therapy Association, 2005.

BOX 1-5 | *Model Pledge for Physical Therapy*

As I enter the profession of physical therapy to practice as a physical therapist, I solemnly and willingly pledge the following:

I will respect the rights and dignity of all individuals and will provide compassionate care. (1)

I will be trustworthy towards my patients and clients and in all other aspects of physical therapy practice. (2)

I will place the welfare of my patients and clients above my own self-interest. (7)

I will provide accurate and relevant information to patients and clients about their care and to the public about physical therapy services. (8)

I will exercise sound judgment and comply with laws and regulations that govern physical therapy and protect the public from unethical, incompetent, and illegal acts. (4, 3, 9)

I will maintain professional competence and promote high standards for physical therapy practice, education, and research. (5, 6)

I will address the health needs of society and strive to effect changes that benefit patients, clients, and the community. (10, 3)

I will respect the rights, knowledge, and skills of colleagues and other health care professionals and seek consultation whenever the welfare of the patient or client may be advanced. (11)

Thus, with this pledge, I freely accept the responsibilities that accompany the practice of physical therapy.

Adopted as model February, 2004.

Note: Numbers refer to corresponding elements of the Code of Ethics. They are not meant to be read aloud.

From Model Pledge for Physical Therapy. Alexandria, VA, American Physical Therapy Association. Available at www.aptaeducation.org/Model_Oath.pdf. Accessed March 20, 2006.

HISTORICAL DEVELOPMENT

Examining the origin and development of the profession and practice of physical therapy in the United States will serve to explain some of the current characteristics and conditions. It will also demonstrate how certain positions have changed over time. The reader is referred to resources at the end of this chapter for more detailed historical accounts.

ORIGINS OF PHYSICAL THERAPY

Granger[18] described how physical measures were used in ancient civilizations to relieve pain and improve function. Massage was used by the Chinese in 3000 BC, described by Hippocrates in 460 BC, modified by the Romans, and accepted as a scientific procedure in the early 1800s. Techniques of muscle reeducation developed from this evolution. Hydrotherapy was practiced by the Greeks and Romans through the use of baths and river worship. The development of electrotherapy began in the 1600s with the introduction of electricity and electrical devices.

More modern techniques of physical therapy were practiced extensively in Europe, particularly England and France, before being used in the United States. It took the outbreak of polio epidemics and World War I to bring these techniques to the United States.

IMPACT OF WORLD WAR I AND POLIO

It is unfortunate that the impetus to develop physical therapy in this country was the response to widespread suffering; at the same time, such an origin demonstrates the direct humanitarian motivation that serves as the foundation of physical therapy. First came the epidemics of polio (poliomyelitis or infantile paralysis) in 1894, 1914, and 1916, which left tens of thousands of children paralyzed and in need of "physical therapy." Then, at the outbreak of World War I, the Surgeon General of the United States sent a group of physicians to England and France to learn about physical therapy techniques for the better management of those wounded in war. As a result, the Division of Special Hospitals and Physical Reconstruction was created in 1917.[19] This division was responsible for training and managing **reconstruction aides** (exclusively women) who would provide physical reconstruction to those injured in war. These women were the forerunners of the profession and practice of physical therapy in the United States (Figure 1-2).

During this period, polio epidemics were occurring in Vermont. A statewide program known as the "Vermont Plan" was developed to study the cause and effects of the disease. Under this plan health care teams conducted field visits to provide care for children with polio.[20] These teams consisted of orthopaedic

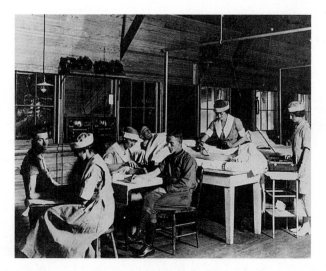

Figure 1-2 ■ Reconstruction aides treating soldiers wounded in World War I at Fort Sam Houston, Texas, in 1919. (From American Physical Therapy Association: Historical Photograph Packet.)

surgeons, public health nurses, **physiotherapists** (commonly known as "physicians' assistants"), brace makers, and stenographers. The physiotherapists became involved in making accurate measurements to determine muscle strength and providing therapy through exercise and massage (Figures 1-3 and 1-4).

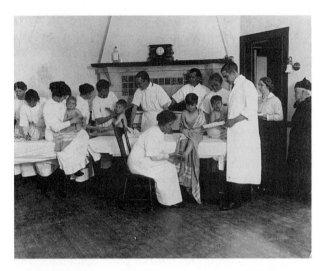

Figure 1-3 ■ Physical therapists and physicians working together to evaluate and treat children at a polio clinic in New England in 1916. (From American Physical Therapy Association: Historical Photograph Packet.)

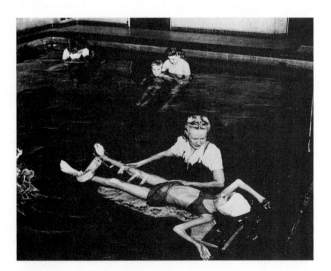

Figure 1-4 ■ Aquatic therapy was very effective for individuals who had polio. (From American Physical Therapy Association: Historical Photograph Packet.)

POST–WORLD WAR I PERIOD

Even after the war, the need for physical therapy continued. Attention shifted from preserving a fighting force to maintaining a working force. Humanitarian interests and the labor requirements of an industrial society resulted in a focus on "crippled children."[21] As the reconstruction aides moved into civilian facilities to address these needs, their titles and practices were plagued by confusion and ambiguity. The time had come to establish a clear identity through a national organization.

The origin of the first national organization representing "physical therapeutics" is traced to a meeting suggested by a military physician. This meeting, on January 15, 1921, at Keen's Chop House in New York City, was attended by 30 reconstruction aides and five physicians. Accomplishments of the first meeting included creation of a national organization, the **American Women's Physical Therapeutic Association,** and election of the first president, Mary McMillan.[22] According to the first constitution, the organization was established to maintain high standards and provide a mechanism for sharing information (Box 1-6).

Mary McMillan was the overwhelming choice for president (Figure 1-5). Trained in England, she is credited with becoming the first "physical therapist" in the United States.[20] As a reconstruction aide she was stationed at Walter Reed General Hospital in Washington, D.C., where she was appointed head reconstruction aide in 1918. Later, while at Reed College in Portland, Oregon, she participated in the largest (over 200 students) of seven emergency training programs for reconstruction aides.

Under the leadership of Miss McMillan, the new organization took immediate action. Two membership categories were established: charter members (reconstruction aides) and active members who "shall be graduates of recognized schools of **physiotherapy** or physical education, who have had

BOX 1-6	*Founding Objectives of the American Women's Physical Therapeutic Association*

1. To establish and maintain a professional and scientific standard for those engaged in the profession of physical therapeutics.
2. To increase efficiency among its members by encouraging them in advanced study.
3. To disseminate information by the distribution of medical literature and articles of professional interest.
4. To make available efficiently trained women to the medical profession.
5. To sustain social fellowship and intercourse upon grounds of mutual interest.

From Beard G: Foundations for growth: A review of the first forty years in terms of education, practice, and research. Phys Ther Rev 41:843-861, 1961.

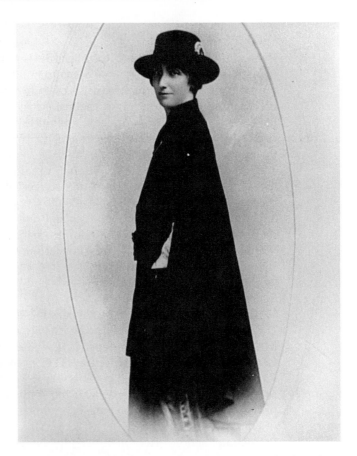

Figure 1-5 ■ Mary McMillan was elected in 1921 as the founding president of the American Women's Physical Therapeutic Association (precursor to the American Physical Therapy Association). (From American Physical Therapy Association: Historical Photograph Packet.)

training and experience in massage and therapeutic exercise, with some knowledge of either electrotherapy or hydrotherapy."[23] An official journal, *P.T. Review,* was established and first published in 1921. Annual meetings were initiated in conjunction with annual meetings of the American Medical Association (AMA) to capitalize on their programs and gain recognition. The name of the organization was changed in 1922 to the **American Physiotherapy Association (APA).** Two men were admitted in 1923. In 1926, the journal was retitled *Physiotherapy Review.* To honor the pioneering work of Mary McMillan, the organization eventually created in her name a lectureship (presented as a major opening event at the Annual Conference) and student scholarship programs that continue today.

Two issues involving physicians took decades to resolve. The first pertained to identity. Physicians perceived these practitioners to be technicians or aides and suggested that this distinction be reflected in their title. Members of the

APA believed that they had a more professional status and objected to that reference. This issue was not settled until the 1940s, when physicians established physical medicine as a medical specialty. These physicians were known as **physiatrists,** and the term "physical therapist" (without adding "technician" or "aide") became acceptable thereafter.[21]

The second issue was more substantive and involved education requirements. No standard educational program existed for a physiotherapist; therefore the APA developed a suggested curriculum and published it in 1928. This was a 9-month program (1200 total clock hours). Entrance requirements included graduation from a school of physical education or nursing.[22] In contrast, most of the students in the 14 training programs for reconstruction aides were physical education teachers or graduates of physical education schools. A committee of the APA visited all institutions offering educational programs for physiotherapists and published a list of 11 approved programs in 1930.

The action by the APA did not fully resolve the issue of education requirements. Greater recognition of education programs and standards was required, so the APA sought assistance from the AMA in 1933. Consequently, the Council on Medical Education and Hospitals of the AMA inspected 35 schools of physiotherapy. Based on this inspection, as well as input from the APA and other related organizations, the AMA adopted the Essentials of an Acceptable School for Physical Therapy Technicians in 1936. Entrance requirements and length of program remained essentially unchanged; however, the curriculum was stated in detail, and other characteristics were stipulated (institutional affiliation, faculty, resources, clinical facilities). Thirteen schools were approved by the AMA in 1936.[22]

IMPACT OF WORLD WAR II AND POLIO

Once again, national and global tragedies combined to expand the need for physical therapy, and as before, the profession responded. To meet the demands of the war, eight emergency 6-month courses were authorized to be offered among the 15 approved full-length programs in physical therapy. These shortened courses were discontinued in 1946 when war-related demands for services dropped.

Unfortunately, polio continued to create a need for therapy. In response to repeated epidemics, the **National Foundation for Infantile Paralysis** (often referred to as **the Foundation**) was established in 1938 for research, education, and patient services.[19] PTs continued to provide vital services for children affected by polio.

The Foundation was a source of substantial support for the profession and practice of physical therapy. Catherine Worthingham, a past president of the APA, accepted the position of Director of Professional Education on the staff of the Foundation in 1944. In the same year, the first national office of the APA was established in New York City and the first executive director was hired. Both these actions were made possible by a grant from the Foundation. Also in 1944, a permanent headquarters and staff for the APA enabled the organization to create the House of Delegates to serve as a policymaking body. Other grants from the Foundation provided scholarships to recruit and retain physical therapy students and faculty, funds to hire a consultant to recruit and assign PTs for emergency work relating to polio, and financial support for training in techniques fostered by Sister Elizabeth Kenny for individuals with polio (early application of moist heat to permit mobilization and prevent contractures).

POST–WORLD WAR II PERIOD

The U.S. Army recognized the need to retain PTs in an organized unit to provide service to military personnel. As a result, the Women's Medical Specialist Corps was established in 1947. It consisted of PTs, occupational therapists, and dietitians. A PT, Emma Vogel, became the first chief of the Corps and was accorded the rank of colonel.[19] In 1955, the Corps became the Army Medical Specialist Corps to allow men and women to serve with commissions in the military.[22]

A major breakthrough in the treatment of polio occurred during this period with the introduction of gamma globulin and the Salk vaccine. Finally the disease could be controlled. PTs played prominent roles during field trials of these medications, which began in 1951.

Name clarification continued as the term "physiatrist" became recognized as the title given to physicians who practiced physical medicine. **Physical therapists** could now practice "physical therapy." This role clarification was reflected in the new name for the national organization, the American Physical Therapy Association, in 1947 and a new title for the journal, *Physical Therapy*, in 1962. It was also demonstrated in the title of the new Essentials, which extensively revised the original document of 1936. The new title, Essentials of an Acceptable School of Physical Therapy, no longer referred to technicians. This document was adopted by the AMA in 1955 and was used to approve new and existing educational programs for over 20 years. The new Essentials established minimum curricular standards, including a program length of 12 months.

1960s THROUGH 1980s

[Note: Many of the issues that occurred in this and the final historical period continue to evolve today. Several of these are described in more detail in subsequent chapters and therefore are only highlighted here.] This three-decade period was characterized by growth and recognition in education, practice, and research. Societal issues of this period included an aging population, health promotion, and disease prevention. Federal legislation funded health care for a variety of populations, which increased the demand for physical therapy. The profession responded with several actions.

First, the APTA adopted policy statements in the 1960s to clarify the preparation and use of PTAs and aides. These positions were necessary to meet the growing demand for services.

The headquarters of the APTA was relocated to Washington, D.C., in 1971 to increase political involvement. Executive operations were further strengthened when an office building was purchased in Alexandria, Virginia, in 1983.

New education programs were developed in an attempt to keep pace with the demand; curricular evolution was inherent as health care in general expanded. This period opened with an APTA policy in 1960 declaring the baccalaureate degree to be the minimum educational requirement for a PT. By the late 1970s, it became clear that a postbaccalaureate degree would be necessary to master the knowledge and skills required for competent practice. Consequently, a critical policy adopted by the APTA in 1979 (amended in 1980) stated that new and existing programs in physical therapy must award a postbaccalaureate degree by December 31, 1990. This requirement had a major impact on curricular development.

This period also saw an evolution in the historical link between the AMA and the APTA (formerly APA) regarding approval (accreditation) of educational programs. The APTA became more actively involved in the accreditation process. In 1974, it adopted the Essentials of an Accredited Educational Program for the Physical Therapist, which represented a dramatic departure from the prescriptions in the 1955 Essentials.[21] In 1977, the Commission on Accreditation in Education (a body separate from, but administratively supported by, the APTA) became recognized by the U.S. Office of Education and Council on Postsecondary Education as an accrediting agency. Standards for Accreditation of Physical Therapy Educational Programs was adopted by the APTA in 1979. In 1983, after contesting the value of the AMA in the accreditation process, the Commission on Accreditation in Education became the sole agency for accrediting education programs for PTs and PTAs. This recognition marked the maturity of the profession.

Growth and development in the areas of practice and research resulted in new organizational units and opportunities. The American Board of Physical Therapy Specialties was created by the APTA in 1978 to provide a mechanism for PTs to become certified and recognized as clinical specialists in certain areas. Direct access to physical therapy services became legal in 20 states by 1988. In 1984, the APTA adopted a policy to recognize diagnosis in physical therapy. The Foundation for Physical Therapy was initiated in 1979 to promote and support research in the profession.

1990S INTO THE 21ST CENTURY

Dramatic changes have occurred since 1990, not only in the traditional areas of practice, education, and research, but also in the role and rights of the PTA and in governance of the organization. During this period the outlook for physical therapy has moved from uncertainty to new growth and a clear vision for deliberate action.

Direct access to physical therapy services continued to expand, becoming legal in 42 states; however, external forces unfavorable to the profession were developing. Skyrocketing costs of health care resulted in significant cost control measures in the private and government sectors. New methods of financing and reimbursing health care, created by the proliferation of managed care and the Balanced Budget Act of 1997, had a direct impact on the delivery of health care services, including physical therapy. Costs were controlled by limitation of the type, number, and reimbursement amounts for services. In part to provide a clear description of the role and services provided by PTs to third party payers, the APTA created the Guide to Physical Therapist Practice.[3] The circumstances of PTs and PTAs deteriorated as job availability and salaries plateaued and then declined in some facilities. This unfavorable situation was compounded by the continued proliferation of education programs. One study predicted a surplus of PTs by the end of the decade.[24] Unemployment suddenly became a real issue. Fortunately, the job market opened again after the turn of the century as the health care industry adjusted to the new reimbursement strategies and the need for services continued.

Practice issues had a domino effect on education. With a tight job market, applications to physical therapist and physical therapist assistant education programs dropped. In fact, many of the programs for assistants closed voluntarily because of limited enrollment. Eventually the APTA established a position recommending against the development of new education programs. The shift to postbaccalaureate education gave rise to several national conferences, which resulted in A Normative Model of Physical Therapist Professional Level Education: Version 2004[25] (current version) to provide guidance to these programs. Subsequently, the document titled Evaluative Criteria for the Accreditation of Physical Therapist Education Programs[11] was revised twice to ensure education programs and faculty were contemporary. Similar activities for physical therapist assistant education programs resulted in parallel documents for these programs.[12,26] The baccalaureate degree was finally phased out for physical therapist education programs, with no further accreditation of these degree level programs after January 1, 2002. As the job market improved, so did the applicant pool and outlook for education programs. The major evolutionary event, however, was the rapid transition to the doctor of physical therapy (DPT) degree fostered by Vision 2020, created in the year 2000 (see below).

While the need for clinical research had been known for decades, the controls imposed by third party payers were a direct call for research that would justify physical therapy services. The Guide provided a comprehensive and detailed description of physical therapy services, but research was needed to substantiate these services. A Clinical Research Agenda for Physical Therapy was established to identify areas where research was needed and feasible. Programs offered by the Foundation of Physical Therapy to fund research were expanded. The developing concept of evidence-based practice (practice based on proof) was promoted through the new Hooked on Evidence program. This provided a user-friendly database of current literature pertinent to the practice of physical therapy. New accreditation criteria for physical therapist education programs increased the expectation regarding faculty scholarship. These new opportunities and expectations created by external and internal forces combined to promote further research activities in the profession.

Through the course of this period, the APTA took a strong leadership role in addressing the issues. Extensive lobbying and rallying of public sentiment resulted in legislation that protected patients' rights in managed care organizations and lifted a major funding cap in the Medicare program for physical therapy services. Several task forces were established to consider the role and governance rights of PTAs. Final reports were instrumental in new policies and positions that clarified their clinical role, education level, continuing education opportunities, recognition of advance proficiencies, and governance rights. In 1998, a separate deliberative body for PTAs, the Representative Body of the National Assembly, was approved. In 2005, after an extensive review of its limited effectiveness, the APTA House of Delegates replaced it with a PTA Caucus, which had its first meeting in 2006. Other mechanisms for direct input from the PTA community into the Board of Directors were also approved.

Notwithstanding the significant actions taken by the APTA in response to important issues, an evolutionary action in 2000 was the adoption of the APTA Vision Sentence for Physical Therapy 2020 (Box 1-7; see Box 4-1 for the shortened version, the Vision Sentence).[13] Commonly cited as **Vision 2020**, it has become a beacon for the profession and has provided a distinct direction for current and future action. Its six key components address the areas of practice, education, and research: (1) autonomous practice, (2) direct access, (3) practitioner of choice, (4) DPT, (5) evidence-based practice, and (6) professionalism. It has been the source for follow-up action by the Board of Directors and House of Delegates to further define these elements and establish goals and actions to achieve

---

BOX 1-7   APTA *Vision Statement for Physical Therapy* 2020

Physical therapy, by 2020, will be provided by physical therapists who are doctors of physical therapy and who may be board-certified specialists. Consumers will have direct access to physical therapists in all environments for patient/client management, prevention, and wellness services. Physical therapists will be practitioners of choice in patients'/clients' health networks and will hold all privileges of autonomous practice. Physical therapists may be assisted by physical therapist assistants who are educated and licensed to provide physical therapist directed and supervised components of interventions.

Guided by integrity, life-long learning, and a commitment to comprehensive and accessible health programs for all people, physical therapists and physical therapist assistants will render evidence-based services throughout the continuum of care and improve quality of life for society. They will provide culturally sensitive care distinguished by trust, respect, and an appreciation for individual differences.

While fully availing themselves of new technologies, as well as basic and clinical research, physical therapists will continue to provide direct patient/client care. They will maintain active responsibility for the growth of the physical therapy profession and the health of the people it serves.

From APTA Vision Sentence for Physical Therapy 2020 and APTA Vision Statement for Physical Therapy 2020, HOD P06-00-24-35. House of Delegates Standards, Policies, Positions, and Guidelines. Alexandria, VA, American Physical Therapy Association, 2005.

them. Other trends have also developed. For example, the rapid transition to DPT programs was a direct result from Vision 2020.

Although the future of physical therapy was uncertain in the early part of this period, changes in the health care industry and the adoption of Vision 2020 have provided realistic goals and actions for moving forward with enthusiasm. Several of the issues that arose in this most recent period continue to evolve. The profession and practice of physical therapy remain responsive to societal needs. Subsequent chapters, in particular those in Part I, provide further description.

SUMMARY

Physical therapy is a profession that enjoys a proud heritage. From the reconstruction aides of World War I to the autonomous practitioners of today, PTs continue to provide services to reduce pain, improve function, and maintain health. As a preamble to the remainder of the text, this chapter provided a definition of physical therapy and the qualities that characterize it as a profession, particularly autonomy of judgment. The history of the profession was traced from its origins in World War I. The influence of poliomyelitis and world wars, relationships with the AMA, development of the APTA, and recognition as a profession were described. In the decades following World War II, growth and development were paramount features of the profession until managed care and other forces for cost control in health care took hold in the 1990s. The millennium ended with a tight job market that had an unfavorable impact on education programs. The 21st century opened with Vision 2020, which set new goals and instigated follow-up action. The job market improved, and this helped lead to the rapid establishment of DPT programs. Research was further promoted by the Hooked on Evidence program and higher expectations of faculty. The profession was on the move to achieve the goals established by Vision 2020.

REFERENCES

1. Hislop HJ: The not-so-impossible dream. Phys Ther 1975;55:1069-1080.
2. Guidelines: Physical Therapist Scope of Practice, BOD G03-01-09-29. Board of Directors Standards, Positions, Guidelines, Policies, and Procedures. Alexandria, VA, American Physical Therapy Association, 2005.
3. Guide to Physical Therapist Practice, revised ed 2. Alexandria, VA, American Physical Therapy Association, 2003.
4. Provision of Physical Therapy Interventions and Related Tasks, HOD P06-00-17-28. House of Delegates Standards, Policies, Positions, and Guidelines. Alexandria, VA, American Physical Therapy Association, 2005.
5. Jette A: Physical disablement concepts for physical therapy research and practice. Phys Ther 1994;74:380-386.
6. Nagi S: Some conceptual issues in disability and rehabilitation. *In:* Sussman M (ed): Sociology and Rehabilitation. Washington, DC, American Sociological Association, 1965.
7. Nagi S: Disability concepts revisited: Implications for prevention. *In:* Pope A, Tarlov A (eds): Disability in America: Towards a National Agenda for Prevention. Washington, DC, National Academy Press, 1991.
8. Physical Therapy as a Health Profession, HOD P06-99-19-23. House of Delegates Standards, Policies, Positions, and Guidelines. Alexandria, VA, American Physical Therapy Association, 2005.
9. Swisher LL, Page CG: Professionalism in Physical Therapy: History, Practice, & Development. St Louis, Elsevier, 2005.

10. Moore WE: The Professions: Roles and Rules. New York, Russell Sage Foundation, 1970.
11. Evaluative Criteria for Accreditation of Education Programs for the Preparation of Physical Therapists. Alexandria, VA, American Physical Therapy Association, 1998. Available at http://www.apta.org/AM/Template.cfm?Section=Home&TEMPLATE=/CM/ContentDisplay.cfm&CONTENTID=25709. Accessed March 20, 2006.
12. Evaluative Criteria for Accreditation of Education Programs for the Preparation of Physical Therapist Assistants, Alexandria, VA, American Physical Therapy Association, 2000. Available at http://www.apta.org/AM/Template.cfm?Section=Home&CONTENTID=28816&TEMPLATE=/CM/ContentDisplay.cfm. Accessed March 20, 2006.
13. APTA Vision Sentence for Physical Therapy 2020 and APTA Vision Statement for Physical Therapy 2020, HOD 06-00-24-35. House of Delegates Standards, Policies, Positions, and Guidelines. Alexandria, VA, American Physical Therapy Association, 2005.
14. Autonomous Physical Therapist Practice: Definitions and Privileges, BOD P03-03-12-28. Board of Directors Standards, Positions, Guidelines, Policies, and Procedures. Alexandria, VA, American Physical Therapy Association, 2005.
15. APTA Core Documents, House of Delegates Standards, Positions, Guidelines, Policies, and Procedures. Alexandria, VA, American Physical Therapy Association, 2005.
16. Model Pledge for Physical Therapy. Alexandria, VA, American Physical Therapy Association. Available at www.aptaeducation.org/Model_Oath.pdf. Accessed March 20, 2006.
17. Professionalism in Physical Therapy: Core Values, BOD 05-04-02-03. House of Delegates Standards, Policies, Positions, and Guidelines. Alexandria, VA, American Physical Therapy Association, 2005.
18. Granger FB: The development of physiotherapy. Phys Ther 1976;56:13-14.
19. Davies EJ: The beginning of "modern physiotherapy." Phys Ther 1976;56:15-21.
20. Davies EJ: Infantile paralysis. Phys Ther 1976;56:42-49.
21. Pinkston D: Evolution of the practice of physical therapy in the United States. *In:* Scully RM, Barnes ML (eds): Physical Therapy. Philadelphia, Lippincott, 1989.
22. Beard G: Foundations for growth: A review of the first forty years in terms of education, practice, and research. Phys Ther Rev 1961;41:843-861.
23. Hazenhyer IM: A history of the American Physiotherapy Association. Physiother Rev 1946;26(1):3-14.
24. Vector Research Inc: Executive Summary, Workforce Study. Alexandria, VA, American Physical Therapy Association, 1997.
25. A Normative Model of Physical Therapist Professional Education: Version 2004. Alexandria, VA, American Physical Therapy Association, 2004.
26. A Normative Model of Physical Therapist Assistant Education: Version 1999. Alexandria, VA, American Physical Therapy Association, 1999.

ADDITIONAL RESOURCES

American Physical Therapy Association: Healing the Generations: A History of Physical Therapy and the American Physical Therapy Association. Lyme, CT, Greenwich Publishing Group, 1995.

Comprehensive and detailed description of the history and evolution of the profession and practice of physical therapy in the United States.

The Beginning: Physical Therapy and the APTA. Alexandria, VA, American Physical Therapy Association, 1979.

Excellent anthology of selected articles that describe the history of physical therapy and the APTA.

Hazenhyer IM: A history of the American Physical Therapy Association: 2. Formative years, 1926-1930. Physiother Rev 1946;26(2):66-74.

Describes the pertinent issues confronting the profession during this period, including the first published curriculum and a review of educational programs, controversy over technicians versus professionals, legislation to regulate practice, and growth of the journal.

Hazenhyer IM: A history of the American Physical Therapy Association: 3. Coming of age, 1931-1938. Physiother Rev 1946;26(3):122-129.

Continues description of issues in previous article as they evolved during this pre–World War II period.

Hazenhyer IM: A history of the American Physical Therapy Association: 4. Maturity, 1939-1946. Physiother Rev 1946;26(4):174-184.

In this final article in the series, the author describes issues involving membership rights, chapter organizations, further curricular changes, impact of the National Foundation for Infantile Paralysis, activities in military service, and the journal.

Mathews JS: Professionalism in physical therapy: Current patterns and future directions. *In:* Mathews JS (ed): Practice Issues in Physical Therapy. Thorofare, NJ, Slack, 1989.

Comprehensive review of aspects that contribute to physical therapy as a profession and to physical therapists as professionals.

www.apta.org

Website for the American Physical Therapy Association. Excellent resource for current information and documents pertinent to the profession.

REVIEW QUESTIONS	1. How does the APTA's "definition" of physical therapy differ from its "philosophical statement"? 2. Explain the differences between the practice and the profession of physical therapy, and identify the documents that describe each. 3. Define "profession" and apply its five characteristics to physical therapy. Is physical therapy a profession? 4. How did polio and World Wars I and II affect the origin and evolution of physical therapy in the United States? 5. What impact has Vision 2020 had on the profession of physical therapy?

All physical therapists, regardless of title or position, function in multiple capacities, shifting from one to another as the situation demands. For example, the clinician serves as a teacher, a supervisor, a negotiator, a clinician researcher, an advocate, and a business administrator. Physical therapists in other positions not only share those functions but may assume additional ones as well.

Geneva R. Johnson, PT, FAPTA

2 Roles and Characteristics of Physical Therapists

Michael A. Pagliarulo

OBJECTIVES

After reading this chapter, the reader will be able to:

- Describe the roles of the physical therapist in primary, secondary, and tertiary care.
- Describe the roles of the physical therapist in prevention and health promotion.
- Describe the components of the patient/client management model.

- Describe general features of tests and measures and procedural interventions used in physical therapy.
- Describe other professional roles of the physical therapist in the areas of consultation, education, critical inquiry, and administration.
- List and describe the demographic characteristics of physical therapists.

In the past two decades, the demand for physical therapists (PTs) and physical therapist assistants (PTAs) and the recognition and reimbursement for services they provide have evolved dramatically. This transformation has resulted from several trends and outside influences, including the aging population, federal legislation entitling children in public schools to health care, a burgeoning interest in personal fitness, and actions taken by insurance companies and the government to contain the rising cost of health care. PTs and PTAs have had to adapt to these rapid and extensive changes, which at times have been frustrating to comprehend and accommodate. A Putnam Investments advertisement aptly summarizes these sentiments: "You think you understand the situation, but what you don't understand is that the situation just changed."[1]

The profession of physical therapy has succeeded and will continue to succeed. We have followed several of the ground rules proposed by Price Pritchett, including becoming quick-change artists, accepting ambiguity, and holding ourselves accountable for our individual actions.[1] To provide a framework for understanding the profession in the context of change, this chapter examines the diverse and shifting roles of PTs, the breadth of services provided, and the variety of employment settings where these services exist. Recent demographic data and information on employment activities and conditions are presented.

ROLES IN THE PROVISION OF PHYSICAL THERAPY

The primary role of a PT involves direct patient care. While PTs engage in many other activities and in some cases no longer participate in clinical practice, patient care remains the predominant employment activity. For this reason, the **Standards of Practice for Physical Therapy** is perhaps the foremost core document approved by the House of Delegates of the American Physical Therapy Association (APTA).[2] The Standards and their accompanying criteria, approved by the Board of Directors of the APTA, identify "conditions and performances that are essential for provision of high-quality physical therapy" (Box 2-1). They address not only the provision of services, but also other professional roles, including administration, education, and research. These roles are described later in the chapter.

BOX 2-1   *Standards of Practice for Physical Therapy*

The *Standards of Practice for Physical Therapy* are promulgated by APTA's House of Delegates; Criteria for the Standards are promulgated by APTA's Board of Directors. Criteria are italicized beneath the Standards to which they apply.

Preamble

The physical therapy profession's commitment to society is to promote optimal health and function in individuals by pursuing excellence in practice. The American Physical Therapy Association attests to this commitment by adopting and promoting the following Standards of Practice for Physical Therapy. These Standards are the profession's statement of conditions and performances that are essential for provision of high quality professional service to society, and provide a foundation for assessment of physical therapist practice.

I. **Ethical/Legal Considerations**
   A. Ethical Considerations
      The physical therapist practices according to the *Code of Ethics* of the American Physical Therapy Association.
      The physical therapist assistant complies with the *Standards of Ethical Conduct for the Physical Therapist Assistant* of the American Physical Therapy Association.
   B. Legal Considerations
      The physical therapist complies with all the legal requirements of jurisdictions regulating the practice of physical therapy.
      The physical therapist assistant complies with all the legal requirements of jurisdictions regulating the work of the assistant.

II. **Administration of the Physical Therapy Service**
   A. Statement of Mission, Purposes, and Goals
      The physical therapy service has a statement of mission, purposes, and goals that reflects the needs and interests of the patients/clients served, the physical therapy personnel affiliated with the service, and the community.
      The statement of mission, purposes, and goals:
      ■ *Defines the scope and limitations of the physical therapy service.*
      ■ *Identifies the goals and objectives of the service.*
      ■ *Is reviewed annually.*
   B. Organizational Plan
      The physical therapy service has a written organizational plan.
      The organizational plan:
      ■ *Describes relationships among components within the physical therapy service and, where the service is part of a larger organization, between the service and the other components of that organization.*
      ■ *Ensures that the service is directed by a physical therapist.*
      ■ *Defines supervisory structures within the service.*
      ■ *Reflects current personnel functions.*
   C. Policies and Procedures
      The physical therapy service has written policies and procedures that reflect the operation, mission, purposes, and goals of the service, and are consistent with the Association's standards, policies, positions, guidelines, and Code of Ethics.

Continued

BOX 2-1	Standards of Practice for Physical Therapy—cont'd

The written policies and procedures:
■ *Are reviewed regularly and revised as necessary.*
■ *Meet the requirements of federal and state law and external agencies.*
■ *Apply to, but are not limited to:*
  ■ *Care of patients/clients, including guidelines*
  ■ *Clinical education*
  ■ *Clinical research*
  ■ *Collaboration*
  ■ *Competency assessment*
  ■ *Criteria for access to care*
  ■ *Criteria for initiation and continuation of care*
  ■ *Criteria for referral to other appropriate health care providers*
  ■ *Criteria for termination of care*
  ■ *Documentation*
  ■ *Environmental safety*
  ■ *Equipment maintenance*
  ■ *Fiscal management*
  ■ *Improvement of quality of care and performance of services*
  ■ *Infection control*
  ■ *Job/position descriptions*
  ■ *Medical emergencies*
  ■ *Personnel-related policies*
  ■ *Rights of patients/clients*
  ■ *Staff orientation*

D. Administration
A physical therapist is responsible for the direction of the physical therapy service.
The physical therapist responsible for the direction of the physical therapy service:
■ *Ensures compliance with local, state, and federal requirements.*
■ *Ensures compliance with current APTA documents, including* Standards of Practice for Physical Therapy and the Criteria, Guide to Physical Therapist Practice, Code of Ethics, Guide for Professional Conduct, Standards of Ethical Conduct for the Physical Therapist Assistant, *and* Guide for Conduct of the Physical Therapist Assistant.
■ *Ensures that services are consistent with the mission, purposes, and goals of the physical therapy service.*
■ *Ensures that services are provided in accordance with established policies and procedures.*
■ *Reviews and updates policies and procedures.*
■ *Provides for training of physical therapy support personnel that ensures continued competence for their job description.*
■ *Provides for continuous in-service training on safety issues and for periodic safety inspection of equipment by qualified individuals.*

Continued

BOX 2-1	*Standards of Practice for Physical Therapy—cont'd*

E. Fiscal Management

The director of the physical therapy service, in consultation with physical therapy staff and appropriate administrative personnel, participates in planning for, and allocation of, resources. Fiscal planning and management of the service is based on sound accounting principles.

The fiscal management plan:

■ *Includes a budget that provides for optimal use of resources.*
■ *Ensures accurate recording and reporting of financial information.*
■ *Ensures compliance with legal requirements.*
■ *Allows for cost-effective utilization of resources.*
■ *Uses a fee schedule that is consistent with the cost of physical therapy services and that is within customary norms of fairness and reasonableness.*
■ *Considers option of providing pro bono services.*

F. Improvement of Quality of Care and Performance

The physical therapy service has a written plan for continuous improvement of quality of care and performance of services.

The improvement plan:

■ *Provides evidence of ongoing review and evaluation of the physical therapy service.*
■ *Provides a mechanism for documenting improvement in quality of care and performance.*
■ *Is consistent with requirements of external agencies, as applicable.*

G. Staffing

The physical therapy personnel affiliated with the physical therapy service have demonstrated competence and are sufficient to achieve the mission, purposes, and goals of the service.

The physical therapy service:

■ *Meets all legal requirements regarding licensure and certification of appropriate personnel.*
■ *Ensures that the level of expertise within the service is appropriate to the needs of the patients/clients served.*
■ *Provides appropriate professional and support personnel to meet the needs of the patient/client population.*

H. Staff Development

The physical therapy service has a written plan that provides for appropriate and ongoing staff development.

The staff development plan:

■ *Includes self-assessment, individual goal setting, and organizational needs in directing continuing education and learning activities.*
■ *Includes strategies for lifelong learning and professional and career development.*
■ *Includes mechanisms to foster mentorship activities.*

I. Physical Setting

The physical setting is designed to provide a safe and accessible environment that facilitates fulfillment of the mission, purposes, and goals of the physical therapy service. The equipment is safe and sufficient to achieve the purposes and goals of physical therapy.

Continued

BOX 2-1   *Standards of Practice for Physical Therapy—cont'd*

The physical setting:
- *Meets all applicable legal requirements for health and safety.*
- *Meets space needs appropriate for the number and type of patients/clients served.*

The equipment:
- *Meets all applicable legal requirements for health and safety.*
- *Is inspected routinely.*

J.   Collaboration

The physical therapy service collaborates with all disciplines as appropriate.

The collaboration when appropriate:
- *Uses a team approach to the care of patients/clients.*
- *Provides instruction of patients/clients and families.*
- *Ensures professional development and continuing education.*

III. Patient/Client Management

A.   *Patient/Client Collaboration*

Within the patient/client management process, the physical therapist and the patient/client establish and maintain an ongoing collaborative process of decision-making that exists throughout the provision of services.

B.   Initial Examination/Evaluation/Diagnosis/Prognosis

The physical therapist performs an initial examination and evaluation to establish a diagnosis and prognosis prior to intervention.

The physical therapist examination:
- *Is documented, dated, and appropriately authenticated by the physical therapist who performed it.*
- *Identifies the physical therapy needs of the patient/client.*
- *Incorporates appropriate tests and measures to facilitate outcome measurement.*
- *Produces data that are sufficient to allow evaluation, diagnosis, prognosis, and the establishment of a plan of care.*
- *May result in recommendations for additional services to meet the needs of the patient/client.*

C.   Plan of Care

The physical therapist establishes a plan of care and manages the needs of the patient/client based on the examination, evaluation, diagnosis, prognosis, goals, and outcomes of the planned interventions for identified impairments, functional limitations, and disabilities.

The physical therapist involves the patient/client and appropriate others in the planning, implementation, and assessment of the plan of care.

The physical therapist, in consultation with appropriate disciplines, plans for discharge of the patient/client taking into consideration achievement of anticipated goals and expected outcomes, and provides for appropriate follow-up or referral.

The plan of care:
- *Is based on the examination, evaluation, diagnosis, and prognosis.*
- *Identifies goals and outcomes.*
- *Describes the proposed intervention, including frequency and duration.*

Continued

BOX 2-1	*Standards of Practice for Physical Therapy—cont'd*

2

■ *Includes documentation that is dated and appropriately authenticated by the physical therapist who established the plan of care.*

D. Intervention

The physical therapist provides, or directs and supervises, the physical therapy intervention consistent with the results of the examination, evaluation, diagnosis, prognosis, and plan of care.

The intervention:

■ *Is based on the examination, evaluation, diagnosis, prognosis, and plan of care.*

■ *Is provided under the ongoing direction and supervision of the physical therapist.*

■ *Is provided in such a way that directed and supervised responsibilities are commensurate with the qualifications and the legal limitations of the physical therapist assistant.*

■ *Is altered in accordance with changes in response or status.*

■ *Is provided at a level that is consistent with current physical therapy practice.*

■ *Is interdisciplinary when necessary to meet the needs of the patient/client.*

■ *Documentation of the intervention is consistent with the* Guidelines: Physical Therapy Documentation of Patient/Client Management.

■ *Is dated and appropriately authenticated by the physical therapist or, when permissible by law, by the physical therapist assistant.*

E. Reexamination

The physical therapist reexamines the patient/client as necessary during an episode of care to evaluate progress or change in patient/client status and modifies the plan of care accordingly or discontinues physical therapy services.

The physical therapist reexamination:

■ *Is documented, dated, and appropriately authenticated by the physical therapist who performs it.*

■ *Includes modifications to the plan of care.*

F. Discharge/Discontinuation of Intervention

The physical therapist discharges the patient/client from physical therapy services when the anticipated goals or expected outcomes for the patient/client have been achieved.

The physical therapist discontinues intervention when the patient/client is unable to continue to progress toward goals or when the physical therapist determines that the patient/client will no longer benefit from physical therapy.

Discharge documentation:

■ *Includes the status of the patient/client at discharge and the goals and outcomes attained.*

■ *Is dated and appropriately authenticated by the physical therapist who performed the discharge.*

■ *Includes, when a patient/client is discharged prior to attainment of goals and outcomes, the status of the patient/client and the rationale for discontinuation.*

G. Communication/Coordination/Documentation

The physical therapist communicates, coordinates and documents all aspects of patient/client management including the results of the initial examination and evaluation, diagnosis, prognosis, plan of care, interventions, response to interventions, changes in patient/client status relative to the interventions, reexamination, and discharge/discontinuation of intervention and other patient/client management activities.

Continued

BOX 2-1	*Standards of Practice for Physical Therapy—cont'd*

Physical therapist documentation:

- *Is dated and appropriately authenticated by the physical therapist who performed the examination and established the plan of care.*
- *Is dated and appropriately authenticated by the physical therapist who performed the intervention or, when allowable by law or regulations, by the physical therapist assistant who performed specific components of the intervention as selected by the supervising physical therapist.*
- *Is dated and appropriately authenticated by the physical therapist who performed the reexamination, and includes modifications to the plan of care.*
- *Is dated and appropriately authenticated by the physical therapist who performed the discharge, and includes the status of the patient/client and the goals and outcomes achieved.*
- *Includes, when a patient/client is discharged prior to achievement of goals and outcomes, the status of the patient/client and the rationale for discontinuation.*

IV. Education

The physical therapist is responsible for individual professional development. The physical therapist assistant is responsible for individual career development.

The physical therapist, and the physical therapist assistant under the direction and supervision of the physical therapist, participate in the education of students.

The physical therapist educates and provides consultation to consumers and the general public regarding the purposes and benefits of physical therapy.

The physical therapist educates and provides consultation to consumers and the general public regarding the roles of the physical therapist and the physical therapist assistant.

The physical therapist:

- *Educates and provides consultation to consumers and the general public regarding the roles of the physical therapist, the physical therapist assistant, and other support personnel.*

V. Research

The physical therapist applies research findings to practice and encourages, participates in, and promotes activities that establish the outcomes of patient/client management provided by the physical therapist.

The physical therapist:

- *Ensures that their knowledge of research literature related to practice is current.*
- *Ensures that the rights of research subjects are protected, and the integrity of research is maintained.*
- *Participates in the research process as appropriate to individual education, experience, and expertise.*
- *Educates physical therapists, physical therapist assistants, students, other health professionals, and the general public about the outcomes of physical therapist practice.*

VI. Community Responsibility

The physical therapist demonstrates community responsibility by participating in community and community agency activities, educating the public, formulating public policy, or providing pro bono physical therapy services.

Continued

BOX 2-1   *Standards of Practice for Physical Therapy—cont'd*

The physical therapist:
- *Participates in community and community agency activities.*
- *Educates the public, including prevention, education, and health promotion.*
- *Helps formulate public policy.*
- *Provides pro bono physical therapy services.*

Glossary Standards and Criteria

Client—Individuals who engage the services of a physical therapist and who can benefit from the physical therapist's consultation, interventions, professional advice, health promotion, fitness, wellness, or prevention services. Clients also are businesses, school systems, and others to whom physical therapists provide services.

Diagnosis—Diagnosis is both a process and a label. The diagnostic process includes integrating and evaluating the data that are obtained during the examination to describe the patient/client condition in terms that will guide the prognosis, the plan of care, and intervention strategies. Physical therapists use diagnostic labels that identify the impact of a condition on function at the level of the system (especially the movement system) and at the level of the whole person.

Evaluation—A dynamic process in which the physical therapist makes clinical judgments based on data gathered during the examination.

Examination—A comprehensive screening and specific testing process leading to diagnostic classification or, as appropriate, to a referral to another practitioner. The examination has three components: the patient/client history, the systems review, and tests and measures.

Intervention—The purposeful interaction of the physical therapist with the patient/client and, when appropriate, with other individuals involved in patient/client care, using various physical therapy procedures and techniques to produce changes in the condition.

Patient—Individuals who are the recipients of physical therapy examination, evaluation, diagnosis, prognosis, and intervention and who have a disease, disorder, condition, impairment, functional limitation, or disability.

Physical therapist patient/client management model—The model on which physical therapists base management of the patient or client throughout the episode of care, including the following elements: examination, evaluation and reexamination, diagnosis, prognosis, and intervention leading to the outcome.

Plan of care—Statements that specify the goals and the outcomes, predicted level of optimal improvement, specific interventions to be used, and proposed duration and frequency of the interventions that are required to reach the goals and outcomes. The plan of care includes the anticipated discharge plans.

Prognosis—The determination of the predicted optimal level of improvement in function and the amount of time needed to reach that level.

Treatment—The sum of all interventions provided by the physical therapist to a patient/client during an episode of care.

From Standards of Practice of Physical Therapy, HOD S06-03-09-10 (*BOD S03-05-14-38*), House of Delegates Standards, Policies, Positions, and Guidelines. Alexandria, VA, American Physical Therapy Association, 2005.

PRIMARY, SECONDARY, AND TERTIARY CARE

Individuals who seek health care may move through multiple levels of providers as they enter the system and may eventually reach a specialist. The first level of care, **primary care,** is defined as the level of health care delivered by a member of the health care system who is responsible for the majority of the health needs of the individual.[3] This level of care usually, but not always, is provided by the first health care provider in contact with the recipient. Family and community members may also provide care at this level. **Secondary care** is provided by clinicians on a referral basis, that is, after the individual has received care at the primary level. In **tertiary care** the service is provided by specialists, commonly in facilities that focus on particular health conditions. These services may also be provided on a referral basis.

PTs are engaged in practice at all three levels of care. Physical therapy is most often delivered by referral as secondary or tertiary care. Tertiary care may be provided in a highly specialized unit, such as a burn care center. The entry point for an individual seeking physical therapy services, however, is shifting to primary care. This is described as **direct access** (also known as "autonomous practice" or "patient's choice"). As Burch states, the phrase "direct access" is preferred to "practice without referral," which implies no regard or interest in the critical services provided by practitioners in other disciplines.[4] In the 42 states where direct access is legal, individuals may obtain physical therapy services without requiring a referral from another health care provider. In this role the PT serves as a gatekeeper for further health care services (see also Chapter 7).

TEAM APPROACH

Regardless of the level of care provided, the PT works in collaboration with other health care professionals, including physicians, nurses, occupational therapists, dentists, social workers, speech-language pathologists, and orthotists/prosthetists. As the public seeks the services of other health care professionals, PTs collaborate with such practitioners as podiatrists, chiropractors, massage therapists, acupuncturists, and osteopaths. In addition, the therapist may communicate with other individuals, such as educators and insurers, for the ultimate benefit of the patient/client.

PREVENTION AND HEALTH PROMOTION

Fortunately, the general public has become more aware of healthy lifestyle habits and is engaging in activities and behavior that promote healthy living. By preventing or limiting dysfunction, individuals have more positive work and recreation experiences. In addition, the need for and cost of health care are reduced.

PTs, by virtue of their extensive education in normal body structure and function, are well qualified to provide services that prevent or limit dysfunction. These services may be categorized as screening or prevention activities.[3] In **screening**, the PT determines whether further services are needed from a PT or other health care professional. A common example is posture analysis of schoolchildren to determine whether scoliosis may be present. In

prevention activities the PT provides services designed to prevent, limit, or reduce pain and dysfunction. These programs generally include several components: a history questionnaire, medical screening and evaluation, consultation, exercise performance, and reassessment.[5] The history questionnaire provides information about general health and related habits. A comprehensive medical and physical evaluation is necessary to establish a baseline and design a program. Consultation is provided individually or in a group to describe the results of the evaluation and compare them with norms. The results of the evaluation are used to design exercise programs, which may be conducted at home, at work, or at a health-related facility. Periodic reassessment ensures program effectiveness and serves as a motivating factor.

Recently the business and health care industries have been cooperating to provide programs that will prevent injury and disease and thereby reduce health care costs while increasing productivity. PTs are directly involved in health promotion activities, both as consultants for establishment of programs and as providers of health care on site or in a health-related facility. The PT may conduct an analysis of **ergonomics** at the work site and perform a **functional capacity evaluation**. Ergonomics is the relationship between the worker, the worker's tasks, and the work environment, whereas a functional capacity evaluation involves an examination of the physical abilities of the worker to perform the required tasks.[6] Based on the evaluation, the therapist may design a **work-conditioning program** or **work-hardening program**. The work-conditioning program focuses on the physical dysfunction, whereas the work-hardening program includes this aspect in addition to behavioral and vocational management.[7] The goal of both programs is to return the individual to work.

PATIENT/CLIENT MANAGEMENT MODEL

The Guide to Physical Therapist Practice[3] has been instrumental in defining and describing what PTs do as clinicians. These activities have been summarized in the patient/client management model (Figure 2-1). This model reflects the process of gathering information, designing a plan of care, and implementing that plan to result in optimal outcomes for the patient/client.

Examination. The first component of the patient/client management model, **examination,** is the process of gathering information about the past and current status of the patient/client. It begins with a **history** to describe the past and current nature of the condition or health status of the patient/client. Sources for this information include the patient/client, caregivers, other health professionals, and medical records. A **systems review** is then conducted to obtain general information about the overall medical and cognitive status of the patient/client in five areas: musculoskeletal, neuromuscular, cardiovascular/pulmonary, integumentary, and communication. This review provides information to determine if referral to other health professionals is necessary. In the final component of the examination, **tests and measures,** the therapist selects and performs specific procedures to quantify the physical and functional status of the patient/client. A list of these tests and measures as

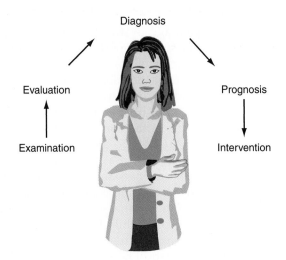

Diagnosis

Evaluation   Prognosis

Examination   Intervention

Figure 2-1 ■ The patient/client management model describes the sequence of events by physical therapists in the process of examination and intervention of individuals who receive care. (Modified from Guide to Physical Therapist Practice, revised ed 2. Alexandria, VA, American Physical Therapy Association, 2003.)

presented in the Guide appears in Table 2-1, and some examples are shown in Figures 2-2 through 2-7. Note that these activities involve observation, manual techniques, simple and complex equipment, and environmental analysis.

Evaluation. After the examination the therapist performs an evaluation as the second component of the patient/client management model. As defined in the Standards of Tests and Measurements in Physical Therapy Practice, an **evaluation** is a *judgment* based on a measurement.[8] The standards further define **assessment** as the *measurement* or assigned value. Therefore an evaluation is a process by which PTs make a clinical judgment based on an assessment.

Diagnosis. Evaluation is essential to establish a **diagnosis,** the next component of the model. The diagnosis is a categorization of the findings from the examination through a defined process. A diagnosis is established in accordance with a policy adopted by the House of Delegates of the APTA (Box 2-2).[9] This policy recognizes the professional and autonomous judgment of the PT and stipulates the responsibility for referral to other practitioners when warranted.

Prognosis. At this point in the model, attention shifts to the future to establish a **prognosis,** or a prediction of the level of improvement and time necessary to reach that level. The therapist also designs a **plan of care** that incorporates the expectations of the patient/client. It identifies short- and long-term goals (alleviation of impairments), outcomes (results of interventions), interventions

Table 2-1
Tests and Measures Used in a Physical Therapy Examination

Test/Measure	Description
Aerobic capacity/endurance	Ability to use the body's O_2 uptake and delivery system
Anthropometric characteristics	Body measurements and fat composition
Arousal, attention, and cognition	Degree of responsiveness and awareness
Assistive and adaptive devices	Equipment to aid in performing tasks
Circulation (arterial, venous, lymphatic)	Analysis of blood and lymph movement to determine adequacy of cardiovascular pump, oxygen delivery, and lymphatic drainage
Cranial/peripheral nerve integrity	Assessment of sensory and motor functions of cranial and peripheral nerves
Environmental, home, and work barriers	Analysis of physical restrictions to functioning in the environment
Ergonomics and body mechanics	Analyses of work tasks and postural adjustment to perform tasks
Gait, locomotion, and balance	Analyses of walking, moving from place to place, and equilibrium
Integumentary integrity	Health of the skin
Joint integrity and mobility	Assessment of joint structure and impact on passive movement
Motor function	Control of voluntary movement
Muscle performance	Analysis of muscle strength, power, and endurance
Neuromotor development and sensory integration	Evolution of movement skills and integration of information from the environment
Orthotic, protective, and supportive devices	Determination of need for fit of devices to support weak joints
Pain	Analysis of intensity, quality, and frequency of pain
Posture	Analysis of body alignment and positioning
Prosthetic requirements	Selection, fit, and use of prostheses
Range of motion	Amount of movement at a joint
Reflex integrity	Assessment of developmental, normal, and pathological reflexes
Self-care and home management	Analysis of activities necessary for independent living at home

Continued

Table 2-1
Tests and Measures Used in a Physical Therapy Examination—*cont'd*

Test/Measure	Description
Sensory integrity	Assessment of peripheral and central sensory processing, awareness of movement, and position
Ventilation and respiration/gas exchange	Assessment of movement of air into and out of the lungs, exchange of gases, and transport of blood to perform activities of daily living and exercises
Work, community, and leisure integration or reintegration	Analyses to determine whether the patient/client can assume a role in community or work

From Guide to Physical Therapist Practice, revised ed 2. Alexandria, VA, American Physical Therapy Association, 2003.

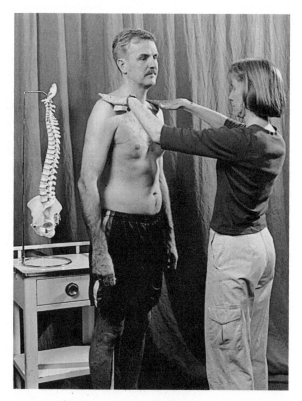

Figure 2-2 ■ Observation is an essential component of a physical therapy examination. In this case the therapist examines the patient's cervical posture. Compare with Figure 2-8. (Courtesy of Dewey Neild.)

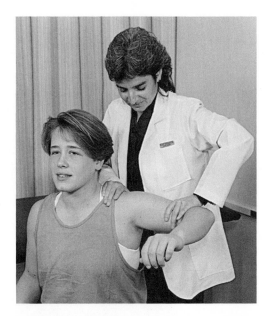

Figure **2-3** ■ Manual techniques such as manual muscle testing are critical in physical examination. Here the therapist is performing a muscle test on the patient's shoulder musculature. (Courtesy of Dewey Neild.)

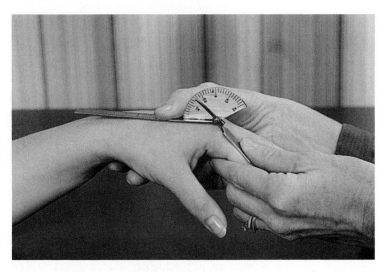

Figure **2-4** ■ Passive range of motion in the joints of the fingers is measured with a simple finger goniometer. (Courtesy of Dewey Neild.)

(type and frequency), and discharge criteria. The **goals** should be measurable, involve the patient/client or family member, and be linked to the impairments, functional limitations, and disabilities.[10] Only after these data-gathering and analysis activities have been completed can interventions begin.

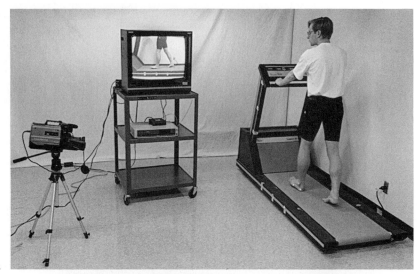

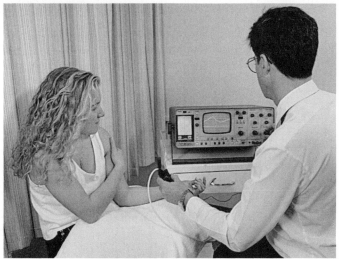

Figure 2-5 ■ The equipment used by physical therapists for examinations can be complex. **A,** In motion analysis of the lower extremity, the patient is videotaped with markers at the joint axes while walking on a treadmill. The videotape is analyzed by computer technology to provide an objective measure of performance. **B,** Electrodiagnostic equipment is used to measure the conduction velocity of nerves. (Courtesy of Dewey Neild.)

Intervention. The last component of the model, **intervention,** occurs when the PT and PTA conduct procedures with the patient/client to achieve the desired outcomes. This component is subdivided into three activities, each of which is described further in the following paragraphs.

COORDINATION, COMMUNICATION, AND DOCUMENTATION. A consistent exchange of information, both orally and in writing, is essential to ensure that all personnel

2

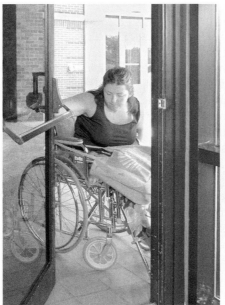
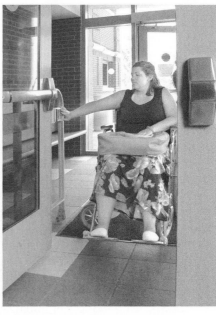

A **B**

***Figure* 2-6** ■ Architectural barriers in the environment, such as doorways that are difficult to manage in a wheelchair, are examined by the physical therapist. **A,** Managing manual doorways can be difficult for individuals in wheelchairs. **B,** Automatic doorways provide excellent accessibility for individuals who use a wheelchair or assistive device. (Courtesy of Dewey Neild.)

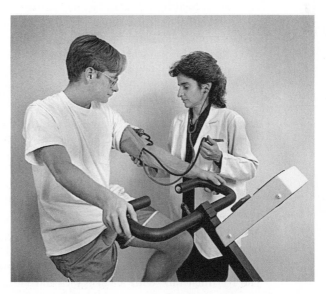

***Figure* 2-7** ■ Physical therapists can conduct cardiovascular and fitness tests with a stationary bicycle. (Courtesy of Dewey Neild.)

BOX 2-2	Diagnosis by Physical Therapists

It is the policy of the American Physical Therapy Association that:

- Physical therapists shall establish a diagnosis for each patient/client.
- Prior to making a patient/client management decision, physical therapists shall utilize the diagnostic process in order to establish a diagnosis for the specific conditions in need of the physical therapist's attention.
- A diagnosis is a label encompassing a cluster of signs and symptoms commonly associated with a disorder or syndrome or category of impairment, functional limitation, or disability. It is the decision reached as a result of the diagnostic process, which is the evaluation of information obtained from the patient/client examination. The purpose of the diagnosis is to guide the physical therapist in determining the most appropriate intervention strategy for each patient/client. In the event that the diagnostic process does not yield an identifiable cluster, disorder, syndrome, or category, intervention may be directed toward the alleviation of symptoms and remediation of impairment, functional limitation, or disability.
- The diagnostic process includes the following: obtaining relevant history, performing systems review, selecting and administering specific tests and measures, organizing and interpreting all data.
- In performing the diagnostic process, physical therapists may need to obtain additional information (including diagnostic labels) from other health professionals. In addition, as the diagnostic process continues, physical therapists may identify findings that should be shared with other health professionals, including referral sources, to ensure optimal patient/client care. When the patient/client is referred with a previously established diagnosis, the physical therapist should determine that clinical findings are consistent with that diagnosis. If the diagnostic process reveals findings that are outside the scope of the physical therapist's knowledge, experience, or expertise, the physical therapist should then refer the patient/client to an appropriate practitioner.

From Diagnosis by Physical Therapists, HOD P06-97-06-19, House of Delegates Standards, Policies, Positions, and Guidelines. Alexandria, VA, American Physical Therapy Association, 2005.

involved in care of the patient/client are well informed about his or her status. This process requires effective oral, written, and nonverbal communication. Although Chapter 4 is entirely devoted to communication, highlights are provided here as they relate to the patient/client management model.

Oral communication is a significant component of physical therapy service. The PT must talk with a variety of individuals, including the patient, family member, referral source, and additional practitioners providing care for the patient. Frequently a combination of oral and written communication is needed to provide a persuasive argument on behalf of the patient. PTs must be skilled communicators to describe their course of action.

Effective written communication is essential in the delivery of physical therapy services. Permanent records provide a baseline for future reference. They must be clear, concise, and accurate. Documentation is required by certain federal and state regulations and all insurance carriers. Fortunately, the APTA has constructed a set of Guidelines: Physical Therapy Documentation for Patient/Client Management[10] to assist PTs in this area.

Written communication can follow many formats. Documentation regarding evaluation and treatment can be written as a narrative. This design allows maximum flexibility but is unstructured. Standardized forms are frequently used as an efficient method of recording information. They are helpful, but the structure of the form may not apply to the particular patient/client situation.

A third format, the **SOAP note,** combines the best attributes of the narrative and standardized form. It is taken from the problem-oriented medical record system introduced by Weed in 1969.[11] The SOAP note is structured, yet adaptable and widely used among health care practitioners. The four components are *S* for subjective (what the patient/client/family member describes), *O* for objective (what the PT observes or measures), *A* for assessment (clinical judgment based on examination; includes goals), and *P* for plan (plan of care). The abbreviations provide an effective and efficient method for outlining and documenting patient information. It should be noted that use of the term "assessment" in this context is not the same as the definition in the Standards of Tests and Measurements in Physical Therapy Practice, but more like the term "evaluation" in the same document.[8]

Computer technology has influenced documentation in health care and has been incorporated into all three of the forms of written communication described above. Some systems simply provide terminals for writing narratives, whereas others use check-off forms on hand-held units. Efficiency in these systems must be balanced by effectiveness to ensure that important information is documented with minimal effort.

An occasionally overlooked mode of communication is nonverbal communication. Facial expressions, body posture, and gestures often convey honest emotions (fear, pain, pleasure) that a person may be suppressing. Mehrabian reported that 55% of the impact of messages comes from facial expression, whereas only 38% comes from the vocal component and 7% from the actual words.[12] PTs and PTAs must always be sensitive to the nonverbal signals displayed by themselves and their patients/clients.

PATIENT/CLIENT-RELATED INSTRUCTION. This activity refers to education and training of the patient/client and caregivers regarding the plan of care and environmental transitions. Instruction may include audiovisual aids, demonstrations, and home programs and should always incorporate the learning abilities and styles of the patient/client and caregiver.

PROCEDURAL INTERVENTION. Procedural intervention is the major therapeutic interaction between the therapist/assistant and patient/client. A list of these interventions, in preferred order of use, is presented in Table 2-2. Figures 2-8 through 2-14 illustrate some examples of these procedural interventions, which

Table 2-2
Procedural Interventions Used in Physical Therapy

Procedural Intervention	Description
Therapeutic exercise	Activities to improve physical function and health status; performed actively, passively, or against resistance
Functional training in self-care and home management	Activities to improve function in activities of daily living and independence in home environment
Functional training in work, community, and leisure integration or reintegration	Activities to integrate or return the patient/client to work
Manual therapy techniques	Skilled hand techniques on soft tissues and joints
Prescription, application, and, as appropriate, fabrication of devices and equipment	Selection (or fabrication), fit, and training in the use of devices and equipment to improve function
Airway clearance techniques	Activities to improve airway protection, ventilation, and respiration
Integumentary repair and protective techniques	Activities to improve wound healing and scar management
Electrotherapeutic modalities	Use of electricity to decrease pain, swelling, and unwanted muscular activity; maintain strength; and improve functional training and wound healing
Physical agents and mechanical modalities	Use of thermal, acoustic, or radiant energy and mechanical equipment to decrease pain and swelling and improve skin condition and joint movement

From Guide to Physical Therapist Practice, revised ed 2. Alexandria, VA, American Physical Therapy Association, 2003.

include manual techniques ("high-touch") and equipment ("high-tech"). At this point a PTA would be involved in a substantial component of the care as delegated by the PT. Further descriptions of procedural interventions can be found in each chapter of Part II of this text.

Throughout the course of the patient/client management model, the PT may periodically conduct reexaminations to determine the effect of the plan of care. If goals and outcomes are not being achieved, the plan, goals, and outcomes may be modified or the patient/client may be referred to other practitioners for services.

Ultimately, physical therapy services will be terminated. This occurs through one of two processes. **Discharge** takes place when the goals and outcomes have

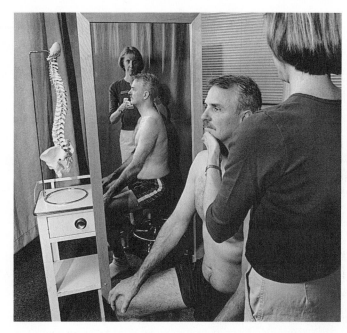

***Figure* 2-8** ■ The physical therapist corrects cervical posture with manual techniques and instruction. Compare with Figure 2-2. (Courtesy of Dewey Neild.)

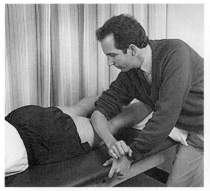
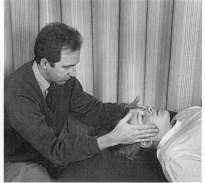

A

B

***Figure* 2-9** ■ Myofascial release techniques are effective, rigorous, and gentle manual stretching techniques for soft tissue. Examples shown are in, **A,** the posterior of the thigh (hamstring muscle) and, **B,** the temporomandibular joint region. (Courtesy of Dewey Neild.)

been achieved, as based on the PT's judgment. **Discontinuation** occurs when (1) the patient/client decides to terminate services, (2) the individual is no longer able to continue because of medical or financial reasons, or (3) the therapist believes that further intervention will not improve the status of the individual. In any case, the PT must plan for the end of services and document

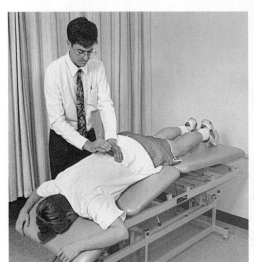 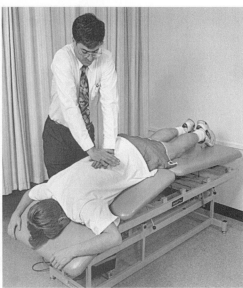

A   **B**

Figure 2-10 ■ Postural drainage involves positioning, percussion, and coughing techniques to remove fluid from specific parts of the lungs. **A,** A cupping technique is applied to the lower ribs in a head-down position to loosen mucus in the lower lobes of the lungs (cupping performed bilaterally). **B,** With outstretched arms the therapist shakes the thoracic cage while the patient exhales to encourage coughing that will remove fluid from the lungs. (Courtesy of Dewey Neild.)

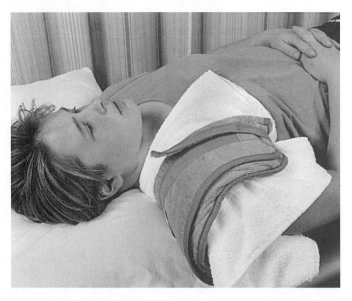

Figure 2-11 ■ Hot packs applied to the shoulder region provide an effective form of superficial heat. (Courtesy of Dewey Neild.)

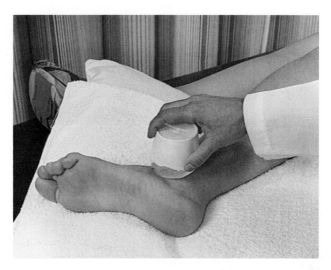

Figure 2-12 ■ An ice massage is administered to the ankle to decrease pain and swelling. (Courtesy of Dewey Neild.)

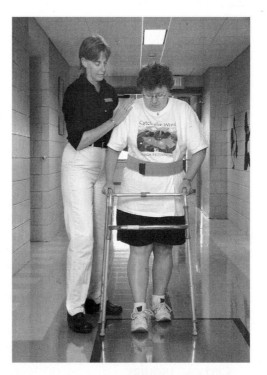

Figure 2-13 ■ A walker is an example of an assistive device used to improve a person's functional abilities, such as ambulation. (Courtesy of Dewey Neild.)

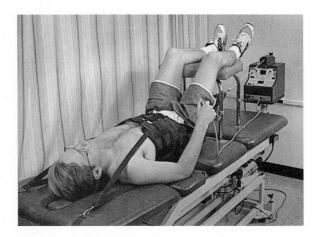

Figure **2-14** ■ Mechanical traction units are used to open disk spaces between vertebrae and reduce pain. (Courtesy of Dewey Neild.)

reasons for termination, status of the patient/client at that time, and any follow-up care that may be necessary.

OTHER PROFESSIONAL ROLES

CONSULTATION

PTs frequently provide consultation that is either patient centered or client centered. In patient-centered consultation the PT makes recommendations concerning the current or proposed physical therapy plan of care. This usually involves an examination but not intervention.

Client-centered consultation refers to the expert opinion or advice given to a client by the PT regarding situations that do not directly involve patient care. Examples include court testimony, architectural recommendations, academic and clinical program evaluation, and suggestions for health care policies.

EDUCATION

PTs and PTAs are continually providing education to a variety of audiences because instruction is an inherent part of patient care activity in physical therapy. Patients and sometimes family members are taught exercises or techniques to enhance function. Such instruction requires knowledge and skills that must be conveyed by the PT or PTA.

Instruction also occurs in the clinical facility when students are supervised during internships. Demonstration, supervision, and feedback are important for practicing and perfecting skills.

PTs and PTAs are involved in academic education. They may teach in a formal academic setting or a continuing education program.

CRITICAL INQUIRY

Critical inquiry in physical therapy is essential for viability of the profession. PTs and PTAs must be healthy skeptics and constantly ask why. They must be able to respond when practitioners and those who pay for their services question them about the choice and efficacy of their interventions. Unfortunately, PTs may not have sufficient answers to these questions. Practice must be based on sound evidence that comes from well-designed research (evidence-based practice). Sound practice is an inherent responsibility of every PT and PTA and is based on the selection of appropriate interventions, complete documentation, and outcomes assessment.

Research is the key to answering critical questions posed by healthy skeptics, within or outside the profession, who challenge the practices of PTs. Experimental and case studies are common methods for answering a research question or describing a technique or outcome. These studies are not necessarily expensive or complex and are usually generated by astute clinical observation and questioning. This type of research may require little more than good documentation and statistical comparison of two different procedural interventions.

ADMINISTRATION

PTs and PTAs may move into a variety of administrative positions. Generally, the promotion ladder in clinical facilities involves more administrative responsibilities at the expense of patient care activities. An individual could also leave the patient care environment and assume an executive position within a health care or related organization. Administrative responsibilities include planning, communicating, delegating, managing, directing, supervising, budgeting, and evaluating. These activities are particularly important when the PT is an owner or partner in an independent practice.

Somewhat related to this role is that of the PT as a case manager. In this scenario, one individual is responsible for managing the health care of the patient/client with regard to the diagnosis. This manager may be a physician, nurse, or other designated health professional, including a PT.[13] Inherent in this model is an agreement by the provider to accept a predetermined fee for the services required for the diagnosis.[14] The case manager has the responsibility and authority for managing the necessary services in a cost-effective manner to achieve the desired outcomes of the plan of care. This role is relatively new for PTs, but one that is important so that the profession can gain more control of reimbursement for necessary services by negotiating appropriate case fees and providing efficient and effective services.

CHARACTERISTICS OF PHYSICAL THERAPISTS

Demographic information on PTs is presented here; comparable information for PTAs is included in Chapter 3. Unless otherwise cited, these data are taken from annual surveys conducted by the APTA based on a sample of members, or for the last year conducted (2004), all members with e-mail addresses.[15]

DEMOGRAPHICS

Gender. Women continue to predominate in the profession of physical therapy. In 2004, they accounted for 68% of the PTs who were members of the APTA. This represents a slight decline in the ratio of women to men from an earlier survey (70:30 in 1999).

Age. The mean age of the respondents in 2004 was 42 years. A modest and progressive increase in this figure has been noted (35 years in 1978)[16]; however, the members of the profession remain relatively young.

Education. The highest earned academic degree of PT members is displayed in Figure 2-15. This represents a continual and significant shift toward the postbaccalaureate degree in comparison with past data. For example, in 1978, 81% of the respondents in a membership survey held the bachelor's degree and only 15% held the master's degree.[16] The recent proliferation and interest in DPT programs are also reflected in these data. Since 1999, the percent of respondents with this degree more than quadrupled, from 1.2% to 6%.

EMPLOYMENT FACILITY

A review of Figure 2-16 reveals that the highest percentage of respondents, 38.9%, are employed in a private office. Regardless of the type of employment facility, the vast majority of respondents, 69%, held full-time positions.

SUMMARY

The roles and activities of PTs have undergone an evolutionary change in response to the recent growth of managed care and mechanisms to control escalating health care costs. Despite these changes, diversity and opportunity remain widespread in physical therapy. Direct patient/client care continues to be the primary activity of PTs. Such care involves examination, evaluation, diagnosis, prognosis, and intervention as outlined in the patient/client management model. PTs also provide services to prevent pain and dysfunction and promote health. Other roles include consultation, education, critical inquiry, and

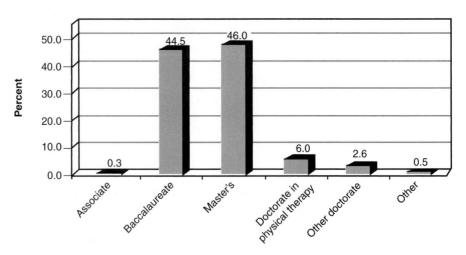

Figure 2-15 ■ Highest earned degree achieved by physical therapists who are members of the APTA (n = 42,107). (From PT: Highest Earned Degree. Alexandria, VA, American Physical Therapy Association. Available at http://www.apta.org/AM/Template.cfm?Section=Demographics& CONTENTID=26306&TEMPLATE=/CM/ContentDisplay.cfm. Accessed March 13, 2006.)

2

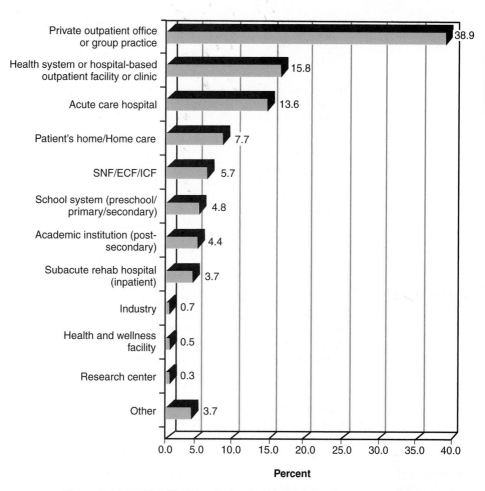

Figure 2-16 ■ Distribution of physical therapists who are members of the APTA by facility of employment (n = 42,864). (From PT: Type of Facility. Alexandria, VA, American Physical Therapy Association. Available at http://www.apta.org/AM/Template.cfm?Section=Demographics&TEMP LATE=/CM/ContentDisplay.cfm&CONTENTID=26309. Accessed March 13, 2006.)

administration. Regardless of the area of activity, PTs must collaborate with other health care providers and communicate effectively in the oral, written, and nonverbal modes.

In terms of demographics, the majority of PTs are female and relatively young. The master's degree predominates as the highest degree, but the number of therapists with a doctoral degree continues to increase. The most common employment facility is a private office.

The characteristics described here indicate that the profession continues to evolve and succeed. Such attributes contribute to the popularity of the profession and the enthusiasm of many individuals for pursuing a career as a PT or PTA.

REFERENCES

1. Pritchett P: The Employee Handbook of New Work Habits for a Radically Changing World. Dallas, Pritchett & Associates, 1994.
2. Standards of Practice for Physical Therapy, HOD S06-03-09-10. House of Delegates Standards, Policies, Positions, and Guidelines. Alexandria, VA, American Physical Therapy Association, 2005.
3. Guide to Physical Therapist Practice, revised ed 2. Alexandria, VA, American Physical Therapy Association, 2003.
4. Burch E: Direct access. *In:* Matthews J (ed): Practice Issues in Physical Therapy. Thorofare, NJ, Slack, 1989.
5. Huhn RH, Volski RV: Primary prevention programs for business and industry. Phys Ther 1985;65:1840-1844.
6. Key GL: Industrial physical therapy. *In:* Gould JA III (ed): Orthopaedic and Sports Physical Therapy, ed 2. St Louis, Mosby, 1990.
7. Resource Guide: Industrial Physical Therapy. Alexandria, VA, American Physical Therapy Association, 1992.
8. Task Force on Standards for Measurements in Physical Therapy: Standards for tests and measurements in physical therapy practice. Phys Ther 1991;71:589-622.
9. Diagnosis by Physical Therapists, HOD P06-97-06-19. House of Delegates Standards, Policies, Positions, and Guidelines. Alexandria, VA, American Physical Therapy Association, 2005.
10. Guidelines: Physical Therapy Documentation of Patient/Client Management, BOD G03-05-16-41. Board of Directors Standards, Positions, Guidelines, Policies, and Procedures. Alexandria, VA, American Physical Therapy Association, 2005.
11. Weed LL: Medical Records, Medical Education and Patient Care. Chicago, Year Book, 1970.
12. Mehrabian A: Silent Messages. Belmont, CA, Wadsworth, 1971.
13. Curtis KA: The Physical Therapist's Guide to Health Care. Thorofare, NJ, Slack, 1999.
14. Nosse LJ, Friberg DG, Kovacek PR: Managerial and Supervisory Principles for Physical Therapists, ed 2. Baltimore, Lippincott Williams & Wilkins, 2005.
15. Physical Therapist Membership Demographic Profile 1999-2004. Alexandria, VA, American Physical Therapy Association. Available at http://www.apta.org/AM/Template.cfm?Section=Demographics&Template=/MembersOnly.cfm&ContentID=25286. Accessed March 27, 2006.
16. American Physical Therapy Association 1987 Active Membership Profile Survey. Alexandria, VA, American Physical Therapy Association, 1987.

ADDITIONAL RESOURCES

Myers RS: Saunders Manual of Physical Therapy Practice, Philadelphia, Saunders, 1995.
   Comprehensive resource text written for experienced practicing physical therapy practitioners.
Pauls JA, Reed KL: Quick Reference to Physical Therapy. Gaithersburg, MD, Aspen, 1996.
   Synopsis of diseases, disorders, and dysfunctions discussed in the physical therapy literature. Extensive references are included.
Scully RM, Barnes ML: Physical Therapy. Philadelphia, Lippincott, 1989.
   A comprehensive text on the profession and practice of physical therapy for advanced level students or practitioners.
www.apta.org
   Website for the American Physical Therapy Association. Excellent resource for current information and documents pertinent to the profession.

REVIEW QUESTIONS

1. Why is the phrase "direct access" preferred over "practice without referral"?
2. You go to a PT for an injury sustained while skiing. Describe what you should expect at the first meeting before intervention begins.
3. Describe the steps in an initial examination.
4. What is included in a plan of care?
5. Discuss how you would decide which documentation format might best suit a PT's needs in any given situation. Show the advantages and disadvantages of each.
6. What is the difference between patient-centered and client-centered consultation?

W*hat matters is not the letters that come after your name, but what you can do.*

Nancy Watts, PT, FAPTA

3 Physical Therapist Assistant

Cheryl A. Carpenter-Davis

OBJECTIVES

After reading this chapter, the reader will be able to:
- Identify historical milestones in the development of the role of the physical therapist assistant
- Differentiate between the role of the physical therapist and the physical therapist assistant in the practice setting
- Define physical therapist assistant educational competencies in the areas of examination, measurement, and intervention
- Identify the rights and privileges of affiliate members in the American Physical Therapy Association

3

The demand for physical therapy services has expanded over the years. An insufficient number of physical therapists to perform the essential physical therapy services has been a problem throughout the history of the profession. As the population ages and medical technology changes, the need for physical therapy services will continue to grow.

The shortage of physical therapy personnel was an observation first made by Catherine Worthingham[1] as a member of a panel discussion on nonprofessional personnel in physical therapy at the 1964 Annual Conference of the American Physical Therapy Association (APTA). The problem identified in that address has been exacerbated as the demand for services has continued to increase. This shortage has led to the need for a new kind of health care team member—one who has knowledge of the life sciences, first aid, and physical therapy techniques and, most important, one who can problem solve to make patient care decisions. The void has been filled by the creation of a formally educated physical therapist assistant (PTA).

DEFINITION

A **physical therapist assistant** is a health care provider who has graduated from an accredited PTA associate degree program (Box 3-1) and whose function is to assist the physical therapist (PT) in the delivery of physical therapy services in compliance with federal and state laws and regulations regarding the practice of physical therapy.[2] Although in all jurisdictions the PTA carries out tasks delegated by the PT, the degree of supervision and autonomy varies by state.

ORIGIN AND HISTORY

The role of the PT and the use of support personnel have been influenced by events occurring over the past few decades. The Hill-Burton Act of 1946 and its amendment in 1954 provided specific funds for the construction of nursing homes, diagnostic and treatment centers, rehabilitation facilities, and chronic disease hospitals.[3] The provision for rehabilitation facilities created a new need for physical therapy.

Increased demands for physical therapy services resulted in a shift from the exclusive use of PTs to the use of support personnel for efficient and cost-effective delivery models of patient care. The anticipated growth of the profession prompted

BOX 3-1   *Definition of the Physical Therapist Assistant*

> The physical therapist assistant is a technically educated health care provider who assists the physical therapist in the provision of physical therapy. The physical therapist assistant is a graduate of a physical therapist assistant associate degree program accredited by the Commission on Accreditation in Physical Therapy Education (CAPTE).

From Direction and Supervision of the Physical Therapist Assistant, HOD P06-05-18-26. House of Delegates Standards, Policies, Positions, and Guidelines. Alexandria, VA, American Physical Therapy Association, 2005.

the 1949 APTA House of Delegates to adopt the first resolution concerning the use of nonprofessional personnel.

During the 1960s, efforts were made to ensure the continued provision of health care in response to the increased demand. The number of employees in the health services industry in 1960 was 2.6 million, a 54% increase over 1950. In 1965, the 89th Congress enacted laws that created Medicare and Medicaid. These laws began to officially recognize the need for innovative trends in health care. It was believed that the establishment and growth of new health care programs would create a need for supportive personnel. Medicare and Medicaid identified categories of these personnel and their relationships to primary care providers.[4]

Changes in the roles and responsibilities of support personnel resulted in a shift in the site of preparation from the work setting (hospital) to the educational setting (campus).[5] Several agencies began to investigate the creation of supportive personnel in physical therapy, including the American Association of Junior Colleges; the U.S. Department of Labor; the U.S. Department of Health, Education and Welfare; vocational schools; proprietary agencies; physician groups; nursing homes; and state health departments. The APTA recognized problems regarding shortages in support personnel and un-regulated education programs. Concern was expressed over the development of training programs without the benefit of physical therapy leadership and input.[6] A task force was established in 1964 to investigate the role of support personnel for the professional PT and the criteria for PTA education programs. In 1967, the task force submitted to the APTA House of Delegates a proposal for guidelines for use of the PTA.

On July 5, 1967, after deliberation, the House of Delegates adopted a policy statement regarding standards for PTA education programs, essentially giving birth to the PTA. The policy statement recommended several actions. The APTA was to establish the standards for the PTA education program, which included some form of accreditation. The profession would define the supervisory relationship between the PT and the PTA. A definition of the assistant would include the types of work PTAs would be allowed to perform. A suggestion was made that mandatory licensure or registration be encouraged and incorporated into existing physical therapy laws. A category of membership would be established in the APTA for PTAs.[7]

A subsequent policy further defined the PTA education program as a 2-year college program offered by an accredited educational institution. For approval, the education program had to provide information to the APTA Board of Directors, which evaluated the program against the standards and curriculum guidelines published by the APTA,[8] similar to the current accreditation process followed by existing PTA programs. Two PTA education programs were created in 1967. Two years later these institutions graduated the first 15 PTAs. The growth and development of new PTA education programs were phenomenal. PTA education programs eventually exceeded the number of PT education programs (Figure 3-1).

In the past decade, several factors combined to reverse the dramatic growth in the number of PTA education programs. The proliferation of managed care

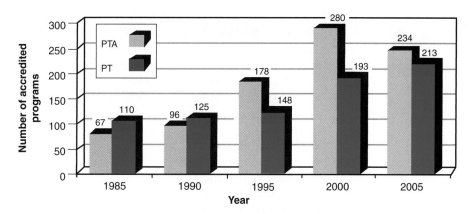

Figure 3-1 ■ Growth of physical therapist assistant and physical therapist education programs. (Data from 2005 Fact Sheet Physical Therapist Education Program and 2005 Fact Sheet Physical Therapist Assistant Education Program. Alexandria, VA, American Physical Therapy Association. Available at http://www.apta.org/AM/Template.cfm?Section=PT_ Programs1&Template=/TaggedPage/TaggedPageDisplay.cfm&TPLID= 132&ContentID=21559 and http://www.apta.org/AM/Template.cfm? Section=Program_Info&Template=/TaggedPage/TaggedPageDisplay.cfm &TPLID=121&ContentID=20582, respectively. Accessed April 16, 2006.)

and the Balanced Budget Act of 1997 led to a tight job market for all health care providers, including PTAs (see Chapter 7). As a result, the applicant pool for PTA education programs decreased significantly and some programs terminated voluntarily (Figure 3-1). Fortunately, the job market has improved and this has increased the number of applicants (see Employment Characteristics).

CURRICULUM AND ACCREDITATION STANDARDS

The curricula for all 2-year associate degree PTA education programs are designed to meet the accreditation standards outlined by the Commission on Accreditation in Physical Therapy Education (CAPTE), the same agency that accredits education programs for the PT.

Many similarities exist in the accreditation criteria for the PTA and the PT, which is indicative of their complementary and interactive roles in the clinical setting. The curricula for both these health care providers must consist of a combination of didactic and clinical learning experiences that reflect contemporary practice.[9,10] A comparison of the similarities and differences in their education programs provides a basis for understanding the tasks appropriate for delegation, supervision, and autonomy in clinical practice.

Educational similarities begin in the core curricula. Both PTA and PT students must complete such courses as anatomy, physiology, biology, and kinesiology, as well as general education courses required for the awarding of the students' respective degrees by the college or university. The difference in the PT's education is the depth of theory and practice provided during mandatory advanced courses in the foundational sciences, clinical sciences, and other areas such as administration and research.

BOX 3-2 Data Collection Skills in Physical Therapist Assistant Curriculum

- Aerobic capacity and endurance
- Anthropometrical characteristics
- Arousal, mentation, and cognition
- Assistive, adaptive, orthotic, protective, supportive, and prosthetic devices
- Gait, locomotion, and balance
- Integumentary integrity
- Joint integrity and mobility
- Muscle performance
- Neuromotor development
- Pain
- Posture
- Range of motion
- Self-care and home management and community or work reintegration
- Ventilation, respiration, and circulation examination

From Evaluative Criteria for Accreditation of Education Programs for the Preparation of Physical Therapist Assistants. Alexandria, VA, American Physical Therapy Association, 2000.

BOX 3-3 Intervention Techniques in Physical Therapist Assistant Curriculum

- Functional training
- Infection control procedures
- Manual therapy techniques
- Physical agents and mechanical agents
- Therapeutic exercise
- Wound management

From Evaluative Criteria for Accreditation of Education Programs for the Preparation of Physical Therapist Assistants. Alexandria, VA, American Physical Therapy Association, 2000.

Courses in the professional portions of the curricula are also similar in content areas. In regard to data collection skills, specific areas must be included in accordance with accreditation criteria (Box 3-2; compare with Table 2-1).[10] Similarly, intervention techniques in specific areas must be addressed (Box 3-3; compare with Table 2-2).[10] As above, the differences lie in the depth of underlying principles and complexity of application. Figure 3-2 illustrates a PTA performing an assessment and an intervention.

Clinical education is a requirement in both curricula. Programs must provide the PTA or PT student with clinical rotations in a variety of settings and with different patient populations. Students have the opportunity to work with numerous

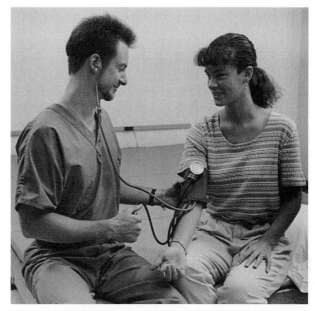

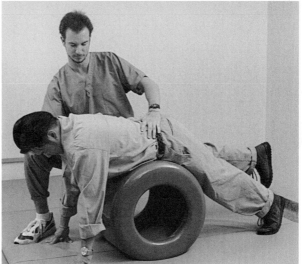

Figure 3-2 ■ Physical therapist assistant performing, **A,** an assessment (blood pressure measurement) and, **B,** an intervention (balance and strengthening exercises).

medical diagnoses in acute care, rehabilitation, outpatient, and school settings while supervised by a clinical instructor. PTAs may supervise PTA students, with additional direction provided by the center coordinator of clinical education or PT at the facility. PTs serve as clinical instructors for both PTA and PT students.

Often, PTA and PT students are involved in clinical affiliations at the same location, which provides an opportunity for students to communicate with one another regarding similarities in the physical therapy education programs. Delegation of tasks and the responsibility for patient follow-up could be simulated with guidance from the respective clinical instructors.

In addition to specific content areas, the accreditation criteria emphasize that PTA program graduates practice in an ethical, legal, safe, caring, and effective manner. The graduate must understand principles of authority and responsibility, planning and time management, the supervisory process, performance evaluations, policies and procedures, fiscal considerations for physical therapy, and quality assurance and must be able to plan for future professional development to maintain practice consistent with acceptable standards. PTA graduates must demonstrate the ability to modify intervention techniques as indicated in the plan of care designed by the PT or as necessitated by acute changes in the client's physiological state. The PTA graduate must also be able to read and interpret professional literature and critically analyze new concepts.

The PTA must be proficient in communication. The graduate must be able to interact with patients and families in a manner that provides the desired psychosocial support; teach other health providers, patients, and families to perform selected intervention procedures; participate in discharge planning and follow-up; document relevant aspects of patient treatment; and promote effective interpersonal relationships. Skill development in these areas requires knowledge and training in written, oral, and nonverbal communication.

UTILIZATION

PHYSICAL THERAPIST ASSISTANT

Although many similarities exist between the PTA and PT, differences in their roles appear soon after they begin employment. In a study conducted on the use of PTAs, Gossett[11] observed that initially new assistant graduates and new physical therapy graduates appeared to function similarly in a clinical setting. Soon after they entered employment, however, the new PT was expected to accept more responsibility in the areas of departmental supervision, patient evaluations, and performance of more complex treatment procedures, setting the therapist apart from the assistant.

Evaluation serves as a clear example of role distinction. The PT is responsible for performing the patient's physical therapy evaluation. This act requires interpreting the results of the examination and using the results as a guide to establish a diagnosis and prognosis, including realistic goals and a plan of care. This process requires understanding and judgment based on the theoretical premises of life sciences that have been provided in the physical therapist curriculum.

Many aspects of the plan of care may be delegated to the PTA. Delegation of patient intervention after the initial evaluation requires supervision and ongoing communication. The exchange of information is crucial to physical therapy practice. These and related responsibilities are delineated in the APTA policy Direction and Supervision of the Physical Therapist Assistant, which states in part, "Direction and supervision are essential in the provision of quality physical therapy services. The degree of direction and supervision necessary for assuring quality physical therapy services is dependent upon many factors, including the education, experience, and responsibilities of the

BOX 3-4   *Direction and Supervision of the Physical Therapist Assistant*

Physical therapists have a responsibility to deliver services in ways that protect the public safety and maximize the availability of their services. They do this through direct delivery of services in conjunction with responsible utilization of physical therapist assistants who assist with specific components of intervention. The physical therapist assistant is the only individual permitted to assist a physical therapist in selected interventions under the direction and supervision of a physical therapist.

Direction and supervision are essential in the provision of quality physical therapy services. The degree of direction and supervision necessary for assuring quality physical therapy services is dependent upon many factors, including the education, experiences, and responsibilities of the parties involved, as well as the organizational structure in which the physical therapy services are provided.

Regardless of the setting in which the service is given, the following responsibilities must be borne solely by the physical therapist:

1. Interpretation of referrals when available.
2. Initial examination, evaluation, diagnosis, and prognosis.
3. Development or modification of a plan of care which is based on the initial examination or reexamination and which includes the physical therapy anticipated goals and outcomes.
4. Determination of when the expertise and decision-making capability of the physical therapist requires the physical therapist to personally render physical therapy interventions and when it may be appropriate to utilize the physical therapist assistant. A physical therapist shall determine the most appropriate utilization of the physical therapist assistant that provides for the delivery of service that is safe, effective, and efficient.
5. Reexamination of the patients/clients in light of their goals, and revision of the plan of care when indicated.
6. Establishment of the discharge plan and documentation of discharge summary/status.
7. Oversight of all documentation for services rendered to each patient/client.

From Direction and Supervision of the Physical Therapist Assistant, HOD P05-06-18-26. House of Delegates Standards, Policies, Positions, and Guidelines. Alexandria, VA, American Physical Therapy Association, 2005.

parties involved, as well as the organizational structure in which the physical therapy services are provided" (Box 3-4).[2]

The factors of education, experience, and responsibilities deserve further analysis. *Education* to become a PTA has been previously reviewed in the Curriculum and Accreditation Standards section. Competency in such areas as therapeutic exercise, goniometry, manual muscle testing, and application of physical agents is a requirement of a PTA graduate. PTAs continue to expand their knowledge base and skills after graduation. Continuing education courses, staff development seminars, and individual in-service training by colleagues take place on an ongoing basis. For example, a PTA may attend an ergonomic seating seminar. Expertise in this area may lend itself to performance of ergonomic assessments for the patient population the PTA is treating. The PT may have included ergonomic instruction as part of the plan of care to be performed based on patient need and, if delegated to the PTA, based on the assistant's ability. If the PT did not delegate this component of care to the PTA, the PT could decide either to conduct the assessment personally or to refer the patient for ergonomic assessment elsewhere.

The degree of delegation and supervision also depends on *experience*. As the PTA continues to work in the clinical environment, this experience reinforces the depth of the knowledge and skill base in repeated areas of work and expands the breadth in new areas. The skills that are mastered become valuable factors for the employment market.

The third factor affecting delegation is *responsibilities*. Part of the APTA policy cited earlier in this section addresses the responsibilities of the PT. Although the PT may delegate all, some, or none of the intervention tasks to the PTA, the ultimate responsibility for the physical therapy services provided to the patient, including evaluations (initial, interim, and final), rests with the PT. Figure 3-3 depicts the delegation of responsibilities and interaction between the PT and PTA as a decision tree.

Delegation and level of responsibility are frequently regulated by PTA/PT ratios. Although PTA/PT ratios are not defined specifically in APTA policies, they may be established in a state physical therapy practice act. When establishing these ratios, the supervising PT, the PTA, and the facility management should be involved. The ratio should take into account the *experience* of the PT and PTA, the *impairment* of the patients, the *patient caseload* per therapist/assistant, and the *accessibility* of the PT by telecommunication. The APTA policy on direction and supervision of the PTA also addresses this issue (Box 3-5).[2]

For example, consider a therapist who is consulting at three clinical facilities in a rural area with one PTA in each facility. The patient load is approximately 15 to 18 patients a day for each PTA. The level of impairment varies from a few patients in intensive care units to patients in the acute care sections of the facilities. In addition, the therapist needs to evaluate 4 or 5 patients per day among the three facilities. The PT carries a beeper and is accessible at all times. Supervision is provided in accordance with the state practice act, which defines it as being available at all times through telecommunication, with weekly on-site visits. In this scenario the therapist is responsible for 45 to 54 patients with varying levels of impairment seen by the PTAs and for 4 or 5 patient evaluations per day. As can be seen from this example, special consideration should be given to establishing appropriate PTA/PT ratios.

Supervision is an inherent component of delegation, and although certain tasks may be delegated to a PTA, as noted earlier, the PT remains ultimately responsible for the patient. The PT must provide supervision, and the PTA should be able to request supervision as needed.

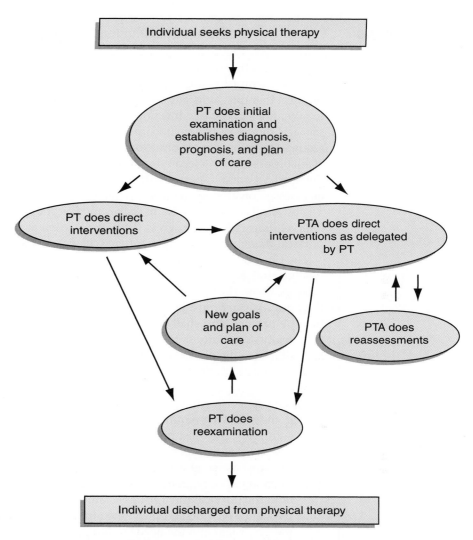

Figure 3-3 ■ Pathways of delegation (decision tree) involving the physical therapist (PT) and physical therapist assistant (PTA).

Delegation in physical therapy cannot rely on myths. As noted by Bashi and Domholdt in 1993,[12] facts to consider are that (1) PTAs are competent to perform many aspects of patient care delegated, including assessment and intervention techniques; (2) PTAs are competent to carry out a plan of care based on well-formulated goals with general instruction from the PT; (3) PTAs do not initially evaluate patients, nor do they diagnose or make a prognosis; (4) PTAs continue to gain expertise through continuing education, specialization, and work-related experience; and (5) PTAs are routinely performing the kinds of procedures that were once believed to be beyond a PTA's comprehension, just as PTs are diagnosing conditions and performing advanced examinations once deemed to be beyond the scope of the practice of physical therapy.

BOX 3-5	*Utilization of the Physical Therapist Assistant*

The physical therapist is directly responsible for the actions of the physical therapist assistant related to patient/client management. The physical therapist assistant may perform selected physical therapy interventions under the direction and at least general supervision of the physical therapist. In general supervision, the physical therapist is not required to be on-site for direction and supervision, but must be available at least by telecommunications. The ability of the physical therapist assistant to perform the selected interventions as directed shall be assessed on an ongoing basis by the supervising physical therapist. The physical therapist assistant makes modifications to selected interventions either to progress the patient/client as directed by the physical therapist or to ensure patient/client safety and comfort.

The physical therapist assistant must work under the direction and at least general supervision of the physical therapist. In all practice settings, the performance of selected interventions by the physical therapist assistant must be consistent with safe and legal physical therapy practice, and shall be predicated on the following factors: complexity and acuity of the patient/client's needs; proximity and accessibility to the physical therapist; supervision available in the event of emergencies or critical events; and type of setting in which the service is provided.

When supervising the physical therapist assistant in any off-site setting, the following requirements must be observed:

1. A physical therapist must be accessible by telecommunications to the physical therapist assistant at all times while the physical therapist assistant is treating patients/clients.
2. There must be regularly scheduled and documented conferences with the physical therapist assistant regarding patients/clients, the frequency of which is determined by the needs of the patient/client and the needs of the physical therapist assistant.
3. In those situations in which a physical therapist assistant is involved in the care of a patient/client, a supervisory visit by the physical therapist will be made:
   a. Upon the physical therapist assistant's request for a reexamination, when a change in treatment plan of care is needed, prior to any planned discharge, and in response to a change in the patient's/client's medical status.
   b. At least once a month, or at a higher frequency when established by the physical therapist, in accordance with the needs of the patient.

Continued

BOX 3-5 | *Utilization of the Physical Therapist Assistant—cont'd*

---

c. A supervisory visit should include:
1. An on-site re-examination of the patient/client.
2. On-site review of the plan of care with appropriate revision or termination.
3. Evaluation of need and recommendation for utilization of outside resources.

From Direction and Supervision of the Physical Therapist Assistant, HOD P05-06-18-26. House of Delegates Standards, Policies, Positions, and Guidelines. Alexandria, VA, American Physical Therapy Association, 2005.

As the physical therapy profession progresses, the personnel within it will be required to adapt to the changes. Although correct use of the title physical thera*pist* assistant implies that ultimate responsibility for physical thera*py* services rests with the PT, partnership is a key ingredient to success in the changing environment of physical therapy. (See also Chapter 7 for recent APTA decisions that affect the role of the PTA.)

PHYSICAL THERAPY AIDE

As the role and utilization of the PTA continue to evolve, confusion remains regarding the role and utilization of the **physical therapy aide**. In part, this uncertainty is due to the variety of state laws that regulate or are silent on the physical therapy aide. To provide clarity and consistency, the APTA adopted a position in 2000 to address the definition and utilization of the physical therapy aide (Box 3-6).[13] The position indicates that the scope of support services is very limited and that direct personal supervision must be continuous throughout each session. In some jurisdictions, supervision may be provided by the PTA.

STATE REGULATION

Physical therapy practice is regulated in all 50 states by practice acts (see Chapter 5). These practice acts define not only physical therapy, but also the qualifications required for use of the title and practice. As an example, each PT must be licensed by the state in which practice is being conducted. The purpose of licensure is to provide standards and protect the public from harm.

Practice acts also address the PTA. Variations in practice acts across the United States give rise to some of the confusion regarding use of PTAs. For instance, PTAs are regulated by licensure, registration, or certification in 43 states and U.S. territories.[14] Where these statutes exist, the PTA is most often defined as a graduate of an accredited PTA program. Although some states do not regulate PTAs, supervisory requirements may be delineated in the physical therapy rules and regulations for support personnel. Many state regulations specify that the PT may delegate aspects of physical therapy care to appropriately trained individuals. This policy directly affects the manner in which the PTA is used and supervised.

BOX 3-6   *Provision of Physical Therapy Interventions and Related Tasks*

Physical therapists are the only professionals who provide physical therapy interventions. Physical therapist assistants are the only individuals who provide selected physical therapy interventions under the direction and at least general supervision of the physical therapist.

Physical therapy aides are any support personnel who perform designated tasks related to the operation of the physical therapy service. Tasks are those activities that do not require the clinical decision making of the physical therapist or the clinical problem solving of the physical therapist assistant. Tasks related to patient/client management must be assigned to the physical therapy aide by the physical therapist, or where allowable by law, the physical therapist assistant, and may only be performed by the aide under direct personal supervision of the physical therapist, or where allowable by law, the physical therapist assistant. Direct personal supervision requires that the physical therapist, or where allowable by law, the physical therapist assistant, be physically present and immediately available to direct and supervise tasks that are related to patient/client management. The direction and supervision is continuous throughout the time these tasks are performed. The physical therapist or physical therapist assistant must have direct contact with the patient/ client during each session. Telecommunications does not meet the requirement of direct personal supervision.

From Provision of Physical Therapy Interventions and Related Tasks, HOD P06-00-17-28. House of Delegates Standards, Policies, Positions, and Guidelines. Alexandria, VA, American Physical Therapy Association, 2005.

These interstate variations result in a broad range of responsibilities and considerable confusion. For example, a state might mandate that the PT be available at all times via telecommunication while the PTA is providing patient care. This requirement would allow a PT to be off-site when a PTA is treating a patient as long as the PT is available by telecommunication. In contrast, if the practice act defines supervision as on-site, the PT must be within the same facility while a PTA is providing patient care.

The state physical therapy practice act provides the legal basis for physical therapy practice. It is imperative that the PT and PTA be familiar with the rules and regulations that pertain to their roles and practice in physical therapy (see Chapter 5).

CHARACTERISTICS OF PHYSICAL THERAPIST ASSISTANTS

Demographic characteristics and information regarding the current primary employment position of PTs were described in Chapter 2. Similar data were obtained from renewal applications by PTAs. The following two subsections are based on the most recent data available (2005) from the APTA website.[15]

DEMOGRAPHICS

Gender. Females accounted for 79% of the respondents. This degree of dominance exceeded that for physical therapist members of the APTA, which was 68%.

Age. Fifty-eight percent of the PTAs surveyed were under 40. Most survey respondents reported being between the ages of 30 and 34 years.

Education. The associate degree was the highest academic degree earned by 70% of the respondents (Figure 3-4), which reflects the degree requirement. A substantial number, 26%, held a bachelor's degree, and 4% held a master's degree.

EMPLOYMENT FACILITY

For PTAs, the primary employment patterns were similar to those for PTs (Figure 3-5), that is, just over one third were employed in a private office. On a percentage basis, twice as many PTAs (16%) as PTs (8%) were employed in an extended care facility. This difference in employment indicates the important role that PTAs perform in tasks delegated by PTs in these facilities. It also provides a context for studying the levels of responsibility of the PT and adequate supervision (see the preceding Utilization section). The current transition to a cost containment environment may play a role in economic decisions regarding the

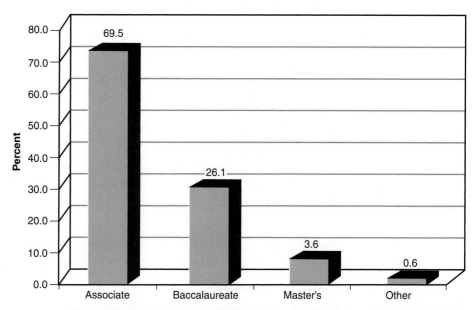

Figure 3-4 ■ Highest earned academic degree of physical therapist assistants (n = 3048). (From PTA: Highest Earned Degree. Alexandria, VA, American Physical Therapy Association. Available at http://www.apta.org/AM/Template.cfm?Section=Demographics&CONTENTID=26276&TEMPLATE=/CM/ContentDisplay.cfm. Accessed April 17, 2006.)

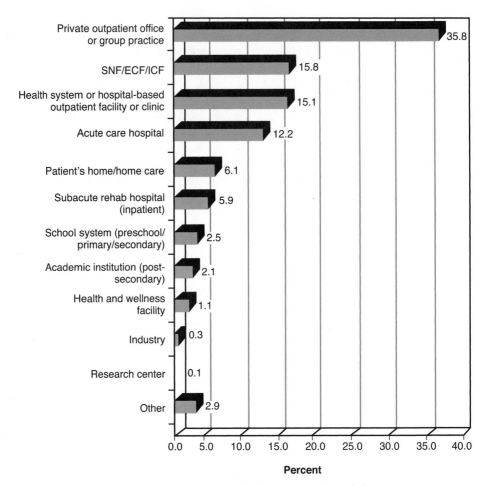

Figure 3-5 ■ Type of facility or institution where physical therapist assistants work (n = 3222). Compare with Figure 2-16 for physical therapists. (From PTA: Type of Facility, Alexandria, VA, American Physical Therapy Association. Available at http://www.apta.org/AM/Template.cfm? Section=Demographics&TEMPLATE=/CM/ContentDisplay.cfm&CONT ENTID=26279. Accessed April 17, 2006.)

relative staffing mix of PTAs and PTs in these settings. Regardless of the employment setting, the majority of respondents held full-time positions (78%).

CAREER DEVELOPMENT

When choosing a career, students consider the profession of physical therapy for a variety of reasons, the most common being that they want to work with patients. When considering a career as a PTA versus a PT, applicants must take into account many factors, such as finances, family, location of the education program, and future career goals.

In the job market, demand varies in accordance with society's need for the service. The need for physical therapy personnel has resulted in a favorable job market for the PTA. According to the U.S. Bureau of Labor Statistics, physical therapist assistant will be among the occupations showing faster than average growth through the year 2012.[16] Licensed PTAs can enhance the cost-effective provision of physical therapy services.

The variety of positions in physical therapy departments provides many opportunities for advancement. Like the PT, a PTA may have previous work experience in such areas as public relations, business, or education. Individual characteristics may include organizational skills, in-depth knowledge of reimbursement and documentation guidelines, and strategic planning skills. All these characteristics can be used in a physical therapy department in a variety of capacities, such as utilization coordinator, center coordinator of clinical education, or in-service coordinator. To make the greatest use of talented employees, most departments make a concerted effort to use any special skills.

In 1988, the APTA studied the issue of retention by conducting a survey of PTAs and PTs in hospital settings. The results revealed that PTAs remained employed at a facility for an average of 5 to 6 years, in contrast to an average of 1 to 2 years for PTs.[17] PTA respondents who had resigned from acute care settings cited low salary, limited opportunity for advancement, and a "nonflexible administration" as reasons for their decision.

The results of this survey prompted some facilities to begin designing **career ladders** for the PTA similar to career ladders for the PT. Eligibility requirements are based on years of experience and tenure at the facility. Duties describing the three position levels (PTA I, II, III) are categorized as clinical, administrative, teaching, educational, and professional. These career ladders are described in Table 3-1.

Another form of career development for a PTA is to return to an education program to pursue an advanced degree. For example, a degree in business may enable an assistant to become involved in the administrative component of a physical therapy practice.

A PTA may make the choice to pursue a degree as a PT. The reasons commonly cited are greater autonomy, greater responsibility for patient care, and an increase in pay. PTAs choosing to seek a degree as a PT should be aware that the coursework previously completed may not be acceptable in the physical therapist education program. Many of these programs allow the PTA to test out of certain courses, but such is not always the case.

RIGHTS AND PRIVILEGES IN THE APTA

The development of PTA education programs and the definition of utilization of support personnel eventually led to discussion regarding the formation of a class of membership for PTAs in the APTA. Heated debates over whether nonprofessional assistants should join the APTA ensued.

In his 1969 presidential address, Eugene Michels, PT, stated, "I am aware of the reasons given against the extension of voting privileges. Those reasons are insufficient and unconvincing. Some say that students and assistants will not know enough about the issues to vote intelligently. That argument is unsound for two reasons. First, give students and assistants half a chance, and you will soon find out what they do know. Second, every active and life member who

Table 3-1
Career Development for the Physical Therapist Assistant

Duties	Physical Therapist Assistant Level I (new graduate)
Clinical	Assists physical therapist in overall assessment of patient Assists in implementation of patient treatment
Administrative	Knowledgeable regarding department policy and procedures Organizes own schedule Carries a standard caseload Provides appropriate and accurate documentation Participates in quality improvement programs Participates in department administration
Teaching	Teaches appropriate techniques to patients and families Provides in-services to staff Provides educational opportunities to physical therapy students
Educational	Attends continuing education programs Attends facility meetings and orientations Attends departmental in-services Reads professional literature and remains current on physical therapy techniques Possesses current CPR certification
Professional	Demonstrates appropriate verbal communication skills Follows appropriate administrative policy Demonstrates professional behavior Actively participates in administrative meetings Demonstrates a willingness to participate in departmental functions
Duties	Physical Therapist Assistant Level II (2 years of experience, same job description as that of PTA I and additional duties listed below)
Clinical	Performs and interprets the results of selected measurement procedures in consultation with the physical therapist Makes modification in patient treatment based on information for less frequent diagnoses Is knowledgeable about community services and makes recommendations to the team
Administrative	Is familiar with policies and procedures and recommends changes as needed Is cognizant of patient care priorities and facility responsibilities and adapts accordingly Participates on facility committees

Continued

Table 3-1
Career Development for the Physical Therapist Assistant—cont'd

Teaching	Provides facility and community in-services Provides educational opportunities to PTA students of at least 1 full-time affiliation per year
Educational	Attends 3 continuing education programs per year Participates in 1 or more patient or community educational programs per year
Professional	Demonstrates appropriate professional conduct Is supportive of management response to staff
Duties	**Physical Therapist Assistant Level III** **(4 years of experience, same job description as that of PTA II and additional duties listed below)**
Clinical	Is able to interpret and follow the plan of care established by the physical therapist for less frequent diagnoses Assists those at the PTA I and PTA II level with the interpretation of subjective and objective evaluation information Assesses the available community services and makes recommendations to the team May initiate patient care conferences after consulting with the evaluating physical therapist
Administrative	Participates in updating policies and procedures with an awareness of standards of accrediting agencies Provides mentoring of those at the PTA I and PTA II level Investigates and initiates equipment repair and potential replacement
Teaching	Participates in orientation of new staff Provides educational opportunities to PTA students of at least 2 full-time affiliations per year
Educational	Attends 4 continuing education programs per year Participates in APTA activities
Professional	Provides insight to management regarding staff concerns

From Carpenter C: PTA career ladders. PT—Magazine of Physical Therapy 1993;1(1):56-61.
APTA, American Physical Therapy Association; *CPR,* cardiopulmonary resuscitation; *PTA,* physical therapist assistant.

3

currently holds a vote does not know what the issues are. Others fear the consequences of being out-voted by the combined power of students and assistants. If that should ever happen, and it is conceivable, the answers to the following two questions deflate that fear: (1) If it does happen, whose fault will it be? and (2) If it does happen, is it necessarily bad? I find it incredible that we place so little trust in others who, we assume, are perfectly content to place their full trust in us. What a familiar ring that has!"[18]

In 1973, the APTA House of Delegates approved a motion that provided an affiliate membership category for PTAs. The rights and privileges of an **affiliate member** (PTA) were different from those of an **active member** (PT). The affiliate member was entitled to (1) attend all meetings; (2) speak and make motions; (3) hold committee appointments, including chairman, but not any office at the national or component level; (4) serve as a chapter affiliate delegate; (5) assert a one-half vote; and (6) receive the official journal of the APTA.[19]

In 1983, the House of Delegates adopted a motion to support the formation of an Affiliate Special Interest Group to manage the concerns of the affiliate and provide more opportunities within the APTA for interaction. After this action, affiliate leaders began to formalize the **Affiliate Special Interest Group,** later known as ASIG, to identify concerns of affiliate members across the country. Regions were identified and assigned to people within the ASIG, and a chairperson was elected. This person served as the liaison with the APTA Board of Directors. The continued support of PTAs throughout the country made apparent the need for a formalized group within the APTA specifically for the PTA.

The issues surrounding categories of membership continued to plague the association. In even-numbered years, when amendments to the bylaws were proposed, topics from the past continued to be presented and defeated. The APTA Board of Directors responded by creating an organizational task force, which studied the issue for 2 years and presented its findings to the 1989 House of Delegates. Among the proposals was the formation of an assembly, whose purpose was to provide a means for members of the same class to meet, confer, and promote the interests of their class. This proposal was adopted in 1989, along with formation of the first assembly, the Affiliate Assembly.

The **Affiliate Assembly** was an officially recognized component of the APTA. The officers were PTAs elected by their peers. The Assembly officers were the affiliate's formal liaisons with the APTA officers and staff. Their mission was to promote the role of the PTA within the Association in keeping with the goals and objects of the Association.

One year after the Affiliate Assembly was created, the House of Delegates approved the **Student Assembly** (1990). The Student Assembly is composed of PT and PTA students. This networking ability will continue to provide a forum in which PTA and PT students can better understand their roles and responsibilities in physical therapy practice.

In 1992, a motion was proposed to the House of Delegates to allow PTAs to hold office at the component level (chapter and section) with the exception of the office of president. This motion was passed in 1992 and amended in 1994 to specify that the PTA could not hold an office that was in direct succession to the presidency of the component.

This motion provided additional rights and privileges to affiliate members. The adoption of such motions further builds on the mission of the APTA to meet the needs and interests of its membership. Over the past 5 years, great strides have been made in enabling PTAs, as members of the APTA, to assume a role in the leadership of physical therapy.

In 1998, the House of Delegates passed the controversial motion RC-1, which created the **National Assembly of Physical Therapist Assistants**, called simply the National Assembly. That body included all affiliate members automatically. In addition to officers, the National Assembly had regional directors who served geographical locations. Although this action excluded affiliates as voting members of the House of Delegates, it provided for the creation of a separate deliberative body unique to PTAs. This group, the **Representative Body of the National Assembly (RBNA),** had its first meeting in 1999. Its structure was similar to that of the House of Delegates and consisted of affiliate representatives from all chapters. The issues put forth in the RBNA dealt solely with issues that affected PTAs. Issues passed by the RBNA were sent to the House of Delegates for final approval. Two National Assembly delegates attended the House of Delegates and were allowed to speak, debate, and make and second motions, but they were not allowed to vote. In addition, three National Assembly board consultants attended sessions of the House to answer questions posed by the speaker of the House of Delegates.

Because the changes in the governance structure of affiliate members were so monumental, the House of Delegates that approved them also adopted a motion to study their effects and issue a final report in 2004. In 2003, the Task Force on National Assembly Governance was created. Findings from the "RC 40 TF" (a task force to study the future role of the PTA; see Chapter 7), although not directly related to governance, were also incorporated into the discussions. It was noted that the National Assembly structure created an opportunity for PTAs to serve as officers in the Assembly and as chapter delegates to the RBNA, but input into the decision-making process continued to be limited. Concerns cited in the final report included (1) limited decision-making abilities of the RBNA, (2) lack of a structural link between the APTA Board of Directors and the RBNA, and (3) absence of a structural link between the APTA Board of Directors and the National Assembly Board of Directors. After widespread input and discussion, the Task Force submitted several changes to the governance structure. These recommendations were enacted by actions of the House of Delegates and APTA Board of Directors in 2005. The House of Delegates amended the Bylaws of the Association, dissolved the National Assembly and RBNA, and formed a **PTA Caucus**. The PTA Caucus was organized to serve purposes as prescribed and published by the APTA Board of Directors. It consists of representatives who are physical therapist assistant, life physical therapist assistant, or retired physical therapist assistant members and are elected or selected at the chapter level. The purpose of the PTA Caucus is to represent the interests of PTAs in each chapter; to meet, confer, and provide recommendations on issues important to PTAs; and to elect the five PTA delegates to the House of Delegates. The five PTAs are elected to serve as nonvoting delegates to the APTA House of Delegates and are allowed to speak and debate in both the House of Delegates and the Caucuses.

Subsequent action by the APTA Board of Directors created an Advisory Panel of Physical Therapist Assistants consisting of five PTAs. An advisory panel is an established structure and an effective method to provide direct input to the APTA Board of Directors and thereby influence decisions. The Board of Directors appoints panel members to provide input regarding issues pertinent to the PTA. PTAs are also appointed to selected panels, including the Advisory Panels on Education and Practice based on nominations from components. Questions remain as to the exact operation of the PTA Caucus, but the overall changes allow PTAs to have a more direct say in Association issues.

TRENDS

Trends in health care will continue to influence the way in which PTs and PTAs are prepared and function in the provision of service. PTA education programs will continue to adapt their curricula to meet the needs of contemporary physical therapy services; on recommendation from the RC 40 TF, however, the House of Delegates reaffirmed the associate's degree as the minimal educational requirement for the PTA.[20] Continued growth in academic and clinical programs will result in greater use of PTAs in education programs as instructors, academic coordinators of clinical education, and program directors. PTAs in the clinic will continue to be directly involved in the supervision of PTA students during clinical rotations where the PTAs' advanced clinical expertise can be put to maximum use and allow them to be positive role models.

Clinical research is another area in which PTAs will play a greater role. To a large extent, the credibility of physical therapy will depend on continued research related to physical therapy outcome studies and provision of effective and efficient models of patient care. Such studies are continually needed to prove the worth of physical therapy services and thus ensure reimbursement for services rendered by all levels of physical therapy professionals.

The diversity of physical therapy services and society's need for these services, from prevention to the provision of care for the aging population, will create new demands for physical therapy practitioners. PTAs can provide the opportunity for PTs to spend additional time performing patient evaluation, diagnosis, prognosis, reevaluation, and research, which is not to say that the PTA can replace the therapist in patient care. Certain patient impairment levels will continue to require the presence of a PT.

PTAs will also continue to advance their skills and knowledge and become involved in departmental activities such as community education to facilitate health and wellness. Advanced clinical skills will lead to PTA specialization and an expanded need for PTA continuing education courses. As noted in Chapter 7, Recognition of Advanced Proficiency for the PTA was recently created and the first recipients were recognized at the APTA Annual Conference in 2005.

It should be no surprise, in view of all this growth, that developments affecting PTAs will continue at all levels within the APTA. The debate over governance issues that began at the inception of the PTA will continue. We should expect to see PTA members forming groups at the state level to focus on regional concerns, addressing issues of member rights and privileges at meetings of the House of Delegates, and serving more frequently as component officers and committee chairs, and perhaps on the APTA Board of Directors. Current and future PTAs must continually investigate options that will be most beneficial for meeting the needs of PTAs.

SUMMARY

Many turning points have occurred in the growth and development of the PTA. The APTA responded positively to an early need by creating the position of PTA in 1967. As a result, the profession has reaped the benefits of extending its influence and thereby expanding the provision of services to more people.

As PTs became involved in conducting more complicated evaluations and establishing diagnoses, the role of the PTA was advanced to include assessment and measurement activities and selected interventions as delegated by the PT. Education programs for the PTA proliferated and exceeded the number of educational programs for the PT. Governance opportunities for the PTA have continually been an issue, and the most recent revision was the creation of an Advisory Panel of Physical Therapist Assistants and PTA Caucus.

Physical therapy services continue to evolve in variety and mechanism of provision. Greater understanding regarding the personnel who provide these services will lead to more effective and efficient health care. This evolution will result in a profession that is empowered and prepared to face the challenges of tomorrow.

CASE STUDIES

The following case studies illustrate just two examples of the roles PTAs can take in the practice setting.

CASE STUDY ONE

Physical Therapist Assistant I (Novice)

Jackie, a PT working in a private practice setting, recently hired Don, a new graduate PTA. Before assigning patients, Jackie speaks with Don regarding his course work and the physical therapy experience he had during his clinical rotations.

Shortly after this conversation, Jackie reviews with Don the diagnosis, plan of care, and precautions for a new patient with the diagnosis of a frozen shoulder (adhesive capsulitis). After the patient's third treatment, Jackie questions Don on the patient's progress. Don reports that the treatment has consisted of the exercise program Jackie had suggested but that the patient continues to have difficulty moving his arm in the correct patterns.

Jackie asks Don to suggest an exercise that may work better. Don mentions that the patient tends to compensate with his body during pulley activities. He adds that the corrections made to the patient's position have not worked very well. Instead, he would like to try diagonal movement patterns with verbal cueing. Jackie suggests positioning the patient supine (lying face up) and using some of the diagonal patterns with verbal and physical cueing. Don agrees that positioning the patient supine would provide better trunk stability and decrease the compensatory patterns of the trunk. Jackie makes plans to work with Don and the patient during the next exercise session to problem solve together.

CASE STUDY TWO

Physical Therapist Assistant III (Senior)

Eric, a PT in a rural community hospital, has been working with the same PTA, Cindy, for 6 years. After a patient evaluation, Eric confers with Cindy regarding a patient with the diagnosis of a cerebrovascular accident (stroke). He asks Cindy to review the evaluation and address any questions with him before beginning treatment in the afternoon. He requests that Cindy see the patient twice daily.

Cindy reviews the evaluation and notes that the short-term goals of treatment are for the patient to sit unsupported for 5 minutes and transfer three of five times with standby assistance. Eric's long-term goal is for this patient to ambulate with an appropriate assistive device (e.g., cane, walker). Cindy also notes the patient's previous history of a myocardial infarction and coronary artery disease. Cindy determines that she will need to monitor blood pressure and pulse throughout the patient's treatment. Treatment sessions will be limited by the patient's endurance.

Later, Cindy walks into the patient's room, where she finds him sitting in a wheelchair at bedside. She introduces herself as a PTA on staff at the hospital. She reminds the patient of the PT who examined him in the morning and further explains that the PT has assigned her to work with the patient on movement activities. She explains that she will be taking the patient's blood pressure and pulse throughout the treatment sessions.

After informing the nurse, Cindy wheels the patient around the corner to the physical therapy gym. She transfers him to the mat and assesses his transfer and sitting balance. She uses some of the neurodevelopmental techniques that she learned at the fall conference to decrease the patient's sacral sitting posture. She then incorporates upper extremity activities of weight bearing and crossing the body midline. She monitors the patient's pulse and blood pressure during treatment. At the completion of the session, Cindy transports the patient back to his room and informs the nurse that she did so. After she returns to the physical therapy department, she sees Eric. She tells him that the patient did well during the first session and tolerated 20 minutes of treatment before becoming tired. She provides Eric with information regarding the patient's blood pressure and pulse responses during treatment. The PT concurs with the treatment approach.

After a week of treatment, the patient is able to sit unsupported for 5 minutes and transfers from sitting to standing with standby assistance. Cindy has reported this progress to Eric. After reexamining the patient together, they establish new short-term goals for the patient to stand with standby assistance for 5 minutes in the parallel bars, ambulate in the parallel bars for 5 to 10 feet with minimal to moderate assistance, perform dynamic sitting activities with extended reach, and maintain the appropriate posture three of five times without loss of balance.

The next day, Cindy speaks with the social worker and is advised that the patient has reached his insurance limit for skilled physical therapy services and will be leaving the hospital for an extended care facility. She reports this information to Eric and provides him with data on the patient's functional status, manual muscle test grades, and balance/endurance status. Eric reevaluates the patient with the input from Cindy and develops a discharge summary that includes the necessary equipment and a plan of care for the personnel at the extended care facility to follow. Eric writes the final discharge note based on the patient's last physical therapy treatment while Cindy orders the necessary equipment for the patient to take with him.

REFERENCES

1. Worthingham CA: Nonprofessional personnel in physical therapy. Phys Ther 1965;45:112-115.
2. Direction and Supervision of the Physical Therapist Assistant, HOD P06-05-18-26. House of Delegates Standards, Policies, Positions, and Guidelines. Alexandria, VA, American Physical Therapy Association, 2005.
3. Hill Burton State Plan Data: A National Summary. Washington, DC, US Department of Health, Education and Welfare, January 1962.
4. Blood H: Supportive personnel in the health-care system. Phys Ther 1970;50:173-180.
5. Blood H: Report of the Ad Hoc Committee to study the utilization and training of nonprofessional assistants. Phys Ther 1967;47(11, Part 2):31-39.
6. Hislop H: Man power versus mind power. Phys Ther 1963;43:711.
7. White B: Physical therapy assistants: Implications for the future. Phys Ther 1970;50:674-679.
8. Collopy S, Schenck J, Wood W: Report of a three-year study on the physical therapist assistant. Phys Ther 1972;52:1300-1307.
9. Evaluative Criteria for Accreditation of Education Programs for the Preparation of Physical Therapists. Alexandria, VA, American Physical Therapy Association. Available at http://www.apta.org/AM/Template.cfm?Section=Home&TEMPLATE=/CM/ContentDisplay.cfm&CONTENTID=25709. Accessed March 20, 2006.
10. Evaluative Criteria for Accreditation of Education Programs for the Preparation of Physical Therapist Assistants. Alexandria, VA, American Physical Therapy Association. Available at http://www.apta.org/AMT/Template.cfm?Section=Program_Info&CONTENTID=28816&TEMPLATE=/CM/ContentDisplay.cfm. Accessed April 16, 2006.
11. Gossett R: Assistant utilization: A pilot study. Phys Ther 1973;53:502-506.
12. Bashi HL, Domholdt E: Use of support personnel for physical therapy treatment. Phys Ther 1993;73:421-429.
13. Provision of Physical Therapy Interventions and Related Tasks, HOD P06-00-17-38, House of Delegates Standards, Policies, Positions, and Guidelines. Alexandria, VA, American Physical Therapy Association, 2005.
14. Jurisdictional Licensing Reference Guide. Alexandria, VA, Federation of State Boards of Physical Therapy. Available at http://www.fsbpt.org/publications/ReferenceGuide/. Accessed April 16, 2006.
15. PTA Demographics. Alexandria, VA, American Physical Therapy Association. Available at http://www.apta.org/AM/Template.cfm?Section=Demographics&Template=/TaggedPage/TaggedPageDisplay.cfm&TPLID=10. Accessed April 16, 2006.
16. 2004-05 Occupational Outlook Handbook. Washington, DC, Bureau of Labor Statistics, 2005.
17. Carpenter C: PTA career ladders. PT—Magazine of Physical Therapy 1993;1(1):56-61.
18. Michels E: The 1969 Presidential Address. Phys Ther 1969;49:1191-1200.
19. American Physical Therapy Association Bylaws. Phys Ther 1973;53:1095-1105.
20. Educational Degree Qualifications for Physical Therapist Assistants, HOD P06-03-25-22, House of Delegates Standards, Policies, Positions, and Guidelines. Alexandria, VA, American Physical Therapy Association, 2005.

ADDITIONAL RESOURCES

Canan B: What changes are predicted for the physical therapist assistant in the 1980s? Phys Ther 1980;60:312.
Guest commentary on the role of the PT and the assistant as a health care team.

Carpenter C: Physical therapist assistant issues in the 1980s and 1990s. *In:* Mathew JS (ed): Practice Issues in Physical Therapy: Current Patterns and Future Directions. Thorofare, NJ, Slack, 1989.
Overview of PTA origin, education, licensure, specialization, advancement opportunities, and APTA membership.

Carpenter C: Physical Therapist Assistant Education over the Decades. J Phys Ther Educ 2003;17(13):80-85.
Provides a historical perspective regarding physical therapist assistant education.

Carpenter C: APTA Oral History, June 1999. Available at apta.org.
Audio and videotape account of origin of the Affiliate Assembly and Affiliate Membership in the APTA.

Lovelace-Chandler V, Lovelace-Chandler B: Employment of physical therapist assistants in a residential state school. Phys Ther 1979;59:1243-1246.

Provides an analysis of PTA educational preparation and ethical guidelines to aid in the determination of appropriate utilization within a given facility.

Lupi-Williams F, James S, Murphy P: The PTA role and function. Clin Manage Phys Ther 1983;3(3):35-40.

A three-part overview that includes education, utilization in general practice, and a job description of the PTA in a school setting.

Murphy W: Healing the Generations: A History of Physical Therapy and the American Physical Therapy Association. Alexandria, VA, American Physical Therapy Association, 1995.

The book provides a historical perspective of physical therapy and includes a section regarding the physical therapist assistant.

Robinson A, DePalma M, McCall M: Physical therapist assistants' perceptions of documented roles of the physical therapist assistant. Phys Ther 1995:75(12)1054-1064; discussion 1064-1066.

The study investigated physical therapist assistant perceptions of the documented roles of PTAs and compared the perceptions with those of physical therapists from the 1994 study.

Robinson A, McCall M, DePalma MT, et al: Physical therapists' perceptions of the roles of the physical therapist assistant. Phys Ther 1994;74:571-582.

A longitudinal study that investigated PTs' perception of the roles of the PTA through surveys conducted in 1986 and 1992.

Schunk C, Lippert L, Reeves B: PTA practice: In reality. Clin Manage Phys Ther 1992;12(6):88-92.

A survey of licensed PTAs in Oregon, conducted by the Affiliate Affairs Committee of the Oregon Physical Therapy Association, regarding how PTAs practice, what supervision standards are in effect, and what PTAs believe about their utilization.

Woods: PTA twentieth anniversary. PT—Magazine of Physical Therapy 1993;1(4):34-45.

Describes the evolution of the PTA in relation to the APTA and the profession.

REVIEW QUESTIONS

1. Contrast competencies in a PTA curriculum with those in a PT curriculum.
2. Identify common myths regarding the role and utilization of PTAs. Can you combat these myths with "myth-breaking" facts about PTA competence?
3. Describe the scope of PTA competency in the practice setting.
4. What is the difference between a PTA and a physical therapy aide?
5. Discuss the wide-ranging supervision requirements for using physical therapy aides.
6. How might such skills as in-depth knowledge of reimbursement and documentation guidelines or strategic planning be used in the physical therapy setting?

Therapeutic communication requires learning a new skill, but more than that, it requires unlearning habitual, non-helpful ways of interacting.

Carol M Davis, PT

4 Communication in Physical Therapy in the 21st Century

Helen L. Masin

KEY TERMS

affective domain
beginning professional behaviors
cultural continuum
culture of medicine
developing professional behaviors

entry level professional behaviors
generic abilities
high-context assumptions
internal dialogue
LAMP document
low-context assumptions
matching
post–entry level professional behavior
rapport—cultural, verbal, and behavioral
self-assessment

OBJECTIVES ■

After reading this chapter, the reader will be
able to:
■ Define the components of communication
■ Recognize the role of the affective domain in
communication

■ Use rapport in building effective
communication
■ Recognize effective communication in a
multicultural health care environment
■ Discuss high- and low-context
communication assumptions
■ Recognize the culture of medicine
■ Discuss differences in communication across
generations
■ Respond effectively to patients/clients
with visual or auditory impairments, or both
■ Respond effectively to patients/clients and
their caregivers/families
■ Respond effectively with other members of
the health care team
■ Develop effective communication as a
student in both the classroom and the clinic

Physical therapy practitioners of the 21st century agree that communication
is integral to the successful practice of physical therapy. The purpose of this
chapter is to provide you with both a theoretical and practical background for
developing the communication skills you will need to become an effective
physical therapist (PT) or physical therapist assistant (PTA) in the 21st century.
In the spirit of communication, this chapter is written in a more personal tone.
Reflective questions and actions are embedded throughout the chapter (rather
than placed at the end) to promote a more direct consideration of the theory or
application of the skill and the art of therapeutic communication.

The American Physical Therapy Association has defined a clear vision[1] for the
profession in the 21st century (Box 4-1). This has had an impact on goals and
action in practice, education, and research as well as professional behaviors.

BOX 4-1 APTA *Vision Sentence for Physical Therapy* 2020

Physical therapy will be provided by physical therapists who are
doctors of physical therapy, recognized by consumer and other health
care professionals as the practitioners of choice to whom consumers
have direct access for the diagnosis of, interventions for, and prevention
of impairments, functional limitations, and disabilities related to
movement, function, and health.

From APTA Vision Sentence for Physical Therapy 2020 and APTA Vision Statement for
Physical Therapy 2020, HOD P06-00-24-35, House of Delegates Policies, Positions, and
Guidelines. Alexandria, VA, American Physical Therapy Association, 2005.

Similar values and behaviors are recognized by the Section on Health Policy and Administration of the American Physical Therapy Association (APTA) in the development of Leadership, Administration, Management, and Professionalism (LAMP) skills set forth by the Section.[2] These skills are promoted in a **LAMP document** and annual LAMP Summit meeting. In the core values and beliefs of the 2002 LAMP Summit, all PTs, not just managers, must have LAMP skills to become effective professionals.[2]

In the rapidly changing health care environment, LAMP skills affect the physical therapy profession's ability to influence large organizations such as local, state, and national agencies. LAMP skills are the basis for developing such leadership behaviors as networking and political activism, which promote the growth of the profession.

In the educational environment, LAMP skills can best be integrated into the educational experience when they are woven throughout the curriculum. Academic and clinical faculty can model the LAMP skills in the classroom and thereby provide students with role models for learning these behaviors in both the classroom and the clinic.

A recent Delphi study by Lopopolo, Schaeffer, and Nosse[3] revealed that the top-ranked LAMP skills identified by respondents were communication, professional involvement and ethical practice, delegation and supervision, stress management, reimbursement sources, time management, and health care industry scanning. All of the respondents were experienced managers and members of the American Physical Therapy Association (APTA) who were familiar with the content of the LAMP skills. Of the top-ranked LAMP categories, communication had the highest median score and was therefore the most important category. The findings indicated that beginning PTs need "extensive knowledge" of communication techniques and should be "skilled" in applying these techniques in a clinical environment. These skills are essential in both the clinical management and the patient care aspects of physical therapy. To develop the knowledge and skill essential in communication, you need to appreciate what is involved in effective communication.

WHAT IS COMMUNICATION?

What does communication mean to you? Write down your definition of communication before reading further.

As defined in Webster's II New Collegiate Dictionary,[4] communication is "the act or process of communicating; transmission. To communicate is to make known; to transmit to others; to have an interchange; as of ideas or information." There are many types of communication skills, including skills in verbal and nonverbal interactions or reading, writing, and listening. Communication can occur between individuals, within an individual, or among a group of people.

VERBAL AND NONVERBAL COMMUNICATION

What happens during communication between individuals? Both verbal and nonverbal elements of communication occur simultaneously. You can hear what each person is saying when individuals talk to each other. You can observe their body language and notice whether what they are saying matches their body language. The verbal and nonverbal systems together transmit a message.

Think of a recent conversation you had with a friend. What did the friend say to you? What did his or her gestures and facial expressions convey to you? Were the verbal and nonverbal messages similar? How do you know?

Communication may occur within an individual, and this is called **internal dialogue.**[5] It is "heard" only by the individual himself or herself and may affect his or her nonverbal communication to other people. "Internal dialogue" may occur when the individual is alone, with another person, or in a group of people.

Think of a time when you were meeting with your academic advisor. You were listening to her words, but you also "heard" yourself talking to yourself about what you wanted to do over the weekend. The professor noticed that you were not attending to the conversation, but she did not know what was causing your inattention. Your inattention may affect your interactions with her in future conversations. What assumptions might she have made regarding your inattention? How do you know?

Communication may also occur in a group. In a group interaction, multiple speakers may be conveying information both verbally and nonverbally.

Think of a time when you were listening to a professor lecture about a topic in physical therapy. The professor asks several questions of the class. Some students are enthusiastically raising their hands to answer while others may appear to be dozing. What assumptions do you think the professor might make regarding the differing communications by these students? How do you know?

Communication occurs every time we interact with each other. Communication occurs whether or not words are spoken.

Think of a time when you met someone but did not speak to him or her. What assumptions did you make about that person? What cues did you notice about the person to make those assumptions?

READING

Reading is a critical communication skill that enables you to evaluate professional literature and use the findings in your practice. Your reading and understanding of medical information about your patient/client are essential for developing effective physical therapy evaluations and interventions. In addition, your ability to read, understand, and use information from current literature will enhance the quality of care you provide.

WRITING

Writing is an essential communication skill for clinical care, as well as communication with other professionals and peers. Your accurate writing skills often determine whether you will be reimbursed for your services by third party payers. Claims may be denied because of inadequate documentation. Whether you are writing a clinical evaluation for reimbursement or an article for a peer-reviewed journal, your writing skills reflect your ability to effectively communicate your findings to your readers.

LISTENING

Listening is a foundational communication skill for your success as a professional. Whether you are actively listening when interviewing a client or listening to a colleague request your input, your ability to listen actively will let the speaker know that you have understood his or her intended meaning. According to Davis,[6] active listening requires practice and is not easy. It contains three elements: restatement, reflection, and clarification. Restatement involves repeating the words of the speaker as you have heard them. Reflection involves verbalizing both the content and the implied feelings of the sender. Clarification involves summarizing or simplifying the sender's thoughts and feelings and resolving unclear verbalizations by the sender.

As a physical therapy professional, you can develop skill with all five types of communication. You can benefit from understanding the impact of verbal and nonverbal communication for yourself, your colleagues, your patients, and their families. In addition, you can enhance your skills in reading, writing, and listening. According to Davis,[6] communication by practitioners may enhance or detract from their therapeutic presence in their interactions. As a practitioner, you can learn the communication skills that enhance your therapeutic presence and thereby promote healing.

Visualize yourself as a student at your first clinical internship. You are meeting with your first client for the first time. What types of communication occur between you and this new client? How do you know?

GENERIC ABILITIES AND COMMUNICATION

To better appreciate the communication that occurs during the interaction that you visualized above, refer to the **generic abilities** described by May et al. (Table 4-1).[7] This research was initially conducted by use of a Delphi study with clinical educators from the University of Wisconsin in Madison. These behaviors have also been recommended as essential for the development of LAMP skills for practicing clinicians.[2] Clinical educators were asked to identify the behaviors essential for physical therapy professionals that were not explicitly part of the profession's core of knowledge and technical skills, but were required for success in the profession. Ten essential skills were identified. Each of these behaviors can be related to the development of effective communication skills. Through mastering each of these behaviors, you demonstrate the behaviors of a physical therapy professional and thereby enhance your communication with your clients, their families, and your colleagues.

BUILDING AFFECTIVE COMMUNICATION SKILLS

Three domains of learning have been described. The cognitive domain[8] involves knowledge, application, analysis, synthesis, and evaluation and deals with didactic learning. The psychomotor domain[9] involves perception, guided response, complex overt response, and adaptation and deals with "hands-on" skills. Skills in the **affective domain** are considered among the most difficult to teach because this domain deals with attitudes, values, and character development that influence all the other professional skills.[10] This also applies to communication skills. Communication falls within the affective domain.

Table 4-1
The Generic Abilities

Essential Skill	Description and Examples
Commitment to learning	Commitment to learning refers to your ability to self-assess, self-correct, and self-direct. You will identify the needs and sources for your learning and continually seek new knowledge. For example, you may receive feedback from your clinical instructor that you appear shy when working with patients/clients. You would self-assess your behaviors and use the instructor's feedback to learn how to become more assertive in your communication with patients/clients.
Interpersonal skills	Interpersonal skills refer to your ability to interact effectively with patients/clients, families, colleagues, other health care professionals, and the community and to deal effectively with cultural and ethnic diversity issues. For example, you might be working with a patient/client who speaks a language different from your own. You decide to learn more about the culture of your patient/client by reading about that culture and by learning greetings and basic physical therapy commands in the native language of the patient/client.
Communication skills	Communication skills are related to your ability to communicate effectively for varied audiences and purposes. For examples, your communication may include verbal, nonverbal, reading, writing, and listening skill. Your active listening skills will assist you in working with all of your patients/clients during examination, evaluation, and intervention of the patient/client. When you write a home program, you are demonstrating your writing skills as well as your interpersonal skills. You may need to modify your program if the patient/client is unable to read or has a visual impairment. By recognizing the unique needs of the patient/client, you can create a home program that matches the patient's/client's needs. Communication skill also incorporates your ability to critically read evidence-based literature, as well as write and disseminate evidence-based literature. Your clinical research could be written as a case study or presented as a platform or poster presentation at a local, state, or national physical therapy conference.
Effective use of time and resources	Effective use of time and resources demonstrates your ability to maximize benefit from a minimum investment of time and resources. An example of effective use of time and resources related to communication would be learning essential phrases used during physical therapy in the language of your patient/client.
Use of constructive feedback	Use of constructive feedback demonstrates your ability to identify and seek out sources of feedback and use them effectively for improving personal interaction. An example would be actively listening to constructive feedback from your clinical instructor and then incorporating that feedback to improve your clinical skills.

Continued

Table 4-1
The Generic Abilities—cont'd

Essential Skill	Description and Examples
Problem solving	Problem solving demonstrates your ability to recognize and define problems, analyze data, develop and implement solutions, and evaluate outcomes. An example might be analyzing your findings from examining a patient/client, implementing treatment, and evaluating the outcome. If you discover that the outcome was not successful, you can reevaluate and implement another solution. You will also use effective listening skills when assessing the patient/client and modify your treatment accordingly. You will use your verbal and nonverbal communication skills to explain to your patient/client how you are modifying the treatment to enhance the outcome.
Professionalism	Professionalism is your ability to exhibit appropriate professional conduct and to represent the profession effectively. An example would be demonstrating respect for your patients/clients by greeting them in a culturally appropriate manner. In formal cultures, your patient/client may prefer to be addressed by his/her surname. In informal cultures, the patient/client may prefer to be addressed by his/her first name.
Responsibility	Responsibility is your ability to fulfill commitments and to be accountable for actions and outcomes. An example would be following through on your verbal and written commitments related to patient care, service, and research in the profession.
Critical thinking	Critical thinking demonstrates your ability to question logically, to generate and evaluate elements of an argument, to distinguish facts from assumptions, and to distinguish the relevant from the irrelevant. An example would be the ability to evaluate written resources on the Internet. Your critical thinking skills would enable you to determine if the information was valid. If not, you would be able to identify alternative sources that would be more appropriate.
Stress management	Stress management is your ability to identify sources of stress in yourself and develop effective coping behaviors. An example would be recognizing your own frustration when you have difficulty communicating with a patient/client who speaks a language different from your own. You then need to request a trained medical interpreter to work more effectively with this patient/client.

The mastery of affective behaviors develops over time. May et al.[7] described **beginning, developing, entry level,** and **post–entry level professional behaviors** related to the generic abilities. These ten behaviors have specific behaviors associated with performance at each level of development. Beginning professional behaviors develop during the didactic portion of the curriculum. Developing professional behaviors may be acquired during the first half of each internship experience. As students mature and integrate these professional behaviors into their practice, they enhance their effectiveness in the classroom and the clinical setting and contribute to the growth of the profession. Table 4-2 describes each level of the behaviors related to communication for physical therapy students.

Since many beginning PTs and PTAs are young adults, they are learning attitudes, behaviors, values, and character attributes that lay the foundation for their professional development.[11] According to Davis,[6] when students fail to acquire the behaviors on their own, faculty members should assist them in developing these behaviors. When students face challenges in the affective domain, faculty may assist them in learning professional behaviors through **self-assessment** using the generic abilities and guided discovery during advisory sessions with a faculty member.[12]

Faculty can also assist students in developing their affective communication skills by teaching them how to recognize and use **rapport** in their interactions.

Table 4-2
Levels of Student Affective Behaviors That Relate to the Generic Abilities

Behavior Level	Description and Examples
Beginning level behaviors	Demonstrates understanding of basic English (verbal and written); uses correct grammar, accurate spelling and expression Writes legibly Recognizes impact of nonverbal communication; maintains eye contact, listens actively Maintains eye contact (when appropriate)
Developing level behaviors	Uses nonverbal communication to augment verbal messages Restates, reflects, and clarifies message Collects necessary information from the patient interview
Entry level behaviors	Modifies communication (verbal and written) to meet the needs of different audiences Presents verbal or written message with logical organization and sequencing Maintains open and constructive communication Uses communication technology effectively Dictates clearly and concisely

From May WW, Morgan BJ, Lemke JC, et al: Model for ability-based assessment in physical therapy education. J Phys Ther Educ 1995;9(1):3-6.

When building rapport, the professional must be aware of both verbal and nonverbal components of communication (Table 4-3).[13] These are further described below.

In verbal communication you can recognize a variety of communication patterns by listening to the speaker.[13] The language patterns of the speaker may help you to identify his or her learning style. For example, a speaker may say "That sounds good" when hearing about the prescribed exercise program. This suggests an auditory learning pattern. Auditory learners may prefer to learn the exercises by hearing you describe how to perform them. The pace of the speaker might include long or short pauses between words or thoughts. The tonality of the speaker might be high pitched and nervous or low pitched and calm. The intent of the speaker might be to request help or demand service. The speed of the communication might be fast, slow, or variable. Through paying attention to these patterns, you can build rapport by **matching** the client's verbal pace, tonality, intent, and speed.

In nonverbal communication you can recognize the gestures, postures, haptics, proxemics, and oculesics of the speaker.[13] Haptics demonstrate the use of touch as part of a communication pattern. For some people, touching during speaking is an important cue. Others might consider touching to be rude. Proxemics is the distance between the speaker and the listener. Appropriate distance between speaker and listener varies depending on the cultural background of the speaker. Oculesics is the use of eye contact or gaze aversion. In some groups direct eye contact is a sign of respect for the speaker, whereas in other groups gaze aversion signals respect. As a professional you must learn the nonverbal cues that specifically apply to the patients you serve.

Rapport is an important characteristic of communication. Rapport is defined as an interaction marked by mutual collaboration and respect but not necessarily indicating agreement.[5] When people are in rapport, they have behavioral patterns that become similar in nature.

The first of the three primary types of rapport is cultural rapport, which is established by using the form of dress or greeting appropriate to the setting. For example, you might wear a lab coat in an acute care clinical setting, but a

Table 4-3
Verbal and Nonverbal Components of Communication

Verbal Components	Nonverbal Components
Language	Gesture
Pacing	Posture
Tonality	Haptics
Intent	Proxemics
Speed of communication	Oculesics

polo shirt and khaki pants in an outpatient orthopaedic clinical setting. You might use a traditional greeting style appropriate for the culture of your patient, such as touching the patient's cheek or shaking hands with the patient (Figure 4-1).

Remember a clinical situation in which you thought your clothing was appropriate for the particular clinical setting. How did you know?

The second type of rapport is verbal rapport. This is established when you use the same or similar descriptive phrases and conversation content as the person with whom you are speaking. For example, you might work with a client who asks to "see you do the exercises" before performing them. You might respond by "showing" the patient/client how to do the exercise and

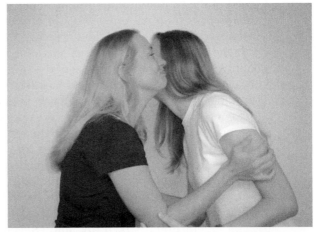

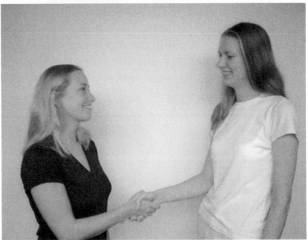

Figure 4-1 ■ Cultural rapport. **A,** Both participants use a common Latin American greeting of touching each other on the cheek. The participants are "in sync" and building rapport with each other. **B,** Both participants use a common North American greeting of shaking hands. The participants are "in sync" and building rapport.

using verbal language patterns related to visual descriptors such as, "How does this look to you?"

Remember a situation in which you were talking with a patient/client and the conversation seemed to flow very easily. What type of language patterns was the patient/client using? What type of language patterns were you using?

The third type of rapport is behavioral. This is established when you mirror the posture and body movements of the person with whom you are speaking. You may also match the person's voice tonality and tempo. For example, you might be working with a toddler in an early intervention program for your pediatric clinical rotation. You could squat or kneel at the eye level of the toddler to build behavioral rapport. Another example might be matching the posture while the person is sitting in a chair (Figure 4-2). To break rapport, you can mismatch the posture of the listener by *not* mirroring it (Figure 4-3).

Remember a situation in which you talked to a patient/client in a wheelchair. Did you change your posture so that you were at the level of the patient/client's eyes? Did changing your posture affect your communication with that patient/client?

Through matching the cultural, verbal, and behavioral patterns of another person, the professional can build rapport in the interaction. Rapport is closely related to the communication process. Studies have shown that people who assume like postures are judged to have a higher rapport with each other than those who do not have similar postures. Through enhancing rapport, the clinician builds a collaborative relationship characterized by mutual respect and harmony. When you coordinate your nonverbal behavior with others, you indicate to them that you are listening to them and want to hear more. Interpersonal interactions with positive emotions and attention enhance the total experience of rapport. Good rapport is often described as harmonious or "in tune," whereas poor rapport is described as awkward or "out of sync" (Figures 4-4 and 4-5).[14]

When students first learn about rapport and matching, they sometimes express concern that the person will notice that they are being matched posturally or verbally. In my experience, individuals are rarely aware of being matched by the professional.

To use matching skills, you need to feel comfortable with yourself. If you are anxious about using these skills, your anxiety may be conveyed to the listener. Therefore you are advised to practice your rapport skills in low-stress situations (at the 1 to 3 level on a scale of 1 to 10 intensity) with classmates, family, and friends before using them with clients. Also practice your matching skills during low-stress communications with your friends and family. Once you feel comfortable with your skills in low-stress situations, you may practice at higher levels. When you feel comfortable using the skill in nonclinical situations, you can apply the skill in the clinical setting. As you become more skilled at recognizing and interpreting verbal and nonverbal patterns in yourself and others, these skills will become more automatic for you.

Students must learn to recognize when to break rapport in a challenging situation. You can mismatch verbal and postural patterns to break rapport when someone is making inappropriate comments or sexual overtures. If you are seated, you might stand and assertively state that the comments of the patient/

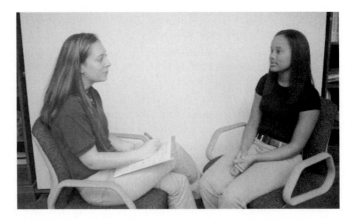

Figure 4-2 ■ Building behavioral rapport. The speaker seated on the left matches the body posture and eye contact of the listener seated on the right. The participants are "in sync" and building rapport with each other.

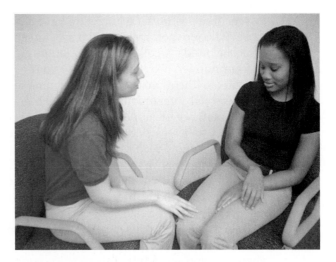

Figure 4-3 ■ Breaking behavioral rapport. The speaker on the left leans forward and touches the listener while the listener on the right leans back in her chair, pulls away, and gazes downward. The speaker is breaking rapport with the listener. They are "out of sync" and rapport is being broken.

client are not acceptable in the clinical environment and that you cannot continue treatment unless the inappropriate comments cease. As you learn to use these communication skills effectively, you will demonstrate your professionalism and maturity when dealing with challenging situations. For example, in a group, you might remain in your seat and avoid eye contact with someone in the group who stands up and makes inappropriate comments during a meeting (Figure 4-6).

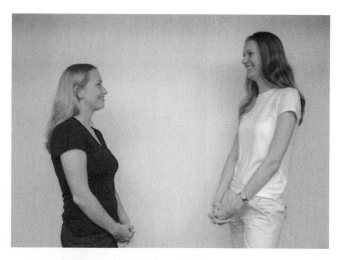

Figure 4-4 ■ Building behavioral rapport. The speaker standing on the left matches the posture, eye contact, and facial expression of the listener standing on the right. They are "in sync" and building rapport.

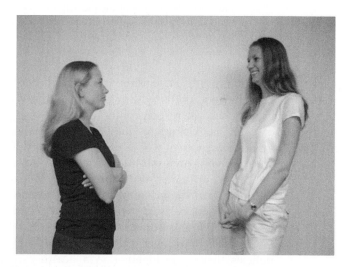

Figure 4-5 ■ Breaking behavioral rapport. The speaker standing on the left breaks rapport by crossing her arms while speaking when the listener on the right is standing with her hands clasped in front. They are "out of sync" and rapport is being broken.

COMMUNICATING EFFECTIVELY IN A MULTICULTURAL HEALTH CARE ENVIRONMENT

As a PT in the 21st century, you will be working with patients/clients and families from a wide variety of ethnicities, generations, religious beliefs, sexual preferences, and socioeconomic backgrounds. Their at-risk status and physical or mental capabilities will differ. Effective communication skills can assist you in working optimally with patients/clients from a diversity of cultures, beliefs, and sociocultural groups.

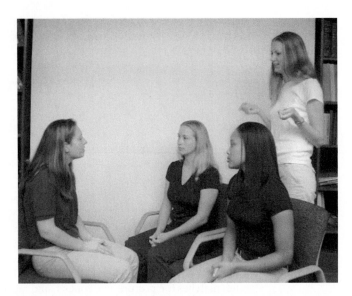

Figure 4-6 ■ Rapport with a group. The speaker seated on the left is matching the posture of the participants seated on the right and mismatching the posture of the participant standing on the right. The speaker is "in sync" with those seated and "out of sync" with the participant who is standing.

According to Pellegrino,[15] the definition of a professional is a person who puts the good of those he or she serves ahead of self-interest. As a professional PT, you assume responsibility for modifying your behavior to meet the needs of your client. Students may find this challenging if they have not lived or worked in settings where there is diversity. To put the good of those served ahead of your own self-interest, you can learn to acknowledge and appreciate the beliefs, attitudes, and behaviors of clients from a variety of backgrounds. You can learn the skills to become culturally competent in your knowledge, attitudes, and behaviors when working with clients and colleagues whose culture is different from your own.

Cultural competence is defined as having the set of behaviors, attitudes, and policies that come together in a health care system, agency, or individual practitioner to function effectively in cross-cultural interactions.[16] In the affective domain this includes awareness of the impact of sociocultural factors, acceptance of responsibility for understanding the cultural dimensions of health and illness, willingness to make clinical settings more accessible to patients of all cultures, appreciation of the heterogeneity that exists within and across cultural groups, recognition of one's own personal biases and reactions, and appreciation of how one's personal cultural values, assumptions, and beliefs affect clinical care.[17] The Vision Statement for Physical Therapy 2020 by the House of Delegates specifically states that PTs and PTAs will "provide culturally sensitive care distinguished by trust, respect and an appreciation for individual differences."[1]

Levels of sensitivity to cultural behaviors have been described as a **cultural continuum.**[18] The cultural continuum is a theoretical model that describes six stages of culturally related behaviors, including (cultural) destructiveness, incapacity, blindness, precompetency, competency, and proficiency (Table 4-4). Students may find themselves at different levels of the cultural continuum as they develop their professional skills.

I have an interesting anecdote regarding the stage of cultural blindness. When I taught the cultural continuum to a group of health care professionals several years ago, one of the participants made an important observation about the term "cultural blindness." As a person who was blind himself, he suggested that the term be changed from cultural blindness to cultural neutral. He pointed out that our use of language itself may indicate our bias or stereotype toward a group of people.

There are indications that the health care community is becoming more sensitive to cultural competency. According to Leavitt, "In my opinion, which is based on my 30 years of experience in this area, many physical therapists—and health care institutions—today are progressing from cultural blindness (neutral) to cultural pre-competence."[19] Health care institutions have begun to recognize the roles that racism and health care disparities play in access

Table 4-4
Stages of the Cultural Continuum

Stage	Description
Cultural destructiveness	People are treated in a dehumanizing manner and denied services on purpose.
Cultural incapacity	Health care systems are unable to work with patients from other cultures effectively, and they treat patients with biases, paternalism, and stereotypes.
Cultural blindness (neutral)	Presumption that all people are the same and that biases do not exist. Services are ethnocentric and encourage assimilation.
Cultural precompetence	Health care system is using appropriate response to cultural differences, weaknesses are acknowledged, and alternatives are sought.
Cultural competence	Cultural differences are accepted and respected. There is continuous expansion of cultural knowledge and resources and services are continuously adapted. There is constant vigilance regarding the dynamics of cultural differences.
Cultural proficiency	Cultural differences are highly regarded. The need for research on cultural differences is acknowledged, and new approaches are developed to promote culturally competent practice.

From Leavitt RL: Cross Cultural Rehabilitation: An International Perspective. London, Saunders, 1994.

to appropriate health care. Indeed, the Office of Minority Health issued 14 Standards for the Provision of Culturally and Linguistically Appropriate Services (CLAS) and made guidelines and recommendations for implementation.[20] These standards are designed to encourage health care organizations and employees to provide more culturally competent services recognizing the needs of culturally and linguistically different individuals and their families.

Reflect on the six stages of cultural competency. Where would you place yourself on the cultural continuum? What skills do you need to learn to enhance your cultural competency? What resources are available to assist you?

COMMUNICATING WITH PEOPLE FROM CULTURES DIFFERENT FROM YOUR OWN

Anthropologists and linguists have long recognized the critical role that culture plays in developing our relationships with those whose culture is different from our own. Anthropologist and linguist Michael Agar stated that "communication in today's world requires culture. Problems in communication are rooted in *who you are* in encounters with a *different mentality, different meanings, a different tie* between language and consciousness. Solving the problems inspired by such encounters inspires culture."[21] As PTs and PTAs, we work with individuals from a diversity of cultures in the broadest sense of culture. This includes individuals with differences in ethnicity, gender, disability, socioeconomic status, sexual orientation, religion, philosophy, and health care expectations. Each of these differences requires us to develop our cultural competence in order to enhance our effectiveness in working with these patients/clients and colleagues.

The first step in enhancing cross-cultural communication is recognizing your own cultural beliefs, attitudes, and behaviors as well as the beliefs, attitudes and behaviors of your profession. You can reflect on your family history and cultural ties and how these affect your life and assumptions about others. For example, your culture may place a high value on direct eye contact or on gaze aversion during verbal interactions with authority figures. You can reflect on the culture of your profession and how this culture influences your behavior as a professional. For example, the biomedical Western culture places high value on direct and linear verbal communication. The second step is educating yourself and appreciating the differences in the cultural community in which you work.

A theoretical tool that can help you appreciate cultural differences is the concept of high-context and low-context cultural assumptions and understanding how these assumptions may influence the beliefs, attitudes, and behaviors of you and your clients.[22] Context in communication refers to what gives "meaning" during a communication. In appreciating contextual assumptions, the clinician learns to appreciate the different cues that create meaning in the culture of the patient/client. For example, in certain cultures direct eye contact conveys respect between the speaker and the listener. In other cultures, gaze aversion by the listener conveys respect for the speaker. These cues vary in different cultural groups. The culturally competent practitioner learns to recognize these verbal and nonverbal cues and how to respond appropriately.

HIGH-CONTEXT ASSUMPTIONS

High-context or collectivistic **assumptions** assume that the group is more important than the individual. The communication style is indirect, and spiral and circular logic is used. Meaning is assumed based on implicit cues, such as where the communication occurs rather than what is said. Nuances in the communication such as posture, eye gaze, and gestures are considered important. The communication is influenced by what the listener already knows rather than what the speaker is saying.

Think about people you know who use high-context assumptions in their communication with you. How do those assumptions affect your communications with them?

LOW-CONTEXT ASSUMPTIONS

Low-context or individualistic **assumptions** assume that the individual is more important than the group. The communication style is direct, linear, and logical. The meaning is based on explicit cues, that is, "what is said is what is meant." Communication is less dependent on contextual cues or nuances. It is influenced by what the speaker is saying rather than what the listener already knows.

Think about people you know who use low-context assumptions in their communication with you. How do those assumptions affect your communications with them?

CULTURE OF MEDICINE

Biomedical Western medicine operates primarily from low-context assumptions in communication. Kleinman,[23] a medical anthropologist and physician, stated that it is the professional's responsibility to understand the family's explanatory model (their beliefs, based on their culture) of the etiology, onset of symptoms, pathophysiology, course of sickness, and treatment for the problem being addressed. He stated that the explanatory model of the family may differ from that of the medical caregivers, which can lead to miscommunication and hamper health care.

If the patient/client being served also operates from low-context assumptions, the chance of miscommunication is reduced. If the patient/client operates from high-context assumptions, however, miscommunication is more likely. The story of Lia Lee in Anne Fadiman's ethnographic book *The Spirit Catches You and You Fall Down*[24] dramatically portrays the life-threatening problems that may result when cross-cultural miscommunication occurs. Lia Lee was a toddler from the Hmong culture in Cambodia who emigrated to California with her parents and older siblings. She was treated for a severe seizure disorder at Merced County Hospital in California. Her physicians prescribed medication to manage her seizures, but her family was not comfortable with administering the drugs to their daughter for a variety of reasons related to Hmong cultural norms.

In the explanatory model of the physicians, the seizures were caused by abnormal electrical discharges in her brain that could be reasonably managed by antiseizure medications. However, in the explanatory model of the family, the seizures were caused when Lia experienced soul loss—a spiritual explanation in the Hmong culture. Because the family viewed the problem from a spiritual perspective, they called on a spiritual healer or shaman to perform healings for Lia in their home. Although the family still administered the antiseizure medications, they had difficulty doing this according to the expectations of the Western medical doctors. For the Lee family, the concept of telling time by the clock was unfamiliar. They were used to telling time by the activity of the day—waking in the morning, working during the day, and eating when hungry rather than using a clock to determine their activities. The biomedical assumptions about a regular schedule for administration of medicine based on clock time were unfamiliar to the family.

Beyond this individual example, the entire Hmong community operated from high-context assumptions. Decisions were made by the extended family and the Hmong community and not just the nuclear family. The medical community operated from low-context assumptions and did not recognize the nuances in communication nor the importance of the extended family and the Hmong community in decision making. Unfortunately, there was little understanding of the explanatory models on either side. Without the acknowledgment and appreciation of these critical differences, Lia's care was compromised. At one point she was removed from her home by the State of California and placed in foster care. For the Lee family this was a terrible blow, since children are deeply adored in the Hmong culture. Because of the high-context or collectivistic orientation of the Hmong culture, removal of a child from her home was a tragedy for the whole community. Her mother became depressed, and other family members suffered emotional distress. Although Lia was eventually reunited with her family, her seizures became worse and severe cognitive and motor deficits developed.

In subsequent interviews by Fadiman with the medical providers, the staff said that they had done everything they could to help Lia and her family. In retrospect, however, they recognized that they had not understood the cultural issues that resulted in continued miscommunications. Since the publication of Fadiman's book in 1997, several educational institutions for medical professionals have made the book required reading to educate students about the critical impact of effective cross-cultural communication in health care.[25]

Through educating yourself and appreciating cultural differences, you can learn to recognize differing explanatory models and differing contextual styles. By recognizing these differences, you may prevent miscommunication that might hamper your delivery of care.

Can you think of a time in which you have experienced a cross-cultural miscom-munication? How did you know? Did you resolve it effectively?

When working with individuals from a culture different from your own, you should avoid stereotyping based on ethnic and cultural expectations. Differences among members of the same ethnic or cultural group may be as great as those among individuals of different ethnic and cultural groups. For example, a client who moves to the United States from Honduras may be similar to or different from another person who arrives from Honduras at the same time. Although they share a nationality, they may differ significantly in such sociocultural variables as religion, socioeconomic status, and sexual orientation. Each individual has a unique cultural experience. As a health care provider, you can use your verbal and nonverbal communication skills to determine how the individual perceives himself or herself and adapt your evaluation and intervention accordingly.

COMMUNICATING WITH PEOPLE WHO SPEAK LITTLE OR NO ENGLISH

Another communication issue that commonly presents problems in health care delivery is language. Whenever possible, you should use a trained medical interpreter to communicate with clients whose language is different from yours. Although younger children in the family may be able to translate, it is preferable *not* to have them translate, since the topics being discussed may contain sensitive health information inappropriate for children.[20] When you do use a medical interpreter to translate, however, you can build rapport with the client by matching the posture and eye contact of the client rather than that of the interpreter. In this way you are building rapport at the nonverbal level with the client even if you are unable to speak his or her language.

Be sure to work with the family decision maker. In some cultures the decision maker may be a family elder or member or the extended family rather than the client.

Be open to working collaboratively with culturally accepted caregivers such as the shaman in the Hmong community. You can build rapport with the patient/client and the family by recognizing and appreciating their cultural norms for healing. By integrating their practices with yours (as long as they are not dangerous to the client), you acknowledge the cultural beliefs of the patient/client and family. As a result, they may be more willing to follow your recommendations.

When working with a medical interpreter, you may notice that the response given by the interpreter is shorter or longer than the statements translated for you. This may be due to the differences in high- and low-context communication styles. If the family uses circular and spiral communication, the medical interpreter may modify the circular communication and provide you with a more linear and logical interpretation, or vice versa for the family.

You may decide to ask the medical interpreter to provide you with the literal translation if you feel that you are not getting the meaning you expect from the interpretation. By watching the body language of the family, you may notice when the information being translated does not reflect the meaning intended by the family and you may ask for a more literal translation.

Remember that language does not equal culture. You may be conversant in a language different from your own, but you may not be aware of cultural norms in different ethnic groups who speak the same language. There may be different cultural interpretations of the same word that would require knowledge of the culture to understand. For example, in British English, the noun "boot" means the trunk of a car. In American English, the noun "boot" means a type of footwear. Because of differences like these, it is optimal to work with a trained medical interpreter who is multicultural as well as multilingual.

COMMUNICATING WITH INDIVIDUALS WHO COME FROM GENERATIONS DIFFERENT FROM YOUR OWN

PTs and PTAs interact with individuals in a diversity of generations from pediatrics to geriatrics. To communicate effectively across generations, you will find it helpful to understand and appreciate the differing traits of each generation.

In the United States today the four primary generations receiving health care are the traditionalists, baby boomers, generation Xers, and millennials. Each generation has characteristics that influence its behaviors and communication styles (Table 4-5).[26]

Traditionalists may be dealing with a wide variety of health disorders, including hearing and visual impairments, hypertension, and heart disease. They may have other chronic diseases that may impair their physical, cognitive, or sensory abilities. They may be taking a variety of medications.[26]

Think of someone you know who could be described as a traditionalist. Does he or she demonstrate the characteristics above? How are they similar to or different from your own?

Boomers are "sandwiched" between their adolescent children and their elderly parents and may be experiencing stress from caregiving as well as coping with age-related disorders themselves.

Table 4-5
Characteristics of Generations in the United States

Generation	Size	Birth Years	Traits	Rewards	Preferred Feedback
Traditionalists	75 million	Before 1946	Patriotic, loyal, fiscally conservative, faith in institutions	Satisfaction of a job well done	No news is good news
Baby boomers	80 million	1946-1964	Competitive, question authority, desire to put their own stamp on things, "sandwiched" (see text)	Money, title, recognition	Once a year whether you need it or not
Generation Xers	46 million	1965-1981	Eclectic, resourceful, self-reliant, distrustful of institutions, highly adaptive, skeptical	Freedom is the ultimate reward	"So, how am I doing?"
Millennials	76 million	1982-2000	Globally concerned, integrated, cyber literate, media savvy, realistic, environmentally conscious	Work that has meaning for me	From a virtual coach with the push of a button

Modified from Lancaster L, Stillman D: Bridging generation gaps in today's workplace. Presented at APTA Combined Sections Meeting, Tampa, FL, 2003.

Think of someone you know who could be described as a boomer. Does he or she demonstrate the characteristics described above? How are they similar to or different from your own?

Generation Xers enjoy being up to date with the latest and greatest technology. They value new learning as a reward.

Think of someone you know who could be described as a generation Xer. Does he or she demonstrate the characteristics described above? How are they similar to or different from your own?

Millennials multitask, doing things simultaneously, and they prefer regular feedback.

Think of someone you know who could be described as a millennial. Does he or she demonstrate the characteristics described above? How are they similar to or different from your own?

As a physical therapy provider, you may be working with individuals from each of these generations. Remember that there are exceptions within each of these categories. Treat each person individually regardless of the category described above. You can recognize the characteristics related to rewards and feedback for each person. You can use that information to enhance your communication when working with individuals from different generations.

COMMUNICATING WITH PEOPLE WHO HAVE VISUAL IMPAIRMENTS

Over 1 million individuals in the United States have visual impairment or low vision, and 800,000 of those are over 65 years old. These impairments can range from mild to severe and may include cataracts, glaucoma, or macular degeneration. As a physical therapy provider, you may have patients/clients with visual impairments.[27]

When speaking or listening to someone who is visually impaired, you can introduce yourself and others by name when you enter the room. When speaking, you can use everyday words, including "see" and "look." You can ask the person if he or she would like assistance if you need to move from one place to another.

If you are writing a home program, the type should be in a large font size with high contrast between the foreground and the background. If the program is handwritten, print or block lettering but not script should be used. Text using both upper- and lower-case letters is easier to read. Check into printing the program in Braille. You can learn about computer technology for the blind and assist your client in accessing the information. Refer your client to services for individuals with visual impairment in your community.

COMMUNICATING WITH PEOPLE WHO HAVE AUDITORY IMPAIRMENTS

Twenty-two million people in the United States have auditory impairments. These may range from mild loss of sensitivity to total hearing loss. The largest group experiencing hearing loss is those over the age of 65.[27] When listening to or speaking with someone who is deaf or hard of hearing, ask what you can do to improve your communication with him or her. You may change your position so that you face the person directly or look directly at the person to provide a clear view of your lips. A light touch on the shoulder will get the person's attention when you want to communicate. Articulate clearly and use

4

natural tones. Shouting may reduce the effectiveness of a hearing aid. If possible, avoid areas that have distracting sounds in the background. Be sure to confirm that the person understood what you said by having the person repeat what was understood in his or her own words.

For written communication, write clearly and simply using everyday words. If the individual has both visual and auditory impairments, use a large font with high contrast between foreground and background. If you recommend instructional videos, make sure they have subtitles.

If you are working with a hearing-impaired patient/client, you can help him or her to access the Text Telephone Delivery (TTY) system for telephone communications. When using interpreters, have a certified deaf interpreter deliver important information and make sure the client feels comfortable with the interpreter.

COMMUNICATING WITH PATIENTS/CLIENTS AND CAREGIVERS/FAMILIES

Remember to create a positive environment for the client and caregivers or family. You can use your verbal and behavioral rapport skills to enhance the communication process. Be sure to introduce yourself and address the client by name. Ask the client whether he or she prefers to be addressed formally by surname or informally by first name.

Limit your teaching objectives and teach only manageable amounts at a time. Ask the patient/client for his or her goals and link those with your goals.

Make your communication clear and simple. Use lay terminology rather than medical jargon. Watch the patient's/client's body language for signs of understanding or lack of understanding. If you notice confusion, ask what is unclear and then explain it in a different way.

Use a variety of ways to get your message across. Some patients/clients prefer written programs, others prefer demonstration, and still others prefer to watch a videotape or DVD. Offer information regarding community agencies and support groups that may assist the patient/client after the physical therapy visit.

Verify that your message was understood by having the patient/client repeat back to you what the person understood in his or her own words. Have the patient/client demonstrate the activities you have taught so that you can offer constructive feedback for improving his or her exercise form or skills.[27]

By incorporating communication skills in your patient/client interactions, you will enhance the quality of the physical therapy services you provide.

COMMUNICATING WITH OTHER MEMBERS OF THE HEALTH CARE TEAM

As a PT or a PTA, you will be interacting with a wide variety of health care providers and will serve as a member of the health care team. You can learn about other disciplines as part of your preservice education, by observing other disciplines at work, or by studying about disciplines other than your own.

PTs not only work closely with PTAs, but also collaborate with occupational therapists, speech-language pathologists, nutritionists, psychologists, nurses, physicians, social workers, audiologists, respiratory therapists, and other professionals. Through collaboration with other disciplines, you learn from other team members about additional information and resources that may enhance the outcome for your client. For example, you may have a client who has been reluctant to participate in physical therapy. Through collaboration with the psychologist, you may learn about psychological barriers that could impede the patient/client from participating in physical therapy. The psychologist may suggest strategies you can use to address those barriers with your client.

Team meetings require good communication skills. Interdisciplinary team meetings are often conducted in hospital and rehabilitation settings. You may be called on to report your findings related to a patient's/client's movement dysfunction. Your verbal and behavioral rapport skills may assist you in promoting communication among all team members. Curtis[28] identified eight behaviors that may assist you in developing effective interdisciplinary collaboration (Box 4-2). When team members follow these guidelines, the patient outcomes may be enhanced as a result of the successful collaboration of the team members.

4

COMMUNICATING THROUGH DELEGATION

As a PT, you will supervise and interact with a wide variety of individuals. They may include PTAs, physical therapy aides, transport staff, and administrative staff.

As a professional, you must know the legal boundaries regarding supervision and delegation in your state. Once you are familiar with the physical therapy practice act in your state, you will be able to delegate accordingly. Since members of the support staff provide service under your supervision and license, your communication skills are critical to the success of your delegation and supervision. You can use your verbal and behavioral rapport skills to enhance the effectiveness of your communication with your support staff.

COMMUNICATING AS A STUDENT IN THE CLASSROOM AND CLINICAL INTERNSHIPS

Development of your professional communication skills begins in the physical therapy classroom. Faculty members model professional behaviors for students in the classroom by demonstrating the generic abilities. They demonstrate commitment to learning by continually seeking new knowledge and understanding through review of current literature and attendance at continuing education

---

BOX 4-2   *Behaviors to Assist in Interdisciplinary Collaboration*

- Making an effort to involve all team members in communication at meetings and in written communications
- Recognizing the perspective of other team members
- Acknowledging the contribution of others
- Scheduling meetings at reasonable times for all members
- Acknowledging your own biases or stereotypes when working with other team members
- Breaking down role conflicts
- Knowing your professional identity
- Focusing on the outcome

From Curtis K: Physical Therapy Professional Foundations. Thorofare, NJ, Slack, 2002.

courses. Interpersonal skills are modeled when they communicate respectfully with students and colleagues in and out of the classroom. Communication skills are modeled when they demonstrate appropriate listening skills while answering questions posed by students and colleagues. Faculty demonstrate appropriate reading and writing skills in their syllabi, course assignments, and research resources. They model appropriate and respectful verbal and nonverbal communication when speaking with students and colleagues. Effective use of time and resources is demonstrated by planning, implementation, and evaluation of their course content. Faculty demonstrate use of constructive feedback by acknowledging student queries regarding exams and assignments in a timely and respectful manner. Problem-solving skills are demonstrated when a variety of possible solutions related to course content are considered and course content is updated based on current research. Faculty show professionalism by dressing appropriately for both classroom and lab sessions. They participate in the APTA and often serve as elected officers in their chosen specialty areas. They model responsibility by being punctual, following through on commitments to students and colleagues, and assuming leadership roles in the profession. They model critical thinking by critiquing hypotheses and ideas and challenging students to think critically in the classroom. Effective stress management is demonstrated when preventive approaches to stress management are used, such as establishing a support network for self and students. By observing these professional behaviors in faculty members, students have an opportunity to recognize the importance of the behaviors and reflect on their own behaviors as compared with their faculty role models.

For students the classroom provides an opportunity to practice their professional skills in a "safe" environment with constructive feedback from both faculty and peers. Through self-assessing your professional behaviors using the generic abilities in your classes and receiving constructive feedback from the faculty and peers, you develop your professional skills from the outset of the curriculum. You may receive grades for your professional behaviors as part of your class participation, your timely completion of assignments, and your affective behaviors during practical exams.[11]

As a student physical therapist or a student physical therapist assistant in the clinical setting, you have an opportunity to apply the professional behaviors learned in the classroom setting in the clinical environment. The student physical therapist is required to practice under the direct supervision of a licensed PT who serves as a clinical instructor (CI). PTAs may serve as CIs for student physical therapist assistants. If you experience challenges with your professional behaviors in the clinical setting, faculty can assist you in modifying these challenging behaviors by having you self-assess using the generic abilities taught in the classroom setting. A faculty advisor may help you to change your challenging behaviors based on your self-assessment and the assessment of your CI. In this way you learn to self-correct and develop your professional behaviors with the guidance of your CI and your faculty advisor.[12]

SUMMARY

PTs are professionals who use a variety of professional communication behaviors that may enhance their effectiveness in the clinical and educational settings.

Several research studies indicate that communication is one of the most important skills used by physical therapy professionals.[2,3] Communication skills include the ability to listen, read, and write effectively. They also include effective verbal and nonverbal skills in interactions with clients, families, colleagues, supervisors, and support staff. Cultural, verbal, and behavioral rapport skills can be learned and implemented in the classroom and the clinic to enhance communication effectiveness. Strategies are discussed for communicating effectively with diverse groups, including:

- Individuals who come from cultures different from your own
- Individuals who speak little or no English
- Individuals who come from a generation different from your own
- Individuals who have visual impairments
- Individuals who have hearing impairments
- Patients/clients and caregivers
- Health care team members
- Support staff
- Faculty and clinical supervisors

Students first learn these professional communication behaviors in their physical therapy classes and apply the behaviors with their faculty and peers. By practicing these behaviors during classroom experiences, students are better prepared to develop them as they proceed from beginning skills as students to post–entry level skills as they become physical therapy providers.

CASE STUDIES

CASE STUDY ONE

You are a physical therapist student working in an early intervention program in Miami, Florida. You have been assigned to evaluate a 2-year-old boy with Down syndrome whose family recently immigrated to Miami from Nicaragua. The family is very concerned because their son is not yet walking. You do not speak Spanish, and you are expected to complete the evaluation with the child and the family.

What professional behaviors will you use to enhance your communication with this family?

Case Study One Answers

1. Request a bicultural and bilingual medical interpreter for the examination and evaluation.
2. Use your behavioral rapport skills with the family when the interpreter is translating.
3. Speak with cultural informants in your clinical setting who are knowledgeable about Nicaraguan culture
4. Seek written or Web resources to learn more about Nicaraguan culture.[29]
5. Learn essential physical therapy phrases in Spanish to help you communicate verbally with the family in subsequent treatment sessions.
6. Contact your CI for assistance if the family has difficulty understanding your examination, evaluation, or intervention suggestions.

CASE STUDY TWO

You are a physical therapist or physical therapist assistant student completing your clinical internship at an inpatient rehabilitation hospital. Your CI has given you feedback at your midterm evaluation that your nonverbal communication indicates that you are disinterested and aloof when working with patients. You are upset because you were not aware that you were conveying disinterest or aloofness toward patients. Your CI stated that she observed you standing about 10 feet away from her patients with your arms folded across your chest when she was treating them. She stated that other staff members had noticed similar nonverbal patterns when you observed their patient treatments.

What professional behaviors will you use to enhance your communication in this situation?

Case Study Two Answers

1. Meet with your CI and ask for specific constructive feedback related to your nonverbal behaviors. Explain that you had not realized how your nonverbal behavior had been perceived.
2. Take responsibility for the behavior and indicate your willingness to modify your behavior appropriately.
3. Contact the academic coordinator of clinical education (ACCE) at your institution and request her assistance in remediation for your nonverbal skills.
4. Complete a self-assessment of your communication and interpersonal skills using the generic abilities.
5. Meet with your CI and the ACCE to compare your self-assessment with the assessment of your nonverbal communication by the CI.
6. Develop a plan for modifying your nonverbal behavior with the assistance of the CI and the ACCE.
7. Modify your behavior by implementing your verbal and behavioral rapport skills.
8. Meet with your CI and ACCE to evaluate your new behavior after a week.

REFERENCES

1. APTA Vision Sentence for Physical Therapy 2020 and APTA Vision Statement for Physical Therapy 2020, HOD P06-00-24-35. House of Delegates Standards, Policies, Positions, and Guidelines. Alexandria, VA, American Physical Therapy Association, 2005.
2. Lopopolo R, Schafer S: Re-conceptualizing the role of leadership, administration, management, and professionalism (LAMP) in physical therapy practice. Health Policy Resource 2004;4(2):1-4.
3. Lopopolo RB, Schafer DS, Nosse LJ: Leadership, administration, management, and professionalism (LAMP) in physical therapy: A Delphi study. Phys Ther 2004;84:137-150.
4. Webster's II: New College Dictionary. Boston, Houghton Mifflin, 1995.
5. Konefal J: Neurolinguistic Psychology Practitioner Manual. Miami, University of Miami, 2002.
6. Davis CM: Patient Practitioner Interaction: An Experiential Manual for Developing the Art of Health Care, ed 3. Thorofare, NJ, Slack, 1998.
7. May WW, Morgan BJ, Lemke JC, et al: Model for ability-based assessment in physical therapy education. J Phys Ther Educ 1995;9(1):3-6.
8. Bloom BJ: Taxonomy of Educational Objectives: The Classification of Educational Goals: Handbook I: Cognitive Domain. New York, David McKay, 1956.
9. Simpson EJ: The Classification of Education Objectives in the Psychomotor Domain. Washington, DC, Gryphon House, 1972.
10. Krathwohl DR, Bloom BS, Masa BB: The need for classification of affective objectives. *In:* Bloom BJ (ed): Taxonomy of Educational Objectives, Handbook II: Affective Domain. New York, David McKay, 1964.

11. Masin HL: Education in the affective domain: A method/model for teaching professional behaviors in the classroom and during advisory sessions. J Phys Ther Educ 2002;16(1):37-45.

12. Masin HL: Integrating the use of the generic abilities, clinical performance instrument, and neurolinguistic psychology processes for clinical education intervention. Phys Ther Case Rep 2000;3(6):258-266.

13. O'Connor J, Seymour J: Introducing Neurolinguistic Programming. London, Aquarian Press, 1993.

14. Bernieri B, Rosenthal R: Interpersonal Coordination: Behavior Matching and Interactional Synchrony. *In*: Fundamentals of Nonverbal Behavior. Cambridge, Eng, Cambridge University Press, 1991.

15. Pellegrino ED: What is a profession. J Allied Health 1983;12(3):168-176.

16. Cross T, Bazron B, Dennis K, et al: Toward a Culturally Competent System of Care. Washington, DC, CAASP Technical Assistance Center, Georgetown University Child Development Center, 1989.

17. Cross Cultural and International Special Interest Group: Draft of Guidelines for Cultural Competency in the Affective Domain. Missoula, MT, American Physical Therapy Association, 2000.

18. Leavitt RL: Cross Cultural Rehabilitation: An International Perspective. London, Saunders, 1994.

19. Leavitt RL: Developing cultural competence in a multicultural world, part I. PT—Magazine of Physical Therapy 2002;10(12):36-48.

20. National Standards for Culturally and Linguistically Appropriate Services in Health Care—Final Report. Rockville, MD, US Dept of Health and Human Services, Office of Minority Health, 2001.

21. Agar M: Language Shock—Understanding the Culture of Conversation. New York, Perennial, 1994.

22. Graham M, Miller D: Cross Cultural Interactive Preference Profile, The 1995 Annual: vol 1, Training. San Diego, CA, Pfeiffer, 1995.

23. Kleinman A: Concepts and a model for the comparison of medical systems as cultural systems. Soc Sci Med 1976;12:85-93.

24. Fadiman A: The Spirit Catches You and You Fall Down—A Hmong Child, Her American Doctors, and the Collision of Two Cultures. New York, Farrar, Strauss, Giroux, 1997.

25. Taylor JS: Confronting culture in medicine's culture of no culture. Acad Med 2003;78:555-559.

26. Lancaster L, Stillman D: When Generations Collide: Who They Are, Why They Clash, How to Solve the Generational Puzzle at Work. New York, Harper Collins, 2002.

27. Osborne H: Overcoming Communication Barriers in Patient Education. Gaithersburg, MD, Aspen, 2001.

28. Curtis K: Physical Therapy Professional Foundations. Thorofare, NJ, Slack, 2002.

29. Ethnomed: Ethnic medicine from Harborview Medical Center 2005, Available at www.ethnomed.org. Accessed August 8, 2005.

ADDITIONAL RESOURCE

Spector RE: Cultural Diversity in Health and Illness, ed 6. Upper Saddle River, NJ, Pearson, Prentice Hall, 2004.

This is a comprehensive text for nursing professionals dealing with the complexities of working with people from diverse cultural backgrounds. It includes resources for developing knowledge, attitudes, and skills related to health and illness in the American Indian and Alaska Native population, black population, Hispanic population, and white population. It includes data resources and networks for selected health organizations.

N*o civilization . . . would ever have been possible without a framework of stability, to provide the wherein for the flux of change. Foremost among the stabilizing factors, more enduring than customs, manners, and traditions, are the legal systems that regulate our life in the world and our daily affairs with each other.*
Hannah Arendt

5

Laws, Regulations, and Policies

Laurie A. Walsh

KEY TERMS

certification
civil law
Code of Ethics
common law
contract
criminal law
law
licensure
malpractice
negligence
policy
practice act
professional misconduct
registration
regulation
risk management
Standards of Ethical Conduct for the Physical Therapist Assistant
statute
tort
vicarious liability

OBJECTIVES

After reading this chapter, the reader will be able to:
- Distinguish among laws, regulations, and policies and how they are made
- Understand basic concepts regarding how various laws, regulations, and policies affect physical therapy practice

■ Identify resources that physical therapists and physical therapist assistants may use to find out more about laws, regulations, and policies that affect physical therapy practice
■ Identify ways in which individuals and groups can effect change in the regulation of physical therapy practice

■ Understand basic issues involved in the various ways that physical therapists and physical therapist assistants can be held legally liable for the care they provide and the consequences of liability

The primary purpose of laws, regulations, and policies affecting the practice of physical therapy is to protect the public by (1) trying to ensure that providers are competent and (2) where services are paid for by government programs, ensuring that taxpayer dollars are being spent appropriately. Laws, regulations, and public policy serve to create, in legal terms, a scope of practice for physical therapy and to distinguish it from other professions. Government regulation is a double-edged sword for physical therapists (PTs) and physical therapist assistants (PTAs): providers receive rights and protection under regulation, but they must also accept responsibilities and limits imposed by regulation. The policies of private organizations may also affect the practice of physical therapy.

A detailed examination of the legal regulation of physical therapy practice is beyond the scope of this chapter, and the reader is referred elsewhere for more detail. As you read this chapter, the following basic principles should be kept in mind:

■ Many of the laws, regulations, and policies that affect physical therapy practice vary from state to state and from program to program. This chapter focuses on general principles, so readers should look to individual state laws, program regulations, and the like for specific information.
■ Various aspects of practice may be governed by both state and federal law. Where they come into conflict, federal law generally prevails.
■ Some laws, regulations, and public policies govern what services PTs and PTAs may legally provide, whereas others may address how these services are reimbursed. The fact that reimbursement may be denied does not necessarily mean that the services cannot legally be provided, only that the therapist must look elsewhere for reimbursement.

STATUTORY, REGULATORY, AND COMMON LAW

Law is "a body of rules of action or conduct prescribed by the controlling authority and hav[ing] binding legal force."[1] *Public* policies are generated by governmental bodies.[2] Public policy may be considered the sum of all of the "law" of a jurisdiction in a particular area, regardless of which body of government is the source. The "law" of a jurisdiction therefore may be composed of laws created by legislatures (called statutes), decrees handed down by courts (common law), or regulations created by government agencies. *Private* policies are developed by private organizations and cannot be enforced in the same ways that laws are. Private policies are discussed later in this chapter.

The various kinds of law may address offenses against society or private wrongs that one individual commits against another. This section addresses the various components of the law and how they affect the practice of physical therapy. This section also discusses the distinctions among three major topic areas in the law: criminal law, civil law, and contract law.

STATUTES

Statutes, as noted above, are a type of law that is "enacted and established by the will of the legislative department of government."[1] Statutes affecting the practice of physical therapy may be enacted at the federal level by Congress or at the state level by the various state legislatures. Provisions of federal and state statutes can be enforced through the state and federal court systems.

Federal Statutes. Federal statutes address those areas the federal government is constitutionally permitted to regulate, such as interstate commerce and taxation. Federal statutes apply consistently to all citizens across state lines and, where they conflict with related state laws, generally supersede state law. A number of federal statutes may affect the provision of physical therapy services, including the following:

- The Americans With Disabilities Act (ADA) requires that goods and services (including health care) available to the public be made accessible to persons with disabilities.[3]
- The Individuals With Disabilities Education Act requires that special education and related services (including physical therapy) be provided at public expense to students with disabilities when needed for students to benefit from an education program (see Chapter 13).[4]
- The Social Security Amendments of 1965 contain, among other provisions, the foundation for (1) the Medicare program, a federally subsidized health insurance program for people 65 years and older, [5] and (2) Medicaid, jointly funded by the state and federal governments as a program designed to provide health care services to the poor. Physical therapy is among the health care services reimbursed under Medicare and Medicaid.[5]
- The Health Insurance Portability and Accountability Act requires that all health care providers who transmit patient information electronically adhere to federal guidelines as to the type of patient information they disclose, to whom they may disclose it, and how they store it in order to protect patient confidentiality.[5]

The consequences for violating federal laws vary. Violations of the ADA may result in fines or injunctions (in this case, court orders requiring defendants to make their businesses more accessible to persons with disabilities). Fraudulent billing of federal benefit programs, such as Medicare, is vigorously prosecuted. One example involved a PT who pled guilty to billing the federal government and private insurance companies $1 million for therapy services that were never provided.[6] The therapist was criminally prosecuted, ordered to repay $125,000, and sentenced to 27 months in a federal penitentiary.

State Statutes.   State statutes are enacted by state legislatures in areas that states are constitutionally permitted to regulate, such as education, professional licensing, and insurance. When no superseding federal law exists, each state is entitled to tailor its laws to meet the needs of its citizens. Consequently, laws in these areas vary from state to state.

State statutes can affect the practice of physical therapy in a number of ways, such as through regulation of the insurance industry, availability of state health care funding for the poor, and state health department requirements. In regard to physical therapy practice, however, the single most important statute is the state physical therapy practice act. The **practice act** is the legal foundation for the scope and protection of physical therapy practice. Among the areas generally covered by practice acts are the state definition of physical therapy practice, identification of providers who may legally provide physical therapy services, identification of tasks that may be delegated (and to which persons they may be delegated), and supervisory requirements. Physical therapy providers are legally permitted to practice only when they comply with their state's practice act, and it is assumed that they are knowledgeable about the provisions of the practice act. The practice act is the final word regarding what is legal physical therapy practice in a given state; it supersedes the provisions of other state practice acts and the guidelines of private organizations, such as the American Physical Therapy Association (APTA). The consequences of violating state practice acts are often stated in the act itself or accompanying regulations. In some states, such as New York, the unlawful practice of physical therapy is a criminal offense.[7]

A copy of a state practice act may be obtained in many ways. The state physical therapy licensing board may have copies available, and most state legislatures now have official websites with all state laws, including practice acts, available online. State practice acts may also be accessed in a variety of places on the World Wide Web.[8] (Note: Although much information on the APTA website is currently available to the public, some information is accessible only to APTA members. In addition, the reader should note that websites often change the links to content, so links current at the time of publication may be changed at a later date.)

Although a great deal of overlap is seen among state practice acts, they also have significant differences. Given that physical therapy providers are legally responsible for knowing their own practice acts, providers must educate themselves and cannot assume that what is legal therapy practice in another state is also legal in their own state. One example is direct access to physical therapy services, which permits a patient to receive services without first obtaining a referral from another provider, usually a physician. As of this writing, 47 states permit evaluation without referral and 42 states permit some form of intervention without referral.[9] Even within direct access states, however, state laws vary, for example, in terms of the amount of experience therapists must have before they can provide services without a referral, or the length of time during which service may be provided before a referral must be obtained.

The manner in which physical therapy providers are regulated also varies from state to state. All 50 states license physical therapists. A license, however,

5

cannot automatically be transferred from one state to another. If a provider moves to another state, that person must apply for a new license according to that state's requirements and procedures. **Licensure** creates a scope of practice, authorizes the individual to practice in a given state, and legally protects use of the professional title.[10] All states require graduation from an accredited program and a passing score on the licensing examination in order to be licensed, but exact procedures, forms, costs, and other requirements vary from state to state. The reader should contact a specific state licensing board to find out what that particular state requires.[8]

The PTA is also recognized under the practice acts of over 40 states and may be licensed, certified, or registered.[11] Functionally, **certification**, like licensure, legally protects the title of the PTA. Unlike licensure, however, it does not create a separate scope of practice or a monopoly to provide a particular service.[10] Requirements, such as passage of the National Physical Therapist Assistant Examination, may vary depending on whether a state offers licensure or certification.[11] **Registration** is the least rigorous form of governmental regulation and requires only that registrants periodically provide the state with updated information on their name, address, and qualifications and pay a registration fee.[10] Individuals who are licensed or certified are generally required to register periodically as well. As with PTs, then, the requirements for PTA practice vary from state to state and PTAs must check with the licensing board of a particular state to determine eligibility requirements.

The reader should not confuse state certification with certification by private organizations. The APTA, for example, has a program to certify practitioners as specialists in particular areas of practice (see Chapter 2). The Neuro-developmental Treatment Association, for example, as well as other organizations, has programs to certify practitioners. These private forms of certification establish that an individual has met the standards of these private organizations in terms of competency in a certain therapeutic approach or specialty area.[10] Unlike state certification, they neither create a legally enforceable professional title nor modify the scope of practice.

With respect to efforts to obtain more consistent physical therapy regulation, there is the Model Practice Act for Physical Therapy (MPA). The MPA is not a statute and does not have the force of law, but it is intended as an "integrated model for the regulation of physical therapy practice" and a guide to assist in the modification of state practice acts.[12] The MPA was developed by the Federation of State Boards of Physical Therapy, a private organization consisting of members of physical therapy licensing boards from all 50 states and the federal territories. The Federation periodically revises the MPA, most recently in 2002.[13] The Federation is also responsible for developing the national licensing examinations for the PT and PTA. More information about the Federation can be obtained from their website (http://www.fsbpt.org).

REGULATIONS

Unlike statutes, regulations are developed by government agencies, not the legislature. Administrative agencies exist at all levels of government and serve to regulate industries and government benefit programs, such as Medicare and

Medicaid. Such agencies are created by legislatures through statutes, for the purpose of regulating a particular industry or programs. Agencies are overseen by the legislative branch and can perform only those duties delegated by the legislature.[14] Unlike legislators, appointees to agencies generally have specific expertise and experience in the industry or program being regulated.

Having been delegated authority in a specific area by the legislature, agencies have the authority to develop regulations and enforce them within a specific industry or program. A **regulation** is a rule controlling the practices of those individuals or organizations under the authority of the agency.[14] For example, regulations may support, clarify, or give further definition to terms in the statutes that created the agency, or they may set forth procedures for programs created by statute. A practice act, for example, may require that a PTA be supervised on-site by a PT. The legislature may then delegate to an appropriate state agency, such as the state's PT board or education department, the responsibility for developing a regulation defining what constitutes appropriate supervision. Consequently, one must be familiar with both the statutes and regulations of a given jurisdiction to have full knowledge of the law governing physical therapy practice.

Federal Regulations   Federal agencies regulate a wide variety of industries and benefit programs. Examples of federal agencies with great impact on the provision of physical therapy services are the Centers for Medicare and Medicaid Services (CMS), part of the federal cabinet Department of Health and Human Services. Formerly known as the Health Care Financing Administration, CMS is responsible for regulation of the Medicare and Medicaid programs. While a detailed discussion of these programs and the role of CMS is beyond the scope of this chapter, CMS regulations determine, for example, to what extent therapists may participate as providers within the Medicare program and how much and for what services they will be reimbursed.[5]

Radical changes have occurred regarding reimbursement within the various aspects of Medicare since the late 1990s, and reimbursement for physical therapy services in many areas has been dramatically reduced.[15] Many of these changes have been driven by congressional amendments to the Medicare legislation; implementation and enforcement of these changes have generally been left up to CMS. One example has been repeated congressional attempts over the years to place an annual monetary "cap" on the amount of reimbursement available for physical therapy services under the Part B section of Medicare (which generally covers outpatient services).[16] Once a patient's Medicare physical therapy expenses under Part B reached the cap, regardless of need, no further Part B Medicare reimbursement for physical therapy services would be available for that year. The APTA has struggled on the behalf of consumers and the profession to restore adequate levels of reimbursement (see Chapter 6). In the case of the Medicare cap, the APTA successfully lobbied for laws placing a moratorium on cap implementation through December 2005. A cap was reinstated on January 1, 2006; therefore physical therapy advocates need to be constantly vigilant regarding this and other efforts to limit physical therapy reimbursement under government programs.

Failure to abide by Medicare regulations may result in denial of reimbursement for services rendered. Federal statutes and regulations also prohibit fraudulent billing; consequently, when evidence of fraud is uncovered, fines and criminal prosecution may follow as noted earlier in this chapter. In the absence of fraud, however, the denial of reimbursement does not mean that services were illegally provided, only that they are not covered by the Medicare program and providers must seek reimbursement elsewhere.

The APTA updates members frequently regarding the activities of CMS and other government agencies through publications such as *PT Bulletin* and *PT—Magazine of Physical Therapy*. The advocacy section of the APTA website also maintains current information and links to government websites. Information specific to CMS may be accessed on their website at http://www.cms.hhs.gov.

State Regulations. State agencies also regulate a variety of industries and programs. Among the most important for the practice of physical therapy is the state physical therapy board. The composition and functions of the physical therapy boards are set by each state's legislature through statutes. While they cannot change the practice acts adopted by the state legislatures, state boards serve many important functions.[17] They may advise the legislature or other government bodies to clarify the scope of practice, as well as provide advice to state-licensed practitioners seeking guidance on practice issues in that state. They also assist in administering the state licensing procedures and are generally at least consulted by prosecutors in professional misconduct cases. More information on the role of a state board can be obtained directly from the licensing board of an individual state and the state practice acts.

Professional misconduct is often regulated by a state disciplinary agency and is a topic that deserves further discussion. **Professional misconduct** involves actions by licensed professionals that demonstrate an inability to meet professional standards and competently perform the duties of a licensed professional.[18] Actions that constitute professional misconduct are defined in the practice act or accompanying regulations and may include physical or sexual abuse of a patient, patient abandonment (discharge of a patient while services are still needed), improper delegation or supervision of treatment activities, provision of unnecessary treatment, fraud, incompetence, and practicing while intoxicated, among other activities. Complaints of unprofessional conduct are typically prosecuted by the state through administrative bodies set up for that purpose, rather than being prosecuted in courts of law. A finding that the PT or PTA has committed professional misconduct may result in a reprimand, fine, requirement to obtain remedial professional education, probation, or suspension or revocation of license.[19]

CREATING STATUTES AND REGULATIONS

Considering the profound effect statutes and regulations can have on the practice of physical therapy (and the consequences of violations), therapists and assistants must remain aware of and be in compliance with the applicable statutes and regulations. When statutes and regulations unnecessarily limit the provision of services to the public, therapists and assistants must work to educate lawmakers to change them. First, however, given that statutes and regulations are created by different government entities, physical therapy providers must educate themselves as to how statutes and regulations are made in order to have an impact on the final outcome.

How Statutes Are Made.   Enacting or amending statutes is often a lengthy process involving negotiation and compromise. It varies somewhat from state to state and between the state and federal governments. In general, however, the process involves introducing a proposed statute (or bill) in one house of the legislature, where it will be referred to at least one legislative committee that has been assigned to address all bills pertaining to a certain topic (i.e., Finance, Education, Appropriations, etc.).[20] Committees gather additional information on the bill, debating and amending it. If passed, the committee's version of the bill is referred to the entire house (or "floor") for debate. If not, the bill "dies" in committee and will have to be reintroduced in the legislature at the next session. If passed by one house of the legislature after a floor vote, the bill is then forwarded to the other house to undergo the same process again. Only when passed by both legislative houses in identical form is a bill forwarded to the executive branch (president or governor) to be signed into law or vetoed.

While the process of enacting statutes is lengthy and complicated, the many steps involved give interested parties, such as physical therapy providers, ample opportunity to contact their legislators to make sure that the interests of the profession and the public are represented. The process of persuading lawmakers, or lobbying, is essential to ensure the well-being of the public and the health of the profession. The APTA is actively involved at both the state and national levels to ensure that the profession's interests are represented. Therapists and assistants must keep abreast of pending legislation that may affect the practice of physical therapy and become involved in lobbying efforts, such as writing to their legislators at various points in the process.

The APTA keeps members updated on current legislative issues through such publications as *PT Bulletin* and *PT—Magazine of Physical Therapy,* as well as through the Advocacy link on the national website. The State Government Affairs link under the advocacy section of the APTA website connects to the members-only Legislative Action Center. This online clearinghouse holds a wealth of information on current physical therapy–related bills before Congress and state legislatures, offers information to quickly identify and contact state and Congressional representatives, and even provides language that can be used in letters to legislators. State chapters also keep members apprised through newsletters, and chapter websites may carry legislative information.

State and federal governments have a number of official publications regarding pending and recent legislation. For example, the Congressional Record publishes a daily record of House and Senate proceedings. The Library of

Congress has extensive federal legislative information available online through its service, THOMAS, at http://thomas.loc.gov. Among the information available at this site are the most recent Congressional Record, bill texts, committee reports, and summaries of the legislative process.

How Regulations Are Made.   Procedures have also been established for promulgating regulations, which also may vary from state to state. In general, though, an agency must first publish a proposed regulation and give interested parties time to comment on it. This "comment period" gives physical therapy providers an opportunity to educate regulatory bodies on the issues and influence the form the final rule takes.[21] At the federal level, proposed and final regulations are published daily in the Federal Register, which can be accessed at http://www.gpoaccess.gov/fr/index.html. State chapter publications and websites often keep members updated about state regulatory activities.

COMMON LAW

The courts serve a number of functions in our legal system, including clarifying and interpreting statutes and regulations. The court system serves as an additional source of law: **common law** is law that has been created by court decisions, written by judges and handed down.[22] Areas of common law evolve as new court decisions are added to the existing body of law in a particular area, and may modify or overrule prior decisions. Certain areas of the law, such as negligence, are governed primarily through common law, although some states have developed statutory definitions of professional negligence.[23] Negligence and malpractice are discussed further in the section on civil law.

CRIMINAL LAW VERSUS CIVIL LAW

The reader should understand that within the law are different areas, or topics. One important distinction is the difference between criminal and civil law. Legal matters may be handled differently, depending on this distinction, and the penalties imposed for a finding of wrongdoing also differ.

CRIMINAL LAW

Criminal law involves prosecution in a court of law for acts "done in violation of those duties which an individual owes to the community."[1] Thus crimes are considered to be infractions committed against society, and the state prosecutes these actions on behalf of the public. Criminal laws are generally found today as state and federal statutes, rather than as part of common law.[1] The consequences of being tried and convicted of, or pleading guilty to, a crime may involve fines, probation, or imprisonment and vary depending on the type of crime committed and the law of the particular jurisdiction involved. For example, the death penalty is legal in certain states, but not others. Criminal prosecution will not directly affect a provider's license but may result in a referral to a state professional disciplinary agency to initiate such an action. Earlier in this chapter, an example was given of a therapist prosecuted criminally for insurance fraud. Other possible sources of criminal liability may involve sexual abuse of patients or, depending on the state law, unlawful practice of a profession.

CIVIL LAW

Unlike criminal law, **civil law** is concerned with wrongs committed among private parties.[1] Civil actions are also prosecuted in courts of law, but in these cases one private citizen brings a lawsuit against another to seek compensation for injuries received.[24] Unlike in criminal cases, persons found liable in civil cases cannot be punished by the state with fines or incarceration; generally, the only remedy available for civil liability is for the defendant to pay money damages to the plaintiff (the person who brings the lawsuit) to compensate that person for injuries shown to be caused by the defendant's actions. A civil lawsuit also cannot affect a person's professional license, but it may, depending on the nature of the wrong, result in a complaint to the state disciplinary agency to initiate a separate action for professional misconduct. Physical therapy providers may be named in civil lawsuits on a variety of grounds, including defamation (saying or writing something untrue that harms another person's reputation) or breach of contract. The most common grounds for civil actions involving physical therapy providers, however, involve claims of negligence or malpractice.

Negligence and Malpractice. Negligence and malpractice are kinds of **torts**: civil injuries for which the injured party can seek legal relief from the courts.[1] **Negligence** is defined as the failure to act as a reasonably prudent person: doing (or failing to do) something that a reasonably prudent person would have done (or would not have done) under similar circumstances.[1] To prove that a therapist was negligent in providing care, a patient would have to prove four things in court[24]:

1. That the therapist owed the patient a legal duty of care; in other words, that a patient-therapist relationship existed at the time of the injury
2. That the therapist failed to provide the appropriate standard of care at the time of the injury
3. That the patient suffered injuries, or damages: physical injuries, financial losses, and so on
4. That the patient's injuries were directly caused by the therapist's failure to provide the appropriate standard of care

An example of negligence in a physical therapy clinic would be failure to mop up water that had been tracked onto the clinic floor, with someone slipping and getting injured. This is considered negligence because any reasonably prudent person would have recognized that the water posed a risk of injury and promptly cleaned it up. **Malpractice**, or professional negligence, on the other hand, is the failure to do (or failure to avoid doing) something that a member in good standing of a profession would have done (or avoided doing), and that causes subsequent injury to the patient.[1] It is a failure to meet a *professional* standard of care, a special kind of negligence. An example of malpractice would be a therapist who excessively mobilizes a joint and thereby causes injury. Why is this not negligence? An ordinary reasonably prudent person would not be expected to know whether or how much to mobilize a joint in a given patient. A therapist, as a professional, however, is held to a higher, professional standard of care and is expected to exercise appropriate clinical judgment to avoid patient injury.

Delegation and Supervision; Vicarious Liability. The legal duty to provide a professional standard of care, and the ultimate responsibility for patient care, *always* remains with the PT. The therapist therefore may be held liable for a patient's injury even if the therapist was not directly providing services at that time. The PT bears this liability because a therapist's professional duty to the patient includes appropriate decision making regarding delegation and supervision of interventions. PTAs or students on affiliation can be held legally liable for their own negligent clinical judgments; however, the therapist may also be liable if tasks were negligently delegated or supervised.[22] If a therapist determines that delegation is appropriate, the therapist should prevent misunderstandings by always advising the patient of the credentials of the person to whom tasks have been delegated.

Similarly, an employer may be held legally responsible for the negligence or malpractice of employees when it is committed within the scope of their employment duties, regardless of whether the employer was involved in rendering care at the time.[22] This form of liability, known as **vicarious liability**, is based on the fact that the employer can control the quality of care rendered by controlling the workplace (policies, hiring, etc.). Thus a therapist who owns a private practice may be held liable for the injuries caused by one of the practice's PTs or PTAs while these employees are treating patients. In contrast, the employer would not be liable for any negligent acts (such as causing a car accident through negligent driving on the way to work) that employees may commit when not performing their professional duties.

Risk Management. **Risk management** involves a coordinated effort by an organization in "recognizing, identifying, and controlling exposures to losses or injuries created by activities of the organization."[2] To decrease the risk of lawsuits, PTs are advised to constantly monitor the quality of the services they provide. In this way they can avoid or minimize the occurrence of activities that increase the risk of patient injuries and other incidents that may impose legal or financial liability. In addition, they are advised to carry professional liability insurance that would cover the costs of legal fees and settlements or judgments arising from civil liability.[25] Under ordinary circumstances, however, liability insurance will not cover legal fees for professional misconduct or criminal actions.

Contract Law. A **contract** is "an agreement between two or more persons which creates mutual obligations to do or not do particular things."[1] Contract law is a subset of civil law, and contractual obligations can be enforced in court. A full discussion of the various types of contracts encountered by physical therapy providers is beyond the scope of this chapter, but a few of the more prominent ones are mentioned here. For example, providers may sign employment contracts with their employers, although most physical therapy providers are employed without having written contracts.[26] Therapists may also contract independently to provide particular services for an agency or facility without becoming actual employees. Providers are advised to thoroughly review any contract, preferably with legal counsel, before signing it. Should a provider breach, or fail to fulfill, an employment contract, the employer may seek to enforce it legally. Although providers cannot be forced to stay at jobs against their will, the employer may be entitled to monetary damages as set forth in the contract.[26] For example, some employers may offer tuition reimbursement or other incentives in return for a provider's agreement to work for the employer for a set period of time. If the provider breaches the agreement by leaving employment early, the employer may be entitled to all or a percentage of the reimbursement provided, with interest.

Therapists may sign agreements with managed care organizations (MCOs) and other payers to become recognized providers for patients enrolled with or covered by those organizations.[27] It is not uncommon for an MCO to refuse to reimburse or limit reimbursement for services rendered to patients enrolled with the MCO if the provider has not signed an agreement with the organization. Where providers have signed agreements with MCOs, the terms may require providers to accept lower rates of reimbursement, or to obtain authorization from the MCO before services are initiated.[27] If a provider does not abide by the terms of the agreement, the MCO can deny reimbursement or, if the breach is severe enough, drop the therapist as a recognized provider. The reader is reminded, however, that contracts regarding reimbursement do not affect the legality of providing services; if state law allows for the provision of interventions, the provider can often seek reimbursement from other sources (including the patient) if the payer denies reimbursement.

POLICIES

As noted earlier, the term "policy" may refer to public policies or the policies of private organizations. The APTA is a private, nongovernmental organization, and its policies do not have the force of law. The APTA defines its **policies** as "Association directives defining operational or administrative activities."[28] Procedures, on the other hand, describe the actions required to achieve a result, such as those needed to implement policies. Private policies affecting physical therapy may be set by other private entities, such as employers and payers. Private policies, unlike laws, cannot be legally enforced unless set forth in a contract. They do, however, represent the consensus of the members of an organization on a given issue. Consequently, private policies related to physical therapy can influence the relationships between physical therapy providers and private organizations, or they can be used to provide some momentum to effect change within private and public organizations.

AMERICAN PHYSICAL THERAPY ASSOCIATION POLICIES

As noted elsewhere in this text, the APTA is the primary professional organization representing the physical therapy profession in the United States. Through the activities of its Board of Directors and the House of Delegates, it establishes and annually reviews policies for its members. Policies of the APTA address a number of areas relating to practice, from documentation to the use of support personnel to national health care policy. Therapists and assistants are encouraged to become active, participating members of the APTA in order to ensure that their voices are heard and their efforts can assist the development of policies affecting current and future practice.

Because the APTA is a private organization, its policies are binding only on members. These policies can, however, have wide-ranging effects as they drive changes in several areas, such as scope of practice (by defining the services provided by a PTA) and reimbursement issues (through lobbying and dialogue with payers).

Certain policies and interpretive guidelines, clustered as core documents, address practice standards and ethical conduct. One example is the Standards of Practice for Physical Therapy,[29] which was discussed in Chapter 2. Two documents that establish standards of ethical conduct for physical therapy providers are the **Code of Ethics** (for physical therapists; Box 5-1) and the **Standards of Ethical Conduct for the Physical Therapist Assistant** (Box 5-2). Companion documents, the Guide for Professional Conduct (for the Code) and the Guide for Conduct of the Physical Therapist Assistant Member (for the Standards), interpret each item in the policies. Copies of each of these documents can be found on the APTA website (www.apta.org).

Violations of these ethical standards by members can be prosecuted by the APTA.[30] A complaint must first be lodged with the state chapter president, who will refer it to the state chapter ethics committee (CEC) for investigation. The member accused of the violation will be notified and given an opportunity to respond. If the investigation shows that the complaint has merit, the CEC will forward the matter to the Ethics and Judicial Committee (EJC) of the national organization. The EJC will then review the matter and impose sanctions ranging from a reprimand to expulsion from the organization. The APTA action can affect only membership; it has no jurisdiction to levy fines or affect the member's license to practice.

PAYER REIMBURSEMENT POLICIES

A full description of reimbursement policies is beyond the scope of this chapter. Different insurance companies, MCOs, government benefit programs, and so forth have different policies regarding such topics as who can be a provider, what services will be reimbursed and for how much, documentation requirements, and procedures for claims review and appeals for claim denials. Physical therapy providers must become familiar with these various policies and adhere to them to be reimbursed for their services. Payer policies may be found in government regulations, insurance company provider agreements, and provider manuals.

Changes in reimbursement policies in recent years have created dilemmas for providers as the temptation exists to allow reimbursement to drive practice. Providers must be actively engaged in dialogue with payers to educate them and ensure that reimbursement is adequate to meet patient needs. Providers must be able to advocate successfully on behalf of patients by using such tools as the Guide to Physical Therapist Practice and research demonstrating the effectiveness of physical therapy. Therapists must also become more

BOX 5-1	*American Physical Therapy Association Code of Ethics*

Preamble

This *Code of Ethics* of the American Physical Therapy Association sets forth principles for the ethical practice of physical therapy. All physical therapists are responsible for maintaining and promoting ethical practice. To this end, the physical therapist shall act in the best interest of the patient/client. This Code of Ethics shall be binding on all physical therapists.

Principle 1

A physical therapist shall respect the rights and dignity of all individuals and shall provide compassionate care.

Principle 2

A physical therapist shall act in a trustworthy manner towards patients/clients, and in all other aspects of physical therapy practice.

Principle 3

A physical therapist shall comply with laws and regulations governing physical therapy and shall strive to effect changes that benefit patients/clients.

Principle 4

A physical therapist shall exercise sound professional judgment.

Principle 5

A physical therapist shall achieve and maintain professional competence.

Principle 6

A physical therapist shall maintain and promote high standards for physical therapy practice, education, and research.

Principle 7

A physical therapist shall seek only such remuneration as is deserved and reasonable for physical therapy services.

Principle 8

A physical therapist shall provide and make available accurate and relevant information to patients/clients about their care and to the public about physical therapy services.

Principle 9

A physical therapist shall protect the public and the profession from unethical, incompetent, and illegal acts.

Principle 10

A physical therapist shall endeavor to address the health needs of society.

Principle 11

A physical therapist shall respect the rights, knowledge, and skills of colleagues and other health care professionals.

From Code of Ethics, HOD S06-00-12-23. House of Delegates Standards, Policies, Positions, and Guidelines. Alexandria, VA, American Physical Therapy Association, 2005.

BOX 5-2   *American Physical Therapy Association Standards of Ethical Conduct for the Physical Therapist Assistant*

Preamble
This document of the American Physical Therapy Association sets forth standards for the ethical conduct of the physical therapist assistant. All physical therapist assistants are responsible for maintaining high standards of conduct while assisting physical therapists. The physical therapist assistant shall act in the best interest of the patient/client. These standards of conduct shall be binding on all physical therapist assistants.

Standard 1
A physical therapist assistant shall respect the rights and dignity of all individuals and shall provide compassionate care.

Standard 2
A physical therapist assistant shall act in a trustworthy manner towards patients/clients.

Standard 3
A physical therapist assistant shall provide selected physical therapy interventions only under the supervision and direction of a physical therapist.

Standard 4
A physical therapist assistant shall comply with laws and regulations governing physical therapy.

Standard 5
A physical therapist assistant shall achieve and maintain competence in the provision of selected physical therapy interventions.

Standard 6
A physical therapist assistant shall make judgments that are commensurate with their educational and legal qualifications as a physical therapist assistant.

Standard 7
A physical therapist assistant shall protect the public and the profession from unethical, incompetent, and illegal acts.

From Standards of Ethical Conduct for the Physical Therapist Assistant, HOD S06-00-13-24. House of Delegates Standards, Policies, Positions, and Guidelines. Alexandria, VA, American Physical Therapy Association, 2005.

involved in clinical research to increase the body of knowledge establishing the effectiveness of physical therapy interventions. (See Chapters 6 and 7 for further description of reimbursement, the Guide, and research).

EMPLOYER POLICIES

Various employment settings also establish policies and procedures that are specific to that facility or organization. These policies and procedures address a wide variety of employment issues, including job descriptions, intervention protocols, documentation requirements, infection control and safety issues, and activities to ensure quality of care. It should be noted that the Standards of Practice for Physical Therapy requires that physical therapy providers have written policies and procedures to ensure the provision of high-quality physical therapy services.[29]

Employer policies generally cannot be legally enforced unless they are contained in an employment contract. They can, however, be grounds for disciplinary actions or firing. In addition, inquiries regarding whether facility policies and procedures were followed are often made during legal actions for negligence or malpractice, as part of the determination regarding whether the appropriate standard of care was met. Employer policies are not, however, a substitute for professional judgment. As professionals, therapists should not blindly follow policies without question, but should be engaged in active dialogue with their employers to ensure that their policies promote ethical, legal, and effective patient care.

SUMMARY

Government oversight of the physical therapy profession provides practitioners with both opportunities and limitations. This oversight occurs through the enactment of statutes by state and federal legislatures and the development of regulations by state and federal agencies, under the authority delegated to them by the legislature, to fill in gaps in statutes or clarify issues raised in a statute. Physical therapy providers must work with legislators and regulatory bodies to ensure that statutes and regulations accurately reflect the current state of practice. Court decisions clarify and interpret statutory language and, in the civil law arena, shape practice through the imposition of liability for acts of malpractice. Policies adopted by private organizations, such as the APTA, can also affect the evolution of physical therapy practice. Examples cited in this chapter indicate how laws, regulations, and policies can have an impact on the practice of physical therapy. Knowledge of and adherence to the applicable laws, regulations, and policies are necessary for safe, legal, ethical, and reimbursable practice.

CASE STUDY

CASE STUDY ONE

You are a PT operating an outpatient clinic that provides services for patients with a wide variety of needs. One of your patients is a 28-year-old construction worker who injured his knee in a work-related accident. He was referred to your clinic after surgery to repair the anterior cruciate ligament. You have completed your examination and evaluation, generated a diagnosis and prognosis, developed a plan of care, and delegated implementation of the intervention plan to an athletic trainer (ATC) who works for you in your clinic. The patient attends routine therapy visits over the next 2 weeks but fails to show up for further visits. Calls to the patient are not returned, and communication with his physician fails to explain the patient's apparent decision to terminate therapy. Several months later, legal papers are served at the clinic indicating that a lawsuit has been filed against you. The patient claims that the treatment received reinjured his knee. You discuss the case with the ATC who, after reviewing his notes, can recall no incidents or complaints involving the patient. From conversations with the patient, the ATC had suspicions that the patient was not adhering to activity precautions appropriate for his stage of recovery. However, the ATC did not believe these suspicions were strong enough to share with you or document in the patient's chart. You immediately contact your malpractice insurance carrier and forward all the legal papers and patient records.

An attorney for the insurance company contacts you to discuss the case. While noting that the patient needs to prove his case to win in court, she states that the failure to follow up on concerns regarding the patient's failure to adhere to precautions will hurt your case. In addition, the attorney advises that she has confidentially contacted a representative of your state's Physical Therapy Board, who has advised her that your state law does not permit delegation of physical therapy interventions to ATCs. Given the problems with this case, she notifies you that she will be recommending that the insurance company settle the case.

Case Study One Questions

1. Can the PT be held liable for the patient's injuries in this case? If so, on what grounds? What penalties can be imposed on the therapist for negligence or malpractice?
2. Assume that the PT's conduct also constitutes professional misconduct in this case. What penalties may be imposed on the basis of professional misconduct?
3. Were any policies implicated in this case? Identify possible areas of policy violations.
4. What actions could the PT have taken to minimize liability risks in this case? Whom could the PT have consulted?

REFERENCES

1. Black's Law Dictionary, ed 5. St. Paul, MN, West, 1990.
2. McGregor D: Health policy. *In*: Shi L, Singh D: Delivering Health Care in America—A Systems Approach. Gaithersburg, MD, Aspen, 2001.
3. Americans with Disabilities Act of 1990, 42 USC 126. Rockville, MD, US Government Printing Office. Available at http://www.access.gpo.gov/uscode/title42/chapter126_.html. Accessed April 18, 2006.
4. Individuals with Disabilities Education Act., 20 USC 33. Rockville, MD, US Government Printing Office. Available at http://www.access.gpo.gov/uscode/title20/chapter33_.html.
5. Nosse J, Friberg D, Kovacek P: Laws relevant to health care business. *In*: Managerial and Supervisory Principles for Physical Therapists, ed 2. Baltimore, MD, Lippincott Williams & Wilkins, 2005.
6. Physical therapist sentenced for billing fraud. PT Bull 1(11):4, 1993.
7. Unauthorized practice a crime, New York State Education Law, Article 130, Subarticle 4, Section 6512. New York State Assembly .
8. See, for example, Directory of State Practice Acts. American Physical Therapy Association. See also Licensing Authorities. Federation of State Boards of Physical Therapy.
9. Georgia Becomes 41st State to Pass Legislation Allowing Direct Access to Physical Therapy Services. Alexandria, VA, American Physical Therapy Association. Available at http://www.apta.org/AM/Template.cfm?Template=CM/HTMLDisplay.cfm&ContentID=30416. Accessed May 17, 2006.
10. Reforming Health Care Workforce Regulation: Policy Considerations for the 21st Century. San Francisco, CA, Pew Health Professions Commissions, 1995.
11. APTA Background Sheet 2006: The Physical Therapist Assistant. Alexandria, VA, American Physical Therapy Association. Available at http://www.apta.org/AM/Template.cfm?Section=Home&TEMPLATE=/CM/ContentDisplay.cfm&CONTENTID=29385. Accessed April 20, 2006.
12. The Model Practice Act for Physical Therapy, ed 2. Alexandria, VA, Federation of State Boards of Physical Therapy, 1997.

13. The Model Practice Act for Physical Therapy, ed 3. Alexandria, VA, Federation of State Boards of Physical Therapy, 2002.
14. Schwartz B: Administrative Law: A Casebook, ed 3. Boston, Little, Brown, 1988.
15. Balanced Budget Act: How It Affects Physical Therapy. Alexandria, VA, American Physical Therapy Association. Available at http://www.apta.org/AM/Template.cfm?Section=Home& TEMPLATE=/CM/ContentDisplay.cfm&CONTENTID=29385. Accessed April 20, 2006.
16. History of Medicare Therapy Caps. Alexandria, VA, American Physical Therapy Association. Available at http://www.apta.org/AM/Template.cfm?Section=Home&Template=/CM/ HTMLDisplay.cfm&ContentID=20959. Accessed April 20, 2006.
17. See, for example, NY Education Law Section 6733, NY State Office of the Professions, California Business and Professions Code Chapter 5.7 Sections 2600-2615, California Physical Therapy Board, and Illinois 225 ILC 90/3 Section 6, Illinois Division of Professional Regulation.
18. Professional Misconduct and Discipline. Albany, NY, New York State Office of the Professions. Available at http://www.op.nysed.gov/opd.htm. Accessed April 20, 2006.
19. See, for example, Penalties for professional misconduct, New York Education Law, Section 6511. NY State Assembly.
20. Legislative process: How a Senate bill becomes a law. US Senate. Available at http://www.senate.gov/reference/resources/pdf/legprocessflowchart.pdf. Accessed April 20, 2006.
21. Wilbanks J: The regulatory branch and you. PT—Magazine of Physical Therapy 1995;3(7):18.
22. Lewis DK: Business Skills in Physical Therapy—Legal Issues. Alexandria, VA, American Physical Therapy Association, 2002.
23. Cowdrey M, Drew M: Basic Law for the Allied Health Professions, ed 2. Boston, MA, Jones & Bartlett, 1995.
24. Lewis DK: General legal requirements and principles. *In*: Nosse LJ, Friberg DG, Kovacek PR: Managerial and Supervisory Principles for Physical Therapists, ed 2. Baltimore, MD, Lippincott Williams & Wilkins, 2005.
25. Lewis DK: Professional liability insurance: Are you covered? PT—Magazine of Physical Therapy 1994;2(7):49-54.
26. Scott RW: Promoting Legal Awareness in Physical and Occupational Therapy. St Louis, Mosby, 1997.
27. Gentry C: Managed care and integrated organizations. *In*: Shi L, Singh D: Delivering Health Care in America—A Systems Approach. Gaithersburg, MD, Aspen, 2001.
28. Standing Rules of the American Physical Therapy Association. Alexandria, VA, American Physical Therapy Association. Available at http://www.apta.org/AM/Template.cfm? Section=Policies_and_Bylaws&TEMPLATE=/CM/ContentDisplay.cfm&CONTENTID=27967. Accessed April 17, 2006.
29. Standards of Practice for Physical Therapy, HOD S06-03-09-10. House of Delegates Standards, Policies, Positions, and Guidelines. Alexandria, VA, American Physical Therapy Association, 2005.
30. Disciplinary Action Procedural Document. Alexandria, VA, American Physical Therapy Association. Available at http://www.apta.org/AM/Template.cfm?Section=Home& TEMPLATE=/CM/ContentDisplay.cfm&CONTENTID=25352. Accessed April 20, 2006.

ADDITIONAL RESOURCES

Scott RW: Legal Aspects of Documenting Patient Care. Gaithersburg, MD, Aspen, 2000.
The text is intended for use by health care students, providers, and administrators as general legal information regarding patient care documentation. The author provides a legal focus on the topic of documentation as an essential part of health care delivery.

Purtilo R: Ethical Dimensions in the Health Professions, ed 4. Toronto, Saunders, 2005.
The text assumes no formal prior study of ethics. It addresses basic concepts of morality and ethics, applies them to specific dilemmas in health care, and includes a process for ethical decision making. It makes extensive use of case studies and study questions.

House of Delegates Standards, Policies, Procedures, and Guidelines. Alexandria, VA, American Physical Therapy Association, 2005.
This document contains standards, policies, and positions adopted by the House of Delegates of the American Physical Therapy Association and is updated annually. It governs the activities of the organization and its members.

Related websites:

www.apta.org

Website of the American Physical Therapy Association. A comprehensive source of information on the profession of physical therapy. Some information is available only to members, but a considerable amount is available to the public, including sections specifically for students and consumers.

www.fsbpt.org

Home of the Federation of State Boards of Physical Therapy, composed of representatives of state physical therapy licensing boards. A free, authoritative source of information on the National Physical Therapy Exam and a clearinghouse for information on licensing within the United States.

www.cms.hhs.gov

Site for the Centers for Medicare & Medicaid Services, the federal agency within the Department of Health and Human Services that, among other duties, administers the Medicare and Medicaid programs. A free, comprehensive source of information on these programs, with specific sections of the site devoted to information for consumers and health care professionals.

http://thomas.loc.gov

Free site maintained by the Library of Congress, with substantial searchable federal legislative information. Information includes the Congressional Record, current bills, and Congressional committee reports, as well as the complete text of all federal statutes and the U.S. Constitution.

http://www.gpoaccess.gov/fr/index.html

Website of the U.S. Government Printing Office. Another free, searchable site with the complete Code of Federal Regulations and Federal Register, as well as the federal statutes and pending bills.

REVIEW QUESTIONS

1. Suggest examples of decisions that would be considered (1) a statute, (2) a common law decision, (3) a regulation, and (4) a policy.
2. Explain the different purposes and effects of a practice act versus federal legislation. Cite examples.
3. Describe how state regulations for professional conduct differ from regulations of the Health Care Financing Administration.
4. Cite major differences between the "code of ethics" and the "standards of practice for physical therapy."

The idea of reimbursement—a physical therapist (PT) provides care to a patient and the patient provides some form of payment to the PT—sounds simple, but unfortunately, it rarely is.

Reimbursement Department, American Physical Therapy Association

6

Financing and Reimbursing Health Care in Physical Therapy

Jennifer Wilson

Medicare
Medicare Advantage
Medicare Fee Schedule
Medicare Modernization Act (MMA)
Medicare Part A—Hospital Insurance
Medicare Part B—Supplementary Medical
    Insurance
Minimum Data Set (MDS)
open enrollment
per diem
pharmaceutical formularies
point-of-service (POS)
preferred provider organization (PPO)
premium
primary care provider (PCP)
prospective payment system (PPS)
provider contracting
provider network (panel)
reimbursement
resource-based relative value scale (RBRVS)
resource utilization groups (RUGs)
retrospective reimbursement
risk
staff model (of HMO)
State Children's Health Insurance Program
    (SCHIP)
subscriber

third party administrator/payer
usual, customary, and reasonable (UCR)
utilization
utilization review (UR)

OBJECTIVES

After reading this chapter, the reader will be able to:

- Discuss the reimbursement process in health care
- Differentiate between retrospective and prospective reimbursement methods
- Discuss how risk and health insurance are related
- Differentiate between indemnity health insurance and managed care plans
- Differentiate among Medicare, Medicaid, and the State Children's Health Insurance Program (SCHIP)
- Discuss how health care is financed
- Define how managed care organizations control health care costs
- State current trends in health care spending
- Discuss the Balanced Budget Act of 1997 (BBA) and its impact on physical therapy reimbursement

In the past two decades, major issues in the health care industry resulted in dramatic changes in how health care is financed, how providers are reimbursed, and ultimately, how health care is delivered. Costs of health care have skyrocketed. In part, this is due to advances in technology and specialization. In addition, the aging of America has put a strain on Medicare, the government-sponsored health insurance program for older adults. In response to the high cost of health care, health insurance companies and the government have imposed limitations on what and how they will reimburse for health care services and goods. Most of these restrictions occurred in the 1990s through the expansion of managed care programs in the private sector and the Balanced Budget Act of 1997 in the government sector. Changes in these programs, however, are continuing at a rapid pace. Providers, including physical therapists (PTs), must abide by the limitations or seek reimbursement directly from the patient/client.

Financing of health care is a source of great frustration for both the provider and the consumer. Words commonly used to describe the contemporary reimbursement experience include *confusing, complex, expensive, competitive, restrictive, exasperating,* and *ineffective.* The *need* for health care has not changed, but the *reimbursement* and *coverage* for these services and goods have changed. Providers must conform to extensive documentation requirements and have altered their delivery of services in order to be reimbursed. Consumers must pay for the services and goods not covered by the insurance industry and in many cases do not have health insurance because of the expensive premiums.

The current status of financing and reimbursement in health care, as well as how and why they evolved to this point, is described in this chapter. Particular attention is given to the impact on the PT and physical therapist assistant (PTA).

HEALTH INSURANCE

Health is unpredictable; it is uncertain if or when a person will become sick or require health care services.[1] The types of health care services a person needs vary greatly from an appointment in a doctor's office to a lengthy hospitalization in an intensive care unit (ICU). The need for catastrophic health care services could obliterate a family's or a person's finances. Therefore people in the United States purchase health insurance to minimize **risk,** defined in health care as the probability of a financial loss. This provides "peace of mind" against the high costs of health care.

Health insurance refers to the variety of policies that can be purchased to cover certain health-related services and goods. Policies range from those that cover the costs of medical, surgical, and hospital expenses to those that meet a precise need, such as covering the costs of long-term care. Typically, to become **insured** (covered by the policy), a **subscriber** (individual who purchases the policy) purchases a health insurance plan from an **insurer** (health insurance company). The subscriber purchases a range of benefits and benefit levels, which are available for a defined period of time, usually 1 year. Benefits are described as **covered services** or those services that are reimbursed by the insurance policy. Some typical covered medical services include inpatient hospital services, outpatient surgery, physician visits (in the hospital), office visits, skilled nursing care, medical tests and x-rays, prescription drugs, physical therapy, and maternity care. Often coverage for some goods, such as **durable medical equipment (DME),** is limited or not provided under the health insurance plan; in this case the patient is completely responsible for payment. Durable medical equipment is medical equipment (such as a wheelchair, hospital bed or ventilator) that a practitioner may prescribe for a patient's use over an extended period.[2]

The need for health insurance developed when, because of technological advances, specialization, and research, hospitals became entrenched as critical centers for health care. Because individuals and families became dependent on hospitals for health care, they could no longer assume the risk that they could pay if or when hospitalization or sophisticated health care services were needed. In addition, hospitals were no longer able to assume the risk that patients admitted and cared for would pay their bills for services rendered. As a result, health insurance companies developed to fill a need in the health care industry.

6

**FINANCING
HEALTH CARE**

Health insurance companies do not finance health care. They were established to offer policies that assume risk and to process health insurance claims; both tasks complicated health care transactions and added administrative expenses to the cost of providing health care. Who then finances health care, or in other words, who pays for these health insurance policies? Figure 6-1 illustrates the relationship between financing and reimbursement in health care and how this has changed dramatically in the United States. In the traditional or first party system, the individual seeking health care (first party) paid the provider (second party) directly. As health care services and costs increased, health insurance companies and the policies they offered became extensive (see above). Individuals could no longer afford to pay for the services or even the policies directly. Employers and the government established programs to contribute to the cost of health insurance. The system shifted to the current or third party system in which health insurance companies (third party) are paid for their policies and then pay for the health care services. Fundamentally, therefore, health care is financed by the individual directly, the employer, or the government.

Figure 6-2 illustrates the percentage of individuals who have insurance provided by each of these sources. Note that this figure is for the nonelderly population, so the impact of Medicare is limited. In addition, note the significant percentage of individuals who are uninsured and the increasing trend for this group. Although health care services may be available, not everyone has **access** to health care, defined as the ability to receive health care services when needed, because of the way the health care system is organized and financed in the United States.

Under the first source of financing health care ("private nongroup" in Figure 6-2), the individual purchases a health insurance policy directly from a health insurance company. Acquiring health insurance this way is expensive and not commonly done. In this direct pay approach the individual pays the **premium**, or cost of the insurance, out of pocket.

The second and most common method of financing health care is in an employment-based arrangement (Figure 6-2). Most employees purchase health insurance through their employers. This is known as **employer-sponsored health insurance,** or group insurance. Employers offer health insurance coverage

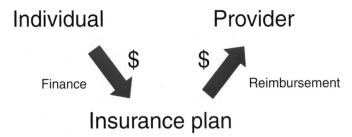

Figure 6-1 ▪ The third party system in the U.S. health care industry incorporates the concepts of finance (who buys insurance) and reimbursement (who pays the provider).

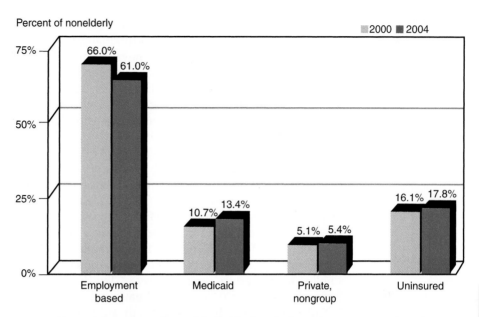

Percent of nonelderly

■ 2000 ■ 2004

Figure **6-2** ■ Percentage of individuals who have insurance purchased by themselves (private nongroup), their employers, the government, or not at all. Note this is for the nonelderly population. In this graph, Medicaid includes the State Children's Health Insurance Program and other state programs. (From Health Insurance Coverage in America: 2004 Data Update. The Kaiser Commission on Medicaid and the Uninsured. Available at http://www.kff.org/uninsured/upload/Health-Coverage-in-America-2004-Data-Update-Report.pdf. Accessed April 19, 2006.)

as a benefit for their employees, typically those who are full time. Employers are given tax incentives to offer health insurance as a benefit. Essentially, in the group model, both employees and employers finance health care. The employers agree to pay all or a certain portion of the premium of a health insurance plan. The employee pays the premiums using payroll deductions combined with the employer's contributions. Each year a period is designated as **open enrollment,** during which an employee has the opportunity to switch to a new health insurance plan based on individual and family needs and health insurance plans available. Once a selection has been made, the subscriber is locked into the choice for a defined period of time, usually 1 year.

Premium costs vary depending on the type of health plan or level of benefits purchased. In addition to the premiums, subscribers are responsible for financing other health care costs incurred at the point of service depending on the type of health insurance plan purchased; usually these costs are paid out of pocket. These cost commitments can include deductibles, copayments ("copays"), and coinsurances. A **deductible** is the amount that the subscriber incurs before a health insurer will pay for all or part of the remaining cost of the covered services. Deductibles may be either fixed dollar amounts, such as $500, or the value of a particular service, such as 2 days of hospital care. Usually, deductibles are linked to some defined time period (e.g., calendar year) over which they must be incurred. Frequently the insured individual can choose a higher deductible to reduce the monthly premiums for the health insurance policy. **Copayments** are flat dollar amounts (e.g., $20) a subscriber has to pay for specific health services (e.g., physician office visit) at the time of service. **Coinsurance,** usually expressed as a percentage, is a cost-sharing obligation under a health insurance policy. The subscriber is required to assume responsibility for a percentage of the costs of the covered services (commonly 20%). Box 6-1 provides an example of how these expenses would occur with a typical office visit.

The third and a major source of financing health care is the government (Figure 6-2). The federal government finances the Medicare program, and the federal and state governments finance Medicaid and the **State Children's Health Insurance Program (SCHIP)** for each state. Approximately 83 million beneficiaries (more than 1 in 4 Americans) received health care coverage through the Medicare, Medicaid, and SCHIP programs in 2004.[3] In addition, the government funds research efforts through the National Institutes of Health (NIH), the Public Health Service, and initiatives. Tax dollars collected from individuals and corporations are allocated to finance these programs and services.

The **Centers for Medicare & Medicaid Services (CMS),** under the Department of Health and Human Services, administers the Medicare program and works with each state to administer Medicaid, SCHIP, and health insurance portability standards. This agency is the largest purchaser of health insurance in the United States, and its policies have a significant impact on the rest of the health insurance industry.

MEDICARE

Medicare is the federally funded health insurance program that was enacted (as an amendment to the Social Security Act) in 1965 to cover the elderly population (age 65 and older), persons with end-stage renal disease, and those who are disabled and entitled to Social Security benefits. Medicare covered approximately 42 million people in 2004.[3] This is an **entitlement** program; that is, Americans 65 years of age and over who have contributed to Medicare

BOX 6-1   *Deductibles, Copayments, and Coinsurance: An Example*

An insured individual is covered under a health insurance policy that requires a $100 deductible, $15 copay, and 80/20 coinsurance. The individual sustained a wrist fracture that required casting and is now coming to physical therapy immediately after removal of the cast. At the time of the visit, and each visit thereafter, the person must pay the $15 copay. The individual's health insurance company is responsible for paying 80% of future covered health care expenses, and the individual will be obligated to pay the remaining 20% for each covered health care expense incurred. This will begin only after the individual has paid the deductible, or $100 in this case, for a specified period of time, usually 1 year.

through taxes or meet other disability eligibility requirements have the right to the benefits of Part A of this program. An individual entitled to Medicare is known as a **beneficiary.**[4]

Medicare Part A—Hospital Insurance provides mandatory coverage for inpatient hospital care, skilled nursing facility services, certain home health services, and hospice care. It is financed by payroll taxes from workers and their employers (each pays 1.45% of the wages; this appears as FICA on the pay stub) and general federal revenues.

Medicare Part B—Supplementary Medical Insurance is a voluntary program. Individuals entitled for Medicare Part A have the option to purchase Medicare Part B. Medicare Part B is funded from beneficiary premium payments, matched by general federal revenues. Medicare Part B helps pay for physician services, outpatient hospital services, select home health services, medical equipment and supplies, and other health services, such as physical therapy.

Medicare Advantage is an optional health plan that recently replaced Medicare+Choice (or Medicare Part C, originally created by the Balanced Budget Act of 1997). Under Medicare Advantage, Medicare beneficiaries gain greater choice and can choose from an array of private health plan options, including managed care arrangements (described below). Approximately 5 million Medicare beneficiaries were enrolled in Medicare Advantage health plans in 2004.[3]

MEDICAID

Medicaid is a health insurance program for the indigent population and is jointly funded by state and federal governments. Essentially, each state has its own Medicaid program. States have the authority to determine eligibility standards, set reimbursement rates, and establish specific benefit levels such as the type, amount, duration, and scope of services. Medicaid covered approximately 43 million people in 2004.[3]

Approximately 6 million people were estimated to be "dual eligibles" in 2004—eligible for both Medicare and Medicaid.[3] These individuals are Medicare beneficiaries who have low incomes and limited resources and may be eligible to receive help paying for their Medicare premiums and out-of-pocket medical expenses through Medicaid.

STATE CHILDREN'S HEALTH INSURANCE PROGRAM (SCHIP)

The federal and state governments finance SCHIP jointly. SCHIP is the program created by the Balanced Budget Act of 1997 to increase access to health care for children in families with incomes up to 200% of the federal poverty level. More that 6 million children were covered by SCHIP in 2004.[3]

TRENDS IN HEALTH CARE SPENDING

Figure 6-3 illustrates the spending for health care in the United States in 2003 by source of funding (*Where It Came From*) and type of service delivered (*Where It Went*).

Health care spending has grown continually for many years. In August 1997, anticipating that Medicare spending would continue to grow at approximately 9% per year while the general economy would grow at 5% per year, President

Where It Came From

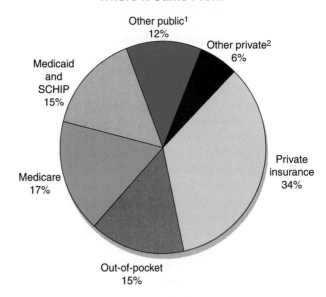

Where It Went

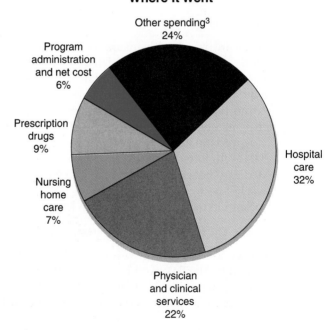

Figure 6-3 ■ Spending for U.S. health care in 2002 by source (where it came from) and service provided (where it went). (From U.S. Health Care System. Rockville, MD, Centers for Medicare & Medicaid Services, Office of the Actuary, National Health Statistics Group. Available at http://www.cms.hhs.gov/TheChartSeries/downloads/sec1_p.pdf. Accessed April 20, 2006.)

Clinton passed the **Balanced Budget Act of 1997 (BBA).**[5] This act eliminated the budget deficit for the first time since 1969. Every segment of the health care industry was affected by the BBA. Many of the cuts in health care spending came as reductions in entitlement spending. For example, some of the imposed reductions—approximately $115 billion for Medicare and $13.6 billion for Medicaid over a 5-year period—reduced Medicare payments to health care providers and hospitals significantly and quickly. Interestingly, the impact on outpatient rehabilitation providers was approximately $1.7 million in reimbursement cuts.[5]

According to CMS, in 2003, the growth of health care spending slowed for the first time in 7 years.[6] Health expenditures in the United States grew 7.7% in 2003 to $1.7 trillion, down from 9.3% growth in 2002. National health expenditures (NHE) continued to rise significantly, however, when measured against several factors. Spending in health care increased to $6280 on a per capita basis (Figure 6-4). Health spending accounted for 16% of the gross domestic product (GDP; the total dollar value of all goods and services produced in a year in the United States) in 2004 (Figure 6-5). Moreover, according to CMS projections, national health expenditures could reach $3.4 trillion in 2013 with these projections, not including the impact of the Medicare Prescription Drug, Improvement, and Modernization Act of 2003. This projection is calculated by use of an estimated average annual growth rate of 7.3% annually during the forecast period 2002-2013. In addition, CMS projects that by 2013, health spending could reach 18.4%

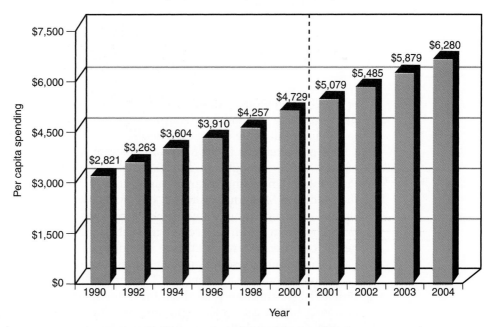

Figure 6-4 ■ Health care spending in the United States per capita from 1990 to 2004. (From Trends and Indicators in the Changing Health Care Marketplace. Menlo Park, CA, Henry J. Kaiser Family Foundation. Available at http://www.kff.org/insurance/7031/index.cfm. Accessed April 20, 2006.)

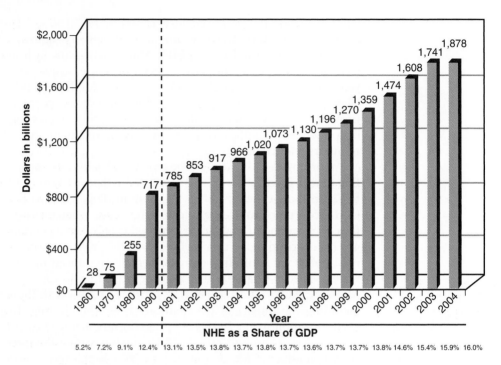

Figure 6-5 ■ Health care spending in the United States as a percentage of the gross domestic product. (From Trends and Indicators in the Changing Health Care Marketplace. Menlo Park, CA, Henry J. Kaiser Family Foundation. Available at http://www.kff.org/insurance/7031/index.cfm. Accessed April 20, 2006.)

of the GDP. Obviously, these projections indicate an urgency and necessity of future ongoing health care reform to control health care spending without sacrificing health care quality and access.

One of the reforms in the Medicare program was controversial in projections of cost versus benefits. In December 2003, Congress passed the Medicare Prescription Drug, Improvement, and Modernization Act (also referred to as the **Medicare Modernization Act,** or **MMA),** which contained the most substantial changes to the Medicare program since 1965.[3] This law provides for more choices in health care coverage (such as Medicare Advantage) and better health care benefits for Medicare beneficiaries. For example, in 2006, new Part D outpatient prescription drug benefits were initiated.

As consumers, we are concerned about the high cost of health care, yet as providers, we are concerned about the limited reimbursement for our services. As rising health care costs continue to be the focus of health policy debate, limitations on reimbursement continue to be set and reimbursement methods change at a brisk pace. Historically, managing the financial side of the PT practice was left to a select few, so PTs and PTAs spent little time in their formal education experiences and during on-the-job training sessions wrestling with the broader issues of health policy, health care spending, health insurance, and reimbursement. In today's health care environment, it is no longer sufficient to simply send a bill after treatment has been delivered and expect it to be paid.[7]

Payment levels are seldom equal to a PT's full charge. Therefore, whether operating in a for-profit or not-for-profit environment, providers must understand the intricacies of the reimbursement process so that they can proactively manage it to ensure that high-quality patient care is delivered and all providers, employees, and staff are paid at the end of the day. More than ever, providers need to work vigorously at maintaining a steady cash flow (by ensuring that the money owed to the practice has been collected) for the PT practice so that practice expenses (e.g., salaries) can be paid.

Currently, many factors can hinder or challenge the reimbursement that a physical therapy practice might receive. Therefore, every PT and PTA should be aware of the patient's coverage at the beginning of each episode of care and, without compromising patient care, integrate any payment limitations into the plan of treatment for the patient.[7]

REIMBURSEMENT METHODS IN HEALTH CARE

To this point the focus has been on how health care is financed, that is, who pays for health insurance. The remainder of the chapter shifts to payments to the provider—how does this person get reimbursed for his or her services? **Reimbursement** in health care is the process by which health care providers receive payment for their health care services. Because of the way health care is organized in the United States, health care providers are commonly reimbursed by a health insurance company functioning as a **third party payer** (see third party system in Figure 6-1). As financing methods in health care evolved in response to escalating costs, so did the methods of reimbursement. This shift is described below.

RETROSPECTIVE METHODOLOGY

Historically, health care providers in the United States followed a **retrospective reimbursement** method in which they were paid *after* health care services were rendered. The insured patient would seek care from the health care provider, the health care provider would provide care to the patient, and then the health care provider would be paid. This method of reimbursement is commonly referred to as **fee-for-services (FFS)**—otherwise known as **indemnity** or traditional health insurance. An indemnity insurance contract usually defines the maximum amounts that will be paid for covered services during a defined period of time.

Health insurers with indemnity policies assumed the risk for health care costs and processed the health care **claims** (forms describing the medical condition, services provided, and bill for services). After services were provided, health care providers submitted claims directly to health insurers for reimbursement. Typically, as long as the fees submitted by health care providers for services rendered fell within the **usual, customary, and reasonable (UCR)** range, the claim was paid in full without dispute. Using data collected through community or state surveys of provider charges, health insurers determined their own UCR—the maximum charge the insurer will reimburse for a particular health care service. This reimbursement process allowed health care providers to establish their own fees, known as a **fee schedule,** for the specific health care services they provided. Providers had little incentive to limit services or costs.

PROSPECTIVE METHODOLOGY

In an attempt to control rising health care costs, health insurance companies shifted to a **prospective payment system (PPS).** Prospective payment refers to various methods of paying hospitals, health systems and organizations, or health care providers in which payments are established in advance. Health care providers are paid these amounts regardless of the costs they actually incur. Prospective payment systems establish some control over cost increases by setting limits on amounts paid during a future period. Some prospective payment systems provide incentives for improved efficiency by sharing savings with health care providers who achieve lower than anticipated costs. In retrospective reimbursement, health care providers are reimbursed for actual expenses incurred, whereas in prospective payment systems they are not.

The federal government had a significant influence in the growth of the PPS. The Social Security Amendments of 1983 created a new PPS for hospital inpatients covered under Medicare Part A. The principle of **diagnostic-related groups (DRGs)** was introduced, in which the patient's diagnosis determines the amount the hospital will be paid; the payment is a fixed amount based on the average cost of treating that particular diagnosis. A measure of **case-mix** for the institution, or composite of the patients in each DRG, is used to determine reimbursement amounts. The hospital is paid the average cost regardless of length of stay or amount of treatment administered. Therefore, if the patient requires less care or fewer days in the hospital than the DRG average, the hospital makes money. Conversely, if the patient stays in the hospital longer or needs more care than the DRG average, the hospital loses money.

Another action taken by the federal government modified the PPS as it applied to physicians paid for services for Medicare beneficiaries under Part B. A new physician reimbursement method was established by the Omnibus Budget Reconciliation Act of 1989 and became effective in 1992. The **resource-based relative value scale (RBRVS)** replaced the fee-for-service system. RBRVS fees were determined based on three components: the total work completed, costs to practice medicine, and an allowance for malpractice insurance expense.[8] Each health care service was assigned a specified number of relative value units (RVUs); these RVUs were multiplied by a national conversion factor and further adjusted to allow for geographical cost variations. This approach had the effect of containing health care costs because the payment for a given health care service was the same regardless of whether it was performed by a generalist or a specialist physician. This system has become the foundation for the **Medicare Fee Schedule,** which lists payments for thousands of services and is frequently used by third party payers for all their subscribers (not just Medicare beneficiaries).

While government intervention had a significant impact on the growth of the PPS, the most influential factor was the development of managed care. Although the principles of managed care are fairly straightforward, the methods of implementation are varied and complex. This reimbursement approach is described in the next section.

MANAGED CARE

With health care costs continuing to rise and with global competition becoming fiercer, employers, health care policymakers, and the government needed to cultivate methods to control health care costs while still ensuring quality health care. In 1973, the Health Maintenance Organization (HMO) Act was passed. This federal legislation empowered health insurance companies to develop new ways to pay for health care services and goods.[8] The law increased control of the delivery of health care by third party payers through government-mandated regulations of health care service. The concept of prepaid or fixed payment under a managed care arrangement escalated.

MANAGED CARE ORGANIZATION

In its simplest form, **managed care** consists of two components: a predetermined payment schedule ("discounted fee schedule") established by the insurance company based on utilization data, and a **provider network (panel)** consisting of providers who contract with the insurance company and agree to accept the payment schedule for their services. Subscribers to these health insurance plans generally pay more for services if they are conducted by providers outside the network. Institutions or groups that employ the managed care principles are called **managed care organizations (MCOs).** Managed care is further characterized by diverse organizational models, distinct methods for reimbursing providers, and various approaches to cost containment. By incorporating these approaches to health care reimbursement, all MCOs restrict access to care in some way. Examples of access restrictions include limits on the types, number, or payment for services covered. Cost of the insurance may also limit access. Figure 6-6 illustrates the percentage of employees who do not accept employer-sponsored health insurance. In theory, employer-sponsored insurance is a way of "managing care"—linking the delivery of and payment for health care, coordinating the delivery of health care cost effectively, and providing prepaid (fixed) health care services within a defined network of health care providers (hospitals, physicians, labs, etc.) to voluntarily enrolled populations. Certainly, fixing payment or the number of visits covered without considering the amounts of actual services provided has shifted how health care services are delivered.

Provider networks in MCOs are developed through a process called **provider contracting.** The provider is deemed "on the provider panel" or a "participating provider" if the provider accepts the terms of the insurer's contract (usually after much negotiation) and after the MCO verifies the provider's credentials (using a process called provider credentialing). Contract terms outline reimbursement methods, including discounted fees and possible incentives, scopes of services allowed for reimbursement, utilization targets, and other stipulations. Participating providers assume responsibility (share financial risk) with health insurers for a population's health care and health maintenance. The contracting process enables insurers to exert influence or decision-making control over the **utilization,** or delivery and cost, of health care services for a defined period of time.

Currently, the three major types of MCOs (commonly referred to as the "triple option") are health maintenance organizations, preferred provider

6

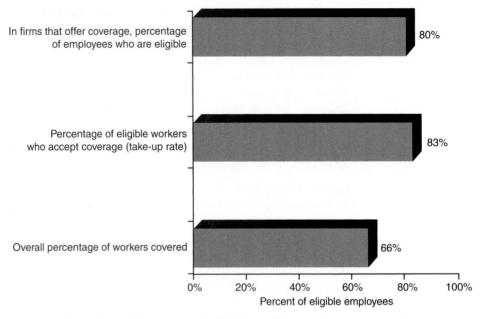

Figure 6-6 ▪ Percentage of eligible employees who accept employer-sponsored health insurance ("take-up rate"). (From Employer Health Benefits: 2005 Annual Survey. Menlo Park, CA, Henry J. Kaiser Family Foundation. Available at http://www.kaisernetwork.org/health_cast/ hcast_index.cfm?display=details&hc=1503. Accessed April 20, 2006.)

organizations, and point-of-service plans. Basically, these models differ in how tightly the provider panels are controlled. Further descriptions of each of these models follow.

Health Maintenance Organization. **Health maintenance organizations (HMOs)** proliferated with the HMO Act of 1973,[8] which provided loans and grants to form these entities. It also stipulated certain outpatient services that had to be provided, and it required that employers with 25 or more employees offer an HMO option if one was available in the area. Two types of HMOs existed originally, the staff and independent practice association models. In the **staff model,** providers are *employed* (not just under contract) by the HMO that also *operates* the facilities where the services are provided. The Kaiser-Permanente Health Care System, established in 1938, remains the foremost example of this model. In the **independent practice association (IPA) model,** individual physicians or physician groups form a legal entity that contracts with the HMO to provide services without operating the facilities where the services are provided.[9] This has predominated over the staff model.

Preferred Provider Organization. The second type of MCO is the **preferred provider organization (PPO).** A PPO is considered an "open managed care model." In this arrangement a health insurer or employer negotiates discounted or lower fees with networks of health care providers (doctors, hospitals, and other health care providers) in return for guaranteeing a certain volume of patients. Enrollees in a PPO can elect to receive treatment outside the network but must pay higher premiums, copayments, or deductibles for it.

Point-of-Service. The third type of MCO, the **point-of-service (POS)** plan, offers both in-network and out-of-network benefits. The greatest level of coverage is available if the insured receives in-network benefits. When an insured receives out-of-network benefits, higher out-of-pocket expenses are incurred. Typically, the insured is responsible for meeting an annual deductible before health care services are reimbursed and for paying a fixed percentage coinsurance amount or copayment for out-of-network services. The insured may also need to pay the difference between the insurer's payment and the actual charges for services received if the out-of-network health care provider's fees exceed the insurer's acceptable in-network contracted rates.

According to the Kaiser Family Foundation, the presence of managed care (including HMOs, PPOs, and POS plans) increased from 27% in 1988 to 93% in 2001 (Figure 6-7).[10] In 2001, 48% of covered workers were enrolled in PPOs, while HMO enrollment had decreased to 23%. Furthermore, traditional fee-for-service enrollment declined from 73% of total enrollment in 1988 to 7% in 2001.

The types of provider panels determine where and how consumers can access health care. For example, traditional HMOs (the oldest form of managed care) require enrollees to choose a **primary care provider (PCP)** from a "closed panel" of participating providers. A PCP is a generalist physician (family practice, general internal medicine, general pediatrics, and sometimes obstetrics/gynecology for women patients) who provides primary care services. Characteristically in an HMO, PCPs become the **gatekeeper**—the primary coordinator who determines whether the patient needs to see a specialist or requires other nonroutine services. The goal of the gatekeeper is to direct the patient to an appropriate level of service while avoiding unnecessary, possibly duplicative, redundant, and costly referrals to specialists or for specialty services. In other words, the gatekeeper restricts access to specialty services in an effort to control costs.

The subscriber must make choices when purchasing the type of managed care plan during open enrollment. These purchasing decisions and the amount of choice purchased directly affect a subscriber's potential future cost-sharing obligations. If the consumer stays *within* the provider network ("in-network") to receive health care, the consumer will not incur additional health care costs outside of the agreed upon copayments and premiums. However, if the consumer desires to purchase the choice to seek health care outside of the network ("out-of-network"), the consumer would be better off purchasing a PPO or POS plan, rather than a tightly controlled HMO plan.

Cost sharing is a reimbursement strategy adopted by most MCOs. By sharing the cost of health care with health care providers and consumers of health care, MCOs spread the risk or burden of trying to limit the potential for financial loss. Deductibles, copayments, and coinsurances are examples of specific cost-sharing strategies.

6

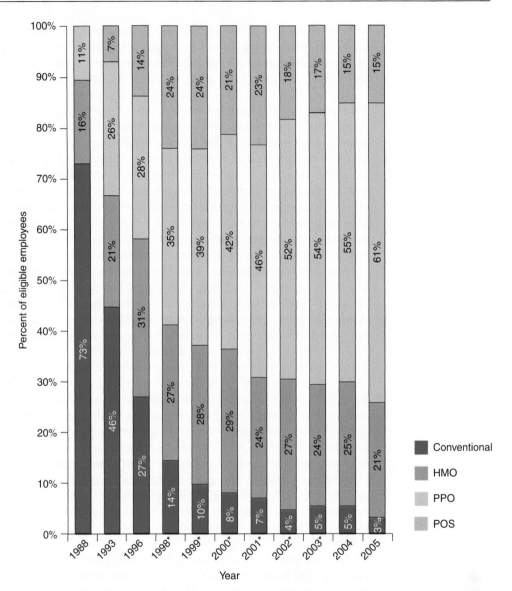

Figure 6-7 ■ Trends in type of health plan enrollment for eligible employees from 1988 to 2005. Figures may not add up to 100% because of rounding. Asterisk indicates that distribution is statistically different from the previous year shown at *p*<.05. (From Employer Health Benefits: 2005 Annual Survey. Menlo Park, CA, Henry J. Kaiser Family Foundation. Available at http://www.kaisernetwork.org/health_cast/hcast_index.cfm?display=detail&hc=1503. Accessed April 20, 2006.)

Most managed care plans, especially HMOs, offer preventive health care benefits. Inherent in the foundation of managed care is the emphasis on maintaining wellness or health (hence the term "health maintenance organizations"). Thus the use of expensive health care services is avoided if a consumer stays healthy (in a state of complete physical, mental, and social well-being).

MCOs use several other strategies to contain costs. These include providing care in the least expensive settings (nursing homes or home care is preferred over hospitals), avoiding the use of expensive emergency rooms in favor of less expensive ambulatory settings such as physicians' offices, and restricting **pharmaceutical formularies.** A pharmaceutical formulary is a list of drugs (usually by generic name) with indications for their use. This list is intended to include a sufficient range of medicines that practitioners can prescribe all "appropriate" medical treatment. A "closed" formulary provides coverage for a limited set of drugs, whereas a "tiered" formulary rewards patients financially for using generic instead of brand-name drugs.[2]

Cost containment strategies also take the form of defined service review mechanisms, such as utilization review and case management, to ensure the services are efficient and effective. **Utilization review (UR)** is defined as the evaluation of the medically necessary, appropriate, and efficient use of health care services, procedures, and facilities.[9] It can be done on a concurrent and retrospective basis. For example, a utilization review of a hospital would include a review of admissions, discharges, and lengths of stay. **Case management** provides monitoring and coordination of treatments rendered to patients to control costs and utilization. Usually patients who have chronic disease(s) (e.g., diabetes) are ideal candidates for case management because they frequently require high-cost or extensive health care services.

Consumer-Driven Health Care Plans

Consumer-driven health plans are new health plan arrangements that are receiving increasing attention from invested stakeholders in health care. Consumer-driven health care reflects a new approach for providing health care benefits that combines employer contributions with increased employee choice and responsibility and increased health plan and provider accountability.[11] Currently, the most prevalent model combines a high deductible (e.g., $1000) with a personal or health savings account option. These accounts permit employers, and sometimes employees, to make pretax contributions, which the employees can use to pay for routine medical care, thereby increasing their choice as to how the money will be spent.[10]

REIMBURSEMENT IN PHYSICAL THERAPY

Policy changes to control health care spending have affected the practice of physical therapy directly and indirectly for many years. The switch from FFS or a retrospective reimbursement methodology to a PPS had a significant impact on the way PTs received payment for their services. This shift in reimbursement forced PTs to look not just at historical costs of providing services (to set fee schedules from year to year), but also at the actual costs of providing care on an ongoing basis. Providers had to implement new approaches to staffing and service delivery to ensure productive, cost-effective care while still maintaining quality.

Managed care has had a dramatic effect on reimbursement and delivery of services in physical therapy. MCOs established limits and other mechanisms to control utilization and cost of health care. In addition to discounted fee schedules, MCOs have required documentation of need ("medical necessity") for physical therapy, a limitation on the number of visits covered, and documentation of functional gains after each physical therapy session. PTs must frequently invest unreimbursable time to advocate for more treatment sessions for individual patients. Documentation requirements across diverse physical therapy practice settings have become more stringent, complex, and labor intensive to improve accountability, causing much friction and sometimes discouragement within the practice of physical therapy. Conflict arises when requirements for documentation become greater and more detailed, yet third party payers (including CMS) do not reimburse the provider for preparation of the documentation.

Besides discounted fee schedules, other payment mechanisms were created to limit reimbursement for services. Private and managed care insurers pay for a large percentage of inpatient hospital stays on a **per diem** (a prenegotiated, per-day, flat/fixed fee) basis. The flat rate covers all services provided in the hospital on a particular day, including physical therapy, regardless of actual time spent with the patient. This payment method requires the provision of care to be time efficient and cost effective.[12] The Balanced Budget Act of 1997 authorized the implementation of a per discharge prospective payment system (PPS) for inpatient rehabilitation facilities (IRFs). The IRF PPS uses information from a patient assessment instrument (IRF PAI) to classify patients into groups based on clinical characteristics and anticipated resource needs. Payments are calculated separately for each group, including the use of case and facility level modifications.[13] Certain HMOs use a capitated payment method. Under **capitation,** a participating health care provider is paid a fixed amount in advance per member per month (PMPM) in anticipation of future services needed by an enrolled patient. This method involves a significant financial risk to the provider and has not been popular among PTs.

The Balanced Budget Act of 1997 had a widespread impact on reimbursement for health care and physical therapy services. The BBA significantly changed Medicare payment policies for rehabilitation services. Beginning January 1, 1999, an annual $1500 per beneficiary cap for physical therapy (including speech-language pathology services) and for occupational therapy was imposed on Medicare beneficiaries receiving outpatient rehabilitation services. After extensive lobbying by the APTA and other professional organizations, a moratorium on the cap became effective on January 1, 2000, and was extended through 2002. On September 1, 2003, a $1590 cap went into effect, followed by a moratorium on the cap beginning December 8, 2003, through December 31, 2005. This most recent moratorium was a result of the Medicare Modernization Act of 2003. The cap went back into effect January 1, 2006.[5] The APTA has advocated strongly against the implementation of this cap, which the APTA believes is insufficient to cover the costs of speech therapy and physical therapy (grouped together under one cap). Furthermore, the APTA contends that it will disrupt the continuum of care by forcing Medicare patients to change treatment settings so they can continue to receive physical therapy. According to the APTA, the development of the $1500 cap (increased to $1740 in 2006) on outpatient rehabilitation services and the skilled nursing facility (Part A) and home health agency (Part B) prospective payment systems have had an unfavorable impact on the ability of Medicare beneficiaries to access high-quality physical therapy services.

Reimbursement for physical therapy services varies greatly depending on the practice setting, creating more confusion and complexity within the profession. PTs are required to use coding systems to cover a variety of situations. For example, in outpatient physical therapy settings, PTs use **Current Procedural Terminology (CPT) codes** (97000 series; CPT is a registered trademark of the American Medical Association) to indicate what physical therapy services are delivered to patients.[14] In contrast, CMS requires PTs in skilled nursing facilities (SNFs) to report rehabilitative therapy minutes on the **Minimum Data Set (MDS).**[14] The MDS is an assessment instrument used in the SNF prospective payment system to classify residents into one of 44 **resource utilization groups (RUGs III)** that categorize patients based on their levels of resources used. The resulting classifications determine payment to the facility. The APTA is actively seeking modifications and clarifications to CPT codes and other coding systems to enhance and justify reimbursement for physical therapy services.

Many of the reimbursement issues created by MCOs have limited access to health care, particularly specialty health care providers. Consequently, PTs faced new challenges, since they have historically been recognized as specialty health care providers. For many years the APTA and PTs nationwide and state by state have been advocating for direct access. Now legal in 42 states, direct access permits PTs to initiate treatment without a referral and positions PTs as primary care providers (see Chapter 7).

Advocating for direct access, however, is not enough. PTs must set patient-centered goals and consider clinical outcomes from the outset. Use of evidence-based practice whenever possible to justify intervention strategies is becoming essential to ensure reimbursement (see Chapter 7). More than ever, practitioners and physical therapy educators are encouraged to conduct clinical research to augment the bank of existing evidence. Furthermore, the APTA has attempted to standardize "preferred practice patterns" through the development of the Guide to Physical Therapist Practice. The adoption of this standardized language by all practitioners nationwide, however, has been slow and tedious.

It is essential that PTs in contemporary practice become acclimated to the impact of reimbursement on physical therapy practice. PTs have to ensure that copays, coinsurances, and deductibles are collected at the time of service. Some PTs are adopting first party payment policies in which they collect payment in full from patients/clients at the time of service, eliminating the need to interface with third party payers. Interestingly, this reimbursement method, generally accepted by consumers for many of the complementary therapies, returns the system to the method so common decades ago. Although the extent of this reimbursement method may never be substantial, it indicates that consumers will pay for what they believe is valuable.

PTs must become invested in the reimbursement process by other means, including the following:

- Developing effective collection strategies
- Using and building evidence-based practice to justify interventions

6

- Using a standardized documentation language that can be understood by multiple stakeholders in the reimbursement process
- Advocating to increase the profession's role as primary care practitioners or practitioners of choice
- Supporting the APTA in its efforts to influence payment and health care policy changes

Furthermore, PTs are encouraged to develop strategies for gaining reimbursement for preventive programs and health care services, an emerging market niche.

SUMMARY

Health care financing and reimbursement originally involved direct transactions between the consumer and provider. Health insurance companies then arose to assume the risk of health care costs. The government entered this arena with the Social Security Act Amendments of 1965, creating the Medicare and Medicaid programs. As health care costs escalated dramatically, new methods of financing health insurance policies and reimbursing health care providers developed. Managed care emerged as the predominant method to control rising health care costs. Managed care organizations (MCOs) took many forms, including HMOs, PPOs, and POS options. Health insurance companies, through MCOs, were empowered to assume responsibility for decision making to coordinate and control utilization of health care services by limiting reimbursement, covered services, and number of covered visits. Legislation by the federal government and related regulation by CMS introduced several significant changes to health care reimbursement. These included DRGs, RBRVS, and a cap on payments for outpatient physical therapy services for Medicare beneficiaries. Payment policy changes made continuously by CMS and third party payers create a sense for health care providers that they are trying to stay afloat amidst a reimbursement tidal wave.

REFERENCES

1. Lee R: Economics for Healthcare Managers. Chicago, Health Administration Press, 2000.
2. Glossary of Terms Commonly Used in Health Care (2004 Edition). Washington, DC, Academy Health. Available at www.academyhealth.org/publications/glossary.pdf. Accessed April 19, 2006.
3. CMS Active Projects Report (annual report). Baltimore, Centers for Medicare & Medicaid Services.
4. Bodenheimer T, Grumbach K: Understanding Health Policy: A Clinical Approach, ed 4. New York, Lange Medical Books/McGraw-Hill, 2005.
5. The Balanced Budget Act: How It Affects Physical Therapy. Alexandria, VA, American Physical Therapy Association. Available at http://www.apta.org/AM/Template.cfm?Section=Home&CONTENTID=22156&TEMPLATE=/CM/Contentdisplay.cfm. Accessed April 19, 2006.
6. Highlights—National Health Expenditures, 2003. Baltimore, Centers for Medicare & Medicaid Services, 2005.
7. What Is Reimbursement? Alexandria, VA, American Physical Therapy Association. Available at http://www.apta.org/AM/Template.cfm?Section=About_Reimbursement&TEMPLATE=/CM/ContentDisplay.cfm&CONTENTID=27184. Accessed May 2, 2006.
8. Sultz H, Young K: Health Care USA: Understanding Its Organization and Delivery, ed 5. Gaithersburg, MD, Aspen Publishers, 2006.
9. Shi L, Sing D: Delivering Health Care in America: A Systems Approach. Sudbury, MA, Jones & Bartlett, 2004.
10. Henry J. Kaiser Family Foundation: Employer Health Benefits: 2004 Annual Survey. Menlo Park, CA, Henry J. Kaiser Family Foundation, 2004.
11. Wojciechowski M: The future of physical therapy as shaped and defined by patients. PT—Magazine of Physical Therapy 2005;13(2):46-52.

12. Payment by Treatment Setting. Alexandria, VA, American Physical Therapy Association. Available at http://www.apta.org/AM/Template.cfm?Section=Reimbursement2&Template=/MembersOnly.cfm&ContentI. Accessed April 19, 2006.
13. Inpatient Rehabilitation Facility PPS Overview. Baltimore, MD, Centers for Medicare and Medicaid, US Department of Health & Human Services. Available at http://cms.hhs.gov/InpatientRehabFacPPS/01_overview.asp. Accessed May 2, 2006.
14. The Reimbursement Resource Book. Alexandria, VA, American Physical Therapy Association, 2005.

ADDITIONAL RESOURCE

Physical Therapy Reimbursement News, APTA.

APTA's newly redesigned, bimonthly newsletter offers analysis of industry developments, provides useful tips for navigating the claims process, and reports changes in legislation, regulations, and policies.

REVIEW QUESTIONS

1. How is prospective reimbursement different from retrospective reimbursement?
2. What does it mean to be "insured" in health care?
3. How does a person become insured for health care in the United States?
4. How is risk in health care linked to health insurance?
5. How has managed care attempted to control health care costs?
6. How has the BBA affected physical therapy reimbursement?
7. What role does the APTA play in physical therapy reimbursement?
8. What strategies can PTs use to enhance reimbursement?
9. What role does the government play in financing health care in the United States?
10. What role does the consumer play in financing his or her own health care?

6

> A*chievement of* Vision 2020's *goal of all physical therapists*
> *completing the* DPT *by that year will ring hollow unless each*
> *practitioner demonstrates integrity, accountability, and excellence, as*
> *defined in* Professionalism in Physical Therapy: Core Values.
>
> Joe Black, Senior Vice President, American Physical Therapy
> Association

7 Current Issues: Physical Therapy in Evolution

Susan E. Bennett

OBJECTIVES

After reading this chapter, the reader will be able to describe:

- The difference between professional and postprofessional education and the need for both in physical therapy
- The doctor of physical therapy degree and the transitional doctor of physical therapy degree
- Three practice issues having an impact on the physical therapist assistant

- The results of the Vector Study
- The development of health care systems and the benefits of continuum of care
- How encroachment may have an impact on physical therapy
- The effects of the Balanced Budget Act of 1997 on the practice of physical therapy
- The importance of evidenced-based practice

The profession of physical therapy constantly evolves to maintain a contemporary approach in the areas of education, practice, and research. As issues arise from external or internal forces, they are addressed for the best interests of the members of this profession and the patients and clients it serves. In the 1990s, practice issues appeared to dominate. These included managed care, the Balanced Budget Act of 1997, and direct access. While the impact of these and additional practice issues continues, the current movement toward the doctorate degree driven by the APTA Vision Statement for Physical Therapy 2020[1] (Vision 2020) presents a major evolution in the area of education. The speed of programmatic transition to the doctorate degree has been a great surprise. Underscoring all these trends are the continuing issue of evidenced-based practice and the developing attention to professionalism. The need to conduct sound research has long been an issue in this profession, but attention to applying the findings to practice has intensified. Professionalism was also derived from Vision 2020 and has become the focus of attention to define, describe, and apply the behaviors to practice.

This chapter examines how issues in education, practice, and research influence the profession of physical therapy. The historical perspective is presented, as appropriate, to demonstrate the longevity and evolution of some of these issues.

EDUCATION

HISTORICAL OVERVIEW

The extent of the educational preparation and degree required to practice physical therapy has been a topic of debate for some time. The physical therapist (PT) evolved from the reconstruction aides established during World War I (see Chapter 1). These reconstruction aides were trained in emergency courses, but the position was phased out at the end of the war. Standards for Schools of Physical Therapy, published in 1928, was the first recommended course of study for physical therapy. The American Physical Therapy Association (APTA), at that time called the American Physiotherapy Association, was closely involved in the development of these programs until 1936, when the American Medical Association (AMA) assumed responsibility for overseeing the educational preparation.[2] This change was initially perceived to be a positive step for the profession, but as it turned out, the AMA limited the input from PTs and never revised or updated the curricula until 1955.

The first discussion of academic degree requirements occurred in 1955, when it was determined that if physical therapy education was integrated with a bachelor's degree program, the graduates could receive a bachelor's degree in physical therapy. This action was formalized in 1960 by the APTA House of Delegates and provided strong support to change the first professional degree in physical therapy from a certificate to a bachelor's degree. In 1977 the APTA was recognized as an independent accrediting agency, and in 1983 the APTA became the only recognized accrediting agency for PT and physical therapist assistant (PTA) education programs. The 1977 action eliminated the conflict created by the AMA's limiting the growth and independence of education programs for physical therapy.[2]

PROFESSIONAL LEVEL EDUCATION

More controversy was to follow. In 1979, the APTA House of Delegates adopted a policy, which was amended in 1980, ruling that "physical therapist professional education be that which results in the awarding of a postbaccalaureate degree" and "that all physical therapist professional education programs and all developing physical therapist professional educational programs shall comply with this policy by December 31, 1990."[3] Postbaccalaureate education moved academic preparation of the PT beyond the bachelor's degree and into the master's degree level. By January 1994, 55% of PT education programs were at or had received approval to move to the postbaccalaureate level. While this figure reflects a substantial transition to postbaccalaureate level education, it also indicates that the policy adopted by the House of Delegates in 1979 could not supersede each state's requirements for education and licensure for PTs. Each state is responsible for establishing and regulating the education and practice of licensed professionals. A national organization, such as the APTA, cannot supersede any rules and regulations set by each state. Awarding of the bachelor's or master's degree remained a controversy for many years.

New terminology was adopted by the House of Delegates in June 1993 to differentiate entry level education from advanced preparation for PTs.[4] **Physical therapist professional education** refers to all academic programs that prepare students to practice physical therapy (*entry level*) regardless of the degree. **Postprofessional education** is *advanced* education (at either the master's or doctoral level) completed by a licensed PT.

In 1993, a policy was to be presented to the House of Delegates to investigate the **doctor of physical therapy (DPT)** as the professional degree. Students in this program, although receiving a doctoral degree, would be entry level graduates in the field of physical therapy. Other doctoral programs had been proposed, but at the postprofessional level (an advanced degree for licensed PTs). This policy did not reach the House floor for discussion; however, it did generate much discussion outside the House of Delegates. As previously noted, the policy adopted in 1979 by the House of Delegates could not mandate a postbaccalaureate degree for physical therapy education, so it was believed that the DPT would meet the same fate. Even discussing a DPT as the professional degree seemed premature to many members of the House of Delegates, especially in view of the status of the postbaccalaureate degree.

EDUCATION TODAY

Two documents, **A Normative Model of Physical Therapist Professional Education**[5] and the **Evaluative Criteria for Accreditation of Education Programs for the Preparation of Physical Therapists**,[6] serve as guidelines and standards, respectively, for existing and developing professional level programs in physical therapy. The Normative Model is a standardized framework for all PT education programs that serves to "translate practice expectations into educational outcomes, identify necessary content strategies, and describe possible strategies to achieve these outcomes based on a conceptual framework that places the curriculum in the context of its immediate settings and the extended environment."[5] The Evaluative Criteria describe the specific components that must be in place for accreditation of professional level programs. These components include the organization of the department and institution that provide the resources to support the program, curriculum development and content, and the means by which the program is continually assessed. The 1998 revisions of the Evaluative Criteria were particularly significant because the document stipulated that accrediting activities for professional level education programs would be limited to those that awarded postbaccalaureate degrees beginning January 1, 2002.

These two documents are reflective of the role that physical therapy plays in health care today. Programs that integrate the Normative Model in the curriculum and meet the Evaluative Criteria graduate students who are ready to enter a health care system as primary care providers. This is the case when patients/clients have direct access to a PT without a physician's referral. This responsibility for patient care has triggered many PTs to provide **evidence-based practice,** which has become another integral component of the educational curriculum. Education programs commonly require a total of 100 or more credits in professional study to complete the requirements for practice as a PT. In the majority of PT programs, students are required to have a bachelor's degree before entering the professional program in physical therapy. At several academic institutions the clinical education component of the professional program is similar to the medical model in that a residency period is required. In the academic programs that require a residency, it is usually scheduled at the completion of the didactic phase of education and is for 6 to 12 months. At one institution the 1-year residency is a paid educational experience supported by the academic institution and clinical facility.

With the expanding autonomy of the PT in health care and the extensive educational preparation required to practice, the move to the DPT is occurring quickly. Part of this rapid transition is driven by the market. Students who are exploring PT education programs have the option to complete a 3-year professional graduate program at one institution and earn a master's degree, or go to another institution for 3 years, complete a similar curriculum, and earn a doctor of physical therapy. The professional doctorate has been described as "the appropriate degree for preparation of practitioners who are competent to meet the broad societal need for physical therapy services now and in the future."[7] The first class of PTs with the designation "DPT" graduated in 1996 from Creighton University in Omaha, Nebraska. Currently, more than 80% of the professional (entry level) programs are either at the DPT level or planning to move to that level.[8]

Will the DPT become the *required* professional degree of our profession? Action taken by the 2000 House of Delegates indicated that the DPT is the degree for the PT of the future. That body endorsed a Vision Sentence stating, "By 2020, physical therapy will be provided by physical therapists who are doctors of physical therapy, recognized by consumers and other healthcare professionals as the practitioners of choice to whom consumers have direct access for the diagnosis of, interventions for, and prevention of impairments, functional limitations, and disabilities related to movement, function, and health."[1] Box 7-1, published on the APTA webpage of Frequently Asked Questions, lists the rationale for moving to a professional DPT degree.

What of the practicing PTs with a bachelor's or master's degree? Do they need to earn a DPT degree, or do they receive the credentials based on years of competent practice? These questions were debated by practicing clinicians as the DPT became the degree awarded by the majority of PT education programs. Part of the debate was based on the experienced clinician having a bachelor's

---

BOX 7-1   *What Is the Rationale for Having Professional (Entry Level) DPT Programs?*

The rationale for awarding the DPT is based on at least four factors:
1. The level of practice inherent to the patient/client management model in the Guide to Physical Therapist Practice requires a breadth and depth in educational preparation not easily acquired within the time constraints of the typical MPT program;
2. Societal expectations are that the fully autonomous health care practitioner with a scope of practice consistent with the Guide to Physical Therapist Practice be a clinical doctor;
3. The realization of the profession's goals in the coming decades, including direct access, "physician status" for reimbursement purposes, and clinical competence consistent with the preferred outcomes of evidence-based practice, will require that practitioners possess the clinical doctorate (consistent with medicine, osteopathy, dentistry, veterinary medicine, optometry, and podiatry);
4. Many existing professional (entry-level) MPT programs already meet the requirements for the clinical doctorate; in such cases, the graduate of a professional (entry-level) MPT program is denied the degree most appropriate to the program of study.

From Doctor of Physical Therapy (DPT) Degree Frequently Asked Questions. Alexandria, VA, American Physical Therapy Association. Available at http://www.apta.org/AM/Template.cfm?Section=Profession_PT&TEMPLATE=/CM/ContentDisplay.cfm&CONTENTID=23597#BM6. Accessed April 23, 2006.

degree and the new graduate earning a doctor of physical therapy degree. Graduates of DPT programs are still challenged by practicing clinicians with a bachelor's or master's degree as to the necessity of the degree and how it is different from the previous degree programs. "The DPT graduate is still a novice clinician," notes Laurie Hack, PT, PhD, MBA, FAPTA, former director of the DPT program at Temple University. "Whatever their degree might be, the DPTs need guidance from experienced clinicians." When a DPT walks into a clinic, Hack says to clinicians she addresses, "it doesn't wipe out all that you know as an experienced clinician. You will indeed need to help guide them—but they can also bring useful knowledge back to you."[9]

Transitional DPT (tDPT) programs were established at academic institutions to enable practicing clinicians to earn a DPT degree in a manner that did not interfere with their full-time clinical practice. "The professional (entry-level) DPT is awarded upon completion of a PT professional education program; the 'transition' DPT is awarded to a licensed PT upon completion of a postprofessional education program and signifies augmented knowledge, skills, and behaviors that are equivalent to current entry-level education standards. This learner-centered augmentation provides the PT with knowledge, skills, and behaviors that have been added to the professional (entry-level) curricula since the learner's year of graduation."[9] As of May 2006, there were 16 academic institutions offering a tDPT requiring on-site participation in class, 16 offering distance learning tDPT academic programs, and 35 offering a combination of on-site and distance learning.[10] Whether a professional DPT degree or a postprofessional transitional DPT is completed, the degree credential is "DPT" and should be preceded by the clinical designator, "PT," recognized by all state licensing boards (e.g., Mary Brown, PT, DPT).

With all the debate over the DPT as the professional degree for physical therapy, one might ask whether advanced degrees are needed at all. According to Rothstein in his May 1998 editorial in *Physical Therapy*, "The DPT prepares an individual for practice, not for a career as an academic. If we substitute the DPT for the PhD, the EdD, the ScD, and the like, we will have abandoned any hope of developing a mature academic enterprise, one that can supply clinicians with the research and scholarship they need to be better practitioners."[11] Sahrmann echoed the sentiment of Rothstein in the 29th Mary McMillan Lecture when she stated, "I believe the development of these postprofessional programs should be encouraged so that the practicing therapist will have the opportunity to be a scholar-clinician, as well as a diagnostician."[12] We have much to learn in our role as movement scientists, and a scientific foundation must be established from which we can justify the effectiveness of interventions we provide.

SUPPLY AND DEMAND

It was not very long ago that graduates of PT and PTA programs had difficulty finding employment after graduation. Within a short span of 4 to 5 years during the mid 1990s, the job market had changed dramatically. Was it because too many education programs were graduating PTs and PTAs? Was the need for physical therapy services dwindling even though the number of individuals 75 years and older continued to increase?

To answer these questions, in 1997 the APTA commissioned Vector Research, Inc., to conduct a study examining the demand for physical therapy services for the years 1995, 2000, and 2005. The results of the study were surprising to many, in that the demand for PTs was projected to be met by 1998, with a mild surplus in 2000 and a large surplus of therapists projected by 2005.[13] Many blamed the surplus on the expansion of existing education programs and development of new programs driven by market demand and the extent of qualified applicants seeking admission to PT and PTA education programs. Others realized that the delivery of physical therapy was changing, as was the reimbursement for services provided. The old model of treating the patient three times a week for 2 to 3 months was no longer being reimbursed. Therapists and employers recognized that they had to do more with less (effects of managed care). The reimbursement rate for services provided had dwindled, and thus therapists were expected to see more patients each day to compensate for the diminished revenue. A projection of the number of visits and frequency of visits per diagnostic condition is described in the Guide to Physical Therapist Practice,[14] but today it is more often dictated by the patient's health insurance. PTs have had to become more efficient in establishing treatment plans and prescribing home programs to actively engage patients in their care and outcome. As of May 2005, the projections that were reported by Vector Research of a large surplus of PTs had not occurred. The APTA did take action in 1999 and 2002 when the House of Delegates endorsed and subsequently revised the position that "the American Physical Therapy Association recommends against the development of new professional PT and entry-level PTA education programs and the expansion of existing programs."[15]

Recent data from the US Department of Labor indicate a positive employment projection for PTs (Box 7-2).[16] Wherever the new graduate in physical

BOX 7-2	*Employment Outlook for Physical Therapists*

Employment of physical therapists is expected to grow faster than the average for all occupations through 2012. The impact of proposed Federal legislation imposing limits on reimbursement for therapy services may adversely affect the short-term job outlook for physical therapists. However, over the long run, the demand for physical therapists should continue to rise as growth in the number of individuals with disabilities or limited function spurs demand for therapy services. The growing elderly population is particularly vulnerable to chronic and debilitating conditions that require therapeutic services. Also, the baby-boom generation is entering the prime age for heart attacks and strokes, increasing the demand for cardiac and physical rehabilitation. Further, young people will need physical therapy as technological advances save the lives of a larger proportion of newborns with severe birth defects.

From Bureau of Labor Statistics, US Department of Labor, Occupational Outlook Handbook, 2004-05 Edition, Physical Therapists.

therapy chooses to practice, the employment opportunities should continue to be strong through 2012. Does our current strong market for PTs and PTAs reflect the response of the education programs to prepare graduates who have time management skills, organization and administrative skills, business skills, program development in wellness and prevention, effective communication skills, and knowledge in marketing? Did the downsizing of enrollment in some PT programs converting to the DPT degree have an effect? Have the health care and insurance industries adjusted to accommodate an increase in demand with more services that are reasonably reimbursed? The answers to these questions are not clear, but one could suspect that the change in academic preparation did affect the employment market in physical therapy.

PHYSICAL THERAPIST ASSISTANT

Evolution of the educational requirement for the PTA (described in Chapter 3) has been less controversial. In 1999, the House of Delegates adopted **A Normative Model of Physical Therapist Assistant Education**,[17] which provides guidelines for the content of these education programs. The document **Evaluative Criteria for Accreditation of Education Programs for the Preparation of Physical Therapist Assistants**[18] is used in the accreditation of PTA programs and was revised in January 2002. The current controversy with PTA education involves three issues: the attendance and participation of PTAs at continuing education courses offered for PTs, restriction of interventions performed by the assistant, and opportunity for recognition of advanced clinical skills. Some may also argue that adoption of the Normative Model for PTA education raises the issue of requiring a bachelor's degree program versus the current associate's degree preparation. The significance of these issues resulted in a task force ("RC 40 TF") to study the future role of the PTA triggered by action of the House of Delegates in 2001.[19] After a 2-year study with widespread input, the final report in 2003 included several motions to the House of Delegates and recommendations for further review. Although specific action was taken, issues remain sensitive as noted below.

Many PTs believe that PTAs should be excluded from attending continuing education courses offered for PTs because the content is beyond the skills of the assistant. If the PTA learns and practices examination and intervention skills in a continuing education course, would the expectation be that the assistant could perform those procedures in the clinic without the direction and supervision of the PT? Should the PTA be restricted from courses that could provide a better understanding of certain techniques without any intention of using them? The problem is magnified by the limited number of continuing education courses specifically offered for the PTA. Regardless of the degree of continuing education completed by the PTA, it is incumbent upon the PT-PTA relationship to delegate and accept responsibilities that are legal and in accordance with APTA policy. Box 7-3 indicates that the APTA supports continuing education for the PTA and also includes guidance on how to use new interventions learned.[20]

Assistants have argued that they are instructed in higher level intervention skills both in their academic preparation and by the supervising therapist.

BOX 7-3   *Position on Continuing Education for Physical Therapist Assistants*

Physical therapist assistants may participate in continuing education that includes and teaches subject matter and interventions that differ from the description of entry-level skills as described in the Normative Model of Physical Therapist Assistant Education. Physical therapist assistants may use the interventions taught in continuing education only as consistent with American Physical Therapy Association [policies, positions, guidelines, standards, and the Code of Ethics] and under the direction and supervision of the physical therapist.

From Continuing Education for the Physical Therapist Assistant, HOD P06-01-22-23. Alexandria, VA, House of Delegates Standards, Policies, Positions, and Guidelines, American Physical Therapy Association, 2005.

Examples include the interventions of mobilization, manipulation, and sharp debridement, which are part of the curricula in several PTA education programs. The APTA addressed this issue through another position and restricted these interventions to the PT (Box 7-4).[21] This position was reaffirmed by the RC 40 TF.

In regard to recognition for advanced clinical skills, PTs have the opportunity to pursue board certification as clinical specialists, yet there is not a parallel option for the PTA. The APTA Board of Directors, in collaboration with the National Assembly of Physical Therapist Assistants, examined the

BOX 7-4   *Procedural Interventions Performed Exclusively by Physical Therapists*

The physical therapist's scope of practice as defined by the American Physical Therapy Association Guide to Physical Therapist Practice includes interventions performed by physical therapists. These interventions include procedures performed exclusively by physical therapists and selected interventions that can be performed by the physical therapist assistant under the direction and supervision of the physical therapist. Interventions that require immediate and continuous examination and evaluation throughout the intervention are performed exclusively by the physical therapist. Such procedural interventions within the scope of physical therapist practice that are performed exclusively by the physical therapist include, but are not limited to, spinal and peripheral joint mobilization/manipulation, which are components of manual therapy, and sharp selective debridement, which is a component of wound management.

From Procedural Interventions Exclusively Performed by Physical Therapists, HOD P06-00-30-36. House of Delegates Standards, Policies, Positions, and Guidelines. Alexandria, VA, American Physical Therapy Association, 2005.

feasibility and need for recognition of advanced achievement by PTAs. A recognition program for the PTA was created in June 2003 when the House of Delegates adopted a Recognition of Advanced Proficiency for the PTA (Box 7-5). The first recipients were recognized at the APTA Annual Conference in June 2005.

In addition to these issues affecting the PTA in the area of education, governance has been an issue since the creation of this position in 1967. The historical and recent significant developments in this area are addressed in Chapter 3.

PRACTICE

BACKGROUND

Health care reform and the distribution of reimbursement dollars have changed the practice of physical therapy. Historically, physical therapy evolved to meet the rehabilitative needs of soldiers from the war and children with polio. Most

---

BOX 7-5   *Recognition of Advanced Proficiency for the Physical Therapist Assistant*

Recognition of Advanced Proficiency for the PTA
Application and instructions
Physical Therapist Assistants who meet the following minimum requirements are eligible for recognition:

- Current member of APTA.
- Five (5) years of work experience that must include a minimum of 2,000 hours total and at least 500 hours in the past year in one of the following categories of advanced proficiency: Musculoskeletal, Neuromuscular, Cardiovascular/Pulmonary, or Integumentary.
- Completion of at least 60 contact hours (6 CEUs) of continuing education in physical therapy within the last five (5) years. Continuing education must include a minimum of:
  - 6 contact hours (.6 CEUs) per year for the five years prior to application
  - 75% or forty-five (45) hours must be in the selected category of advanced proficiency
- Continuing education must be related to physical therapy and within the scope of work of the PTA as defined by APTA standards, policies, and positions and the Guide to Physical Therapist Practice. Continuing education may include topics that are both clinical and non-clinical.
- Consistent, above-average job performance within the PT/PTA team verified through a letter of reference from a supervising physical therapist.
- Evidence of involvement in at least three activities that demonstrate the applicant's leadership abilities and contributions to the community. At least two of these activities must be related to physical therapy or health care.

From Recognition of Advanced Proficiency for the PTA: Application and Instructions. Alexandria, VA, American Physical Therapy Association. Available at http://www. apta.org/AM/Template.cfm?Section=Home&TEMPLATE=/CM/ContentDisplay.cfm& CONTENTID=23501. Accessed April 24, 2006.

of these individuals needing physical therapy were treated in hospitals or long-term care facilities. As the profession has expanded, PTs can be found treating individuals across the life span who display a variety of problems that impair their ability to move and function. PTs evaluate and treat patients/clients in a variety of practice settings, such as hospitals, private practice, home health care services, rehabilitation centers, sports clinics, nursing care facilities, adult daycare programs, outpatient care centers, and schools. In addition to working in a variety of practice settings, PTs have adapted their practices to accommodate the rapidly changing health care system.

MANAGED CARE

Escalating costs of health care resulted in the dramatic growth of managed care during the 1990s. In managed care the insurance company contracts with health care providers to provide health care to consumers who subscribe to the insurance plan (see Chapter 6 for a detailed description of this topic). Managed care also affected the number of funded visits allowed for specific conditions. The frequency of visits for outpatient physical therapy care is regulated by the insurance agency rather than the PT. A maximum number of visits is allocated by the insurance company on the basis of the patient's diagnosis, as well as a limit to the length of time the patient can be treated. For example, it is common to be limited by an insurance carrier to eight treatment visits or 2 months of treatment, whichever comes first. In some instances this amount of treatment can be sufficient, but not in the rehabilitation of a patient who has had a stroke or amputation. As a profession, we have come to realize that treatment "doses" do not correlate with patient response and that in many cases more treatment does not necessarily produce greater functional gains.[22] However, to be denied requests for additional treatment visits that were based on our clinical judgment and the patient's response to treatment hurts the patient, especially when in some cases lack of rehabilitation can contribute to a fall or rehospitalization.

The limited number of physical therapy treatments for a particular diagnosis also has an impact on who provides the care. In the past, when a patient was treated two or three times per week, the PTA, under the therapist's supervision, could provide most of the interventions to the patient, with the therapist reexamining the patient once a week. Now, with limited treatments, the patient may be seen only once a week over an 8-week period. Each visit with the therapist, now once a week, consists of reexamination to determine the change that has occurred over the past week and then progression of the treatment program by the therapist with emphasis on patient education. In this delivery model, the role of the PTA becomes diminished because the majority of the treatment session consists of reexamination and patient education.

AMBULATORY CENTERS

Health care reform and advances in medical technology have caused a shift in the delivery of care to ambulatory settings. An **ambulatory center** is any facility in which health care is provided on an outpatient basis. The patient is able to walk into the facility, receive health care, and walk out of the facility the same day. Health care systems usually have several ambulatory centers in the different geographical regions they serve. Outpatient clinics and health maintenance organizations (HMOs; see Chapter 6 for description) are examples of ambulatory centers. Health care in this environment is less costly to the consumer and the insurance companies overall. Therefore this type of setting is becoming more common. In fact, survey data from the APTA indicate that 38.9% of PTs were practicing in a private office or group practice, whereas only 13.6% of the therapists were practicing in an acute care hospital (see Figure 2-16).[23]

ALLIANCES

In addition to managed care, another major change that occurred in health care reform was the formation of alliances. An **alliance** is a collaboration of several health care facilities and practices. For example, two hospitals could work together as an alliance without formally merging. By aligning, they can share resources, programs, and health care providers and negotiate contracts with the insurance companies as a larger entity. This arrangement makes the two hospitals stronger because of the multitude of services they can provide under the alliance and yet maintain their independence as separate hospital corporations. An alliance could also be formed between a PT private practitioner and a hospital or between a private practitioner and other health care providers. The purpose of forming an alliance is to ensure the stability and quality of services that are provided and to market these services to insurance companies.

Resources have also been shared through formal mergers. Community hospitals have merged with large city hospitals, city hospitals have joined together, and home care agencies have been rolled in as well. The force behind these mergers has been the attempt of the chief executive officers (CEOs) of the hospitals to maintain the hospitals' financial viability. Diminished reimbursement from Medicare and other third party payers has forced CEOs to examine how to provide high-quality comprehensive health care with less financial resources. Mergers have resulted in a decrease in resources for capital expenses by eliminating the duplication of expensive diagnostic equipment for each hospital. They have also provided the opportunity for provision of health care along a continuum that has resulted in more efficient delivery of patient care. This **continuum of care** is important because it enables patients to stay within one system and receive tertiary, secondary, and primary care. Tertiary care is high-tech health care provided at a hospital that treats the most seriously ill patients, such as cardiac transplant recipients and neurosurgical patients. Secondary care, such as by a specialist, is treatment on referral, but this care can be performed at a community hospital or even in an outpatient setting. Primary care is the treatment received from an individual who is responsible for the majority of your health care needs, such as a family doctor, the primary care physician who is responsible for keeping you healthy.

PHYSICAL THERAPISTS IN THE HOSPITAL SETTING

The November 2003 report of the Bureau of Labor Statistics[16] reported that 47,930 PTs were employed in hospitals, which is 0.93% of the total employment of the hospitals. The largest practitioner group in the hospitals is registered nurses at 1,382,860 employees. General practitioners and family physicians number 18,520, and occupational therapists total 25,690. Vacancy rates for specific health care practitioners in hospitals vary from state to state and in urban versus rural communities.

In the hospital setting the role of the PT has evolved to include triage of patients requiring care in the acute setting and clinical decision making to determine discharge status of patients. With limited reimbursement to hospitals, and the high cost of care in a hospital, there is pressure to move patients as quickly as possible to less expensive levels of care (e.g., skilled nursing facilities). It is frequently the PT who advises the attending physician when the patient is ready for discharge based on functional ability, and the PT recommends the level of care needed for discharge. The PT may recommend home discharge for a patient with a stroke who is ambulatory and has help at home, but may advise subacute inpatient rehabilitation for another patient who does not have assistance at home and is not ambulatory. As such, a good part of the therapist's day is spent reexamining patients to determine discharge status and instructing family members or caregivers how to manage the patient at home. The PT's recommendation can also facilitate the patients' involvement in the continuum of care established by the hospital alliance.

GUIDE TO PHYSICAL THERAPIST PRACTICE

During her two terms in office as president of the APTA, Marilyn Moffat, PT, PhD, FAPTA, was instrumental in the development and completion of the **Guide to Physical Therapist Practice**.[14] This document was developed "to help physical therapists analyze their patient/client management and describe the scope of their practice."[14] The Guide is a companion document to A Normative Model of Physical Therapist Education and has been instrumental in educating legislators, as well as insurance companies, on the knowledge base and role of the PT in health care. The Guide has also served as the basis for PTs to define their role as primary care providers or case managers. In many education programs the Guide is a required text for all students.

DIRECT ACCESS

Background. Historically, the reconstruction aide worked closely with the physician and carried out orders for exercise, massage, or therapeutic modalities to be applied to the patient. Prescriptions written by the physician specified the type of exercise to be performed, the modality to be used, and the intensity and duration of the treatment. As education of the PT expanded, so did the knowledge base and hands-on skills. As noted earlier in this chapter, however, the education programs, under the auspices of the AMA, were not updated or revised until 1955.

As the educational preparation of the PT expanded after 1955, the provision of physical therapy to the consumer changed as well. In 1957, Nebraska became the first state to have direct access. Citizens of Nebraska could obtain treatment from a PT without seeing a physician first and then being referred to the therapist. The second state to enact legislation for direct access was California in 1968. Legislation proliferated in the 1980s and early 1990s to enable PTs to practice with direct access in other states. In the states that allow direct access,

PTs examine and evaluate the patient, determine appropriate interventions, and implement a plan of care based on their findings.

Direct Access Today. For PTs across the country, direct access is heralded as a badge of professional autonomy. According to Frank Mallon, APTA CEO, "Achieving this professional autonomy hinges upon the successful realization of a two-pronged strategy: (1) establishing the legality of direct access, and (2) securing its recognition by insurers and other third-party payers."[24] Legislation reintroduced to the 109th Congress (Medicare Direct Access to Physical Therapists Act, HR 1333 & S 647) is designed to eliminate the need for patients to obtain physician referrals for physical therapy reimbursed under Medicare Part B. This federal legislation is a tremendous step in securing recognition by insurers. If passed, it would eliminate the requirement that a Medicare beneficiary obtain a referral from a physician to receive outpatient physical therapy treatment.

As federal legislation is addressed by APTA, chapters must continue their efforts to enact state legislation that changes their practice act to legalize direct access. As of May 2006 the consumer has direct access to a PT in 42 states. The concept behind direct access is important because it enables the consumer to have the *choice* of accessing a PT or a physician. If the PT determines that the patient's problem is outside the scope of practice or that the patient needs further medical evaluation, the patient is referred to a primary care physician. Providing the consumer direct access to a licensed PT contributes to the reduction of health care costs (by eliminating the physician office visit to obtain the referral) and expedites initiation of appropriate treatment. In states without direct access, patients may wait 4 to 6 weeks to see a physician, only to have the physician write a referral for physical therapy without conducting a comprehensive evaluation and then potentially bill for a full office visit. When finally referred to the PT (4 to 6 weeks after injury), the acute problem may have developed into a chronic problem with additional secondary problems (such as protective muscle spasms and contracture).

Direct access has worked effectively in the states in which it has been adopted. In states without such legislation, resistance to direct access has come primarily from the physician professional organizations. Concern has been raised that PTs do not have enough knowledge to diagnose problems that the patient has and, consequently, malpractice suits will result. In reality, no evidence of an increase in the rate of malpractice suits has been seen. Moreover, in states without direct access, a diagnosis is not typically noted on the physician's referral. The majority of patients referred to physical therapy from a physician have on the referral "Evaluate and Treat" or a symptom such as low back pain or knee pain. Neither of these reasons for referral is a diagnosis that would aid the PT in determining a plan of care. The plan of care for the patient is developed after the therapist completes the examination, evaluation, diagnosis, and prognosis.

The other unspoken concern of physicians' professional organizations is that the number of patients in their care will be reduced if the PT has direct access. This concern has not been documented as a problem, or reality, in any of the states with direct access. There is, however, a reduction in health care costs associated with direct access. In a study conducted by Jean Mitchell and

7

Gregory de Lissovoy,[25] the total paid claims for physician-referred physical therapy were 2.2 times higher than paid claims to PTs practicing in direct access states (Box 7-6).

PHYSICIAN-OWNED PHYSICAL THERAPY SERVICE

As previously noted, the physician has in the past been the primary coordinator of the treatment a patient receives. The physician ordered the necessary diagnostic work, requested consultations from other health care providers, and ordered the treatment regimen for the patient. With this responsibility and control, many physicians established clinics where they own all the diagnostic equipment, laboratory equipment, pharmacies, and physical therapy clinics. In this situation, physicians refer their patients to their own clinics. When such "self-referral" occurs, the patient has lost the choice of where to go for diagnostic work or treatment, and the potential for overuse of the services is created.

A **physician-owned physical therapy service (POPTS)** is an example of the overuse that can occur when a physician has a financial investment in a clinic. Two studies conducted in Florida and California demonstrated that when the physician owns physical therapy services, physical therapy care is overused, resulting in overspending of health care dollars.[26,27] These two studies have shown that physicians who have ownership in a physical therapy clinic continue to refer patients for physical therapy care even when the patient has reached a plateau or established goals. Patients have also been *inappropriately* referred and treated in such clinical settings.

The AMA reported in the *American Medical News* that it is unethical for physicians to have a financial investment in a laboratory or clinic to which they refer patients.[28] Federal legislation, specifically "Section 1877 of the Social Security Act (the Act), also referred to as the physician self-referral law (Stark II),

---

BOX 7-6   *Cost Effectiveness of Direct Access to Physical Therapy*

In a study conducted to determine whether direct access to physical therapy services provided by a licensed physical therapist is cost effective, it was found that:

- The total paid claims for physician referral episodes to physical therapists were 123% or 2.2 times higher than the paid claims for direct access episodes. The total paid claims averaged $2236 for "physician referral" episodes as compared to $1004 for direct access episodes. When expressed in terms of actual reimbursements, the difference in total paid claims per episode was $1232.
- Physician referral episodes were 65% longer in duration than direct access episodes.
- Physician referral episodes generated 67% more physical therapy claims and 60% more office visits than direct access episodes.

Data from Mitchell JM, de Lissovoy G: A comparison of resource use and cost in direct access versus physician episodes of physical therapy. Phys Ther 1997;77:10-18.

prohibits a physician from making referrals for certain designated health care services (including physical therapy services) to an entity in which the physician (or an immediate family member of the physician) has a financial relationship (ownership or compensation interest), unless an exception applies."[29]

As the organization representing the profession of physical therapy, the APTA has gone on record in opposition to these employment relations. The House of Delegates passed a resolution in 2003 stating that "the American Physical Therapy Association opposes the ownership of physical therapy services by physicians, and supports federal and state laws and regulations that prohibit physician ownership of physical therapy services."[30]

To avoid the unethical and potentially illegal situation of owning an interest in a physical therapy clinic, many physicians hire PTs as their employees. The same abuse of overutilization of physical therapy care can and does exist in this environment, but employment of a PT to work in the physician's office is currently not restricted in any way.

INFRINGEMENT AND HUMAN RESOURCES

Infringement. **Infringement** is defined in *Webster's New World Dictionary* as "to break (a law or agreement); fail to observe the terms of; violate—infringe on (or upon) to break in on; encroach or trespass on (the rights, patents, etc. of others)."[31] In the health care arena, infringement occurs when one health care provider performs the skills and techniques of another health care provider.

Physical therapy is provided by PTs and PTAs. In the past, the shortage of qualified physical therapy professionals to meet the demands of the consumer led other health care providers to fill the void. This situation occurred most often with athletic trainers and occupational therapists. An example is the rehabilitation of a weekend athlete. If an individual injures a knee in a basketball game and edema (swelling), pain, and restricted mobility develop, that person should be treated by a PT. Because the injury occurred in a sporting event, the athletic trainer might say that the individual should be treated by an athletic trainer. Who is infringing on the other's territory? Both providers should not be providing the same treatment to the patient and receiving reimbursement.

In another example, a PT and occupational therapist (OT) are treating an individual who had a stroke and are instructing the patient in bathtub transfers. Is this duplication of services if both OT and PT receive reimbursement for the treatment provided? Who is infringing on the other health care professional's territory?

Questions of this type continue to be raised as each health care profession strives to maintain its own identity and professional integrity. The answers to some of these questions may differ depending on the different practice acts that regulate and govern health care professionals in each state. The bathtub transfer scenario could be performed by both the OT and PT as long as they are both working on different outcomes for the patient. For example, the PT may be doing the transfer activity for the sole purpose of enabling the patient to be independent in the transfer. The occupational therapy goal would be more global and incorporate the activity of daily care so that the patient will be independent in bathing in the bathtub. To accomplish this goal, the

7

patient must be able to perform the transfer as well as manage bathing activities in the tub.

The example of the weekend athlete with a knee injury may be addressed differently in each state. In New York, for example, the PT would be responsible for the acute rehabilitation of the weekend athlete's knee injury. However, either the athletic trainer or the PT could recondition the individual for return to recreational activities. The treatment provided by the PT would be reimbursed as physical therapy. According to the AMA (which establishes the Current Procedural Terminology [CPT] codes), the treatment provided by the athletic trainer cannot be reimbursed by accessing the examination and reexamination billing codes used by PTs. This situation becomes confusing and misleading to insurance agencies when they examine total expenditures for billing codes usually attributed to PTs. Physicians, podiatrists, and, in the past, athletic trainers have used these billing codes, categorized as physical therapy costs, which has inflated the actual dollars spent for physical therapy care. In some states, APTA chapters have attempted to change insurance regulations to require tracking of providers submitting bills attributed to physical therapy costs, but they have had limited success.

Human Resources. The biggest factor contributing to infringement by different health care professions has been the shortage of professionally trained personnel that may exist in a profession and the resulting inability of that profession to meet the service demands of the public. A critical shortage of PTs existed up through 1997, even with the proliferation of schools graduating PTs. In 1992, physical therapist schools graduated 4850 new therapists, but 7000 vacancies remained in the job market.[32] In June 1994, the APTA reported that there were 85,000 PTs in the United States, 2% of whom were retired or not working, which left approximately 83,300 PTs to fill 90,000 physical therapy jobs. In the years that followed, however, managed care and the Balanced Budget Act of 1997 had a dramatic impact on the job market and limited employment opportunities in health care. Surpluses were suddenly projected (see Supply and Demand).

The concern over a surplus of PTs led many experienced and new graduates to examine other areas in which they could be effective in health care, such as wellness and prevention. When in short supply, therapists were struggling just to meet the rehabilitative needs of those with injuries, illness, or disabilities. Many practitioners did not have time to spend in the area of wellness and prevention. Now, therapists use their creative skills to develop and coordinate community health programs and health screening programs. Developing these skills has enhanced the role that PTs play in the continuum of care and promotion of health and wellness within the community.

Fortunately, the job market improved after the turn of the century. The most recent report of the Department of Labor states, "Physical therapists held about 137,000 jobs in 2002. The number of jobs is greater than the number of practicing physical therapists, because some physical therapists hold two or more jobs. For example, some may work in a private practice, but also work part time in another healthcare facility."[16] The labor statistics remain strong for career opportunities in physical therapy.

The development of the DPT degree may have a positive impact on the job market. It establishes the body of knowledge and profession of physical therapy in a more distinct manner than a bachelor's or master's degree in physical therapy. As more therapists with the DPT degree enter the job market, a clearer distinction of roles and responsibilities is expected, with greater autonomy achieved for the physical therapy profession.

CONTINUOUS QUALITY IMPROVEMENT

Continuous quality improvement/total quality management (CQI/TQM) is "a method of examining and improving processes using data management tools."[33] Simply put, it means using data that are collected every day to improve the quality of a service that is provided. It has been a component of most hospitals for several years and has also been integrated into most physical therapy practice settings. TQM in a physical therapy clinic would consist of continual assessment of both delivery of physical therapy care and patient outcomes. In the early implementation of TQM, PTs documented the number of patient visits, cancellations, and no-shows. Now it has expanded to consider how efficiently the care is delivered, whether the patient achieves the desired outcome, and the patient's satisfaction with the care. **Customer satisfaction,** previously associated with the service received in hotels, restaurants, or stores, is now a major emphasis of health care systems.

As TQM developed in hospitals, it led to the advent of a new patient delivery model called **patient-focused care (PFC).** In this model, all departments in a hospital are decentralized and professional staff members are assigned to work on multidisciplinary teams. Instead of having the physical therapy department on one floor and transporting all the patients to it, the therapist is stationed on a nursing unit with other health care providers to provide treatment to a core group of patients with similar problems. A good example is a PT working on a multidisciplinary team for orthopaedic surgical patients. All members of the team are on the floor with the patients, and all services the patients need are brought to them. This system has decreased the wasted time that health care providers spend trying to find a patient because the individual left the nursing floor for tests or other reasons. The team coordinates the treatment to be provided to each patient at the beginning of every day, and responsibilities are shared among members of the team. Trained technicians are part of the team and carry out much of the basic care for the patient after instruction from the PT. Such care may include transfers of the patient and ambulation.

The PFC model also brought with it the controversy of **cross-training** of health care professionals. This concept sent a shock wave through most of the physical therapy professional community. Through cross-training PTs might do some physical therapy care, occupational therapy care, and nursing care for the patient. The concept of cross-training grew out of the inadequate supply of PTs available to work in hospitals, necessitating the training of occupational therapists and nurses to perform some of the physical therapy services. Cross-training affects not only physical therapy, but all other health care professions. Skills from a variety of professions would be integrated to be provided by members of a multidisciplinary team.

7

The PFC model does introduce some cross-training of the members of the multidisciplinary team, but many PTs working in this model say that the important evaluative and treatment components of physical therapy have been retained by the PT. In many settings, therapists report that members of the multidisciplinary team have a better understanding of and appreciation for the knowledge base of the PT.

A positive development of the PFC model was the development of **critical pathways,** defined by Woods as "a guideline for patient care during hospital stay using 'milestones' to progress patients; a guide based on consensus, including only those aspects of care provided to affect patient outcomes."[33] The critical pathway is a planned sequence of treatment progression that is based on the patient's response and recovery. Initiating physical therapy treatment is an established part of the critical pathway, so that a delay in receiving a physician's orders does not occur. The physical therapy progression of the patient is also a component of the pathway. Some therapists who use the system report that critical pathways are clearly defining the parameters of physical therapy practice and the role the PT should play in rehabilitation of the patient.

RESEARCH

The evolution to a doctoring profession, autonomous practice, and direct access requires evidence to support the validity and reliability of standardized assessments and the effectiveness of interventions.

Demonstrating improved patient outcomes as a result of physical therapy intervention will ensure the identity and integrity of the profession. Physical therapy is an art and a science, but clinically based research is needed to substantiate the science component of the profession.

The major emphasis of physical therapy research has been in two areas: (1) establishment and utilization of measurement tools that are valid and reliable and measure patient outcomes and (2) the efficacy of physical therapy treatment.[34] This supports the contemporary approach to health care termed evidence-based practice, which assures the health care consumer that the treatment received is based on scientific research and evidence to substantiate outcomes. In response to evidence-based practice, the APTA developed a "grassroots" program to establish a database containing current research evidence on the effectiveness of physical therapy interventions. The Hooked on Evidence program was motivated by a concern that clinicians lacked access to the knowledge available from current research, thus hindering evidence-based practice.[35] The objectives of the program are listed in Box 7-7.

The best environment for evidenced-based practice is the physical therapy clinic. Clinicians who work with patients every day are an excellent source of data for studying treatment outcomes and can contribute to Hooked on Evidence. Stronger collaboration of physical therapy faculty with clinicians can facilitate clinically based research. Another means to address this issue is to foster students in postprofessional physical therapy education programs to carry out clinically based research in conjunction with clinicians. To support postprofessional education, the Foundation for Physical Therapy has developed the program Doctoral Opportunities for Clinicians and Scholars (DOCS). The DOCS program has a new investigator scholarship award program and a three-level doctoral

BOX 7-7 | *Objectives of Hooked on Evidence Program*

- Allow members to search a database of article extractions relevant to the field of physical therapy to build support for evidence-based practice
- Allow members to contribute extractions of the peer-reviewed literature to the database
- List useful web resources and other information consistent with evidence-based practice
- Disseminate clinical practice guidelines based on systematic reviews of the literature

From Coyne C: Getting hooked on "Hooked on Evidence." PT—Magazine of Physical Therapy 2002;10(6):34-39.

studies program. In 1999, the Foundation awarded more than $300,000 in the DOCS program to PTs in postprofessional education. The research center established by the Foundation for Physical Therapy is another excellent example of advancing research in measurement and treatment efficacy. The University of Iowa was awarded a 3-year grant from the Foundation to establish a research center focusing on total hip and knee replacements and ultrasound treatment. The University of Pittsburgh received a 3-year grant from the Foundation in 1997 to examine PT interventions for the prevention and treatment of low back pain. In the fall of 2002, the research center chose *PTClinResNet* at the University of Southern California to receive a $1.5 million, 3-year contract. The focus of this large multicenter investigation is to "assess the effects of strengthening exercises designed to improve muscle performance and movement skill in the following patients with physical disabilities: adults post-stroke, children with cerebral palsy, shoulder pain in adult paraplegics with spinal cord injury, and orthopedic/low back pain. There is also a coordinated effort to compare treatments, facilitated by the use of a common valid set of outcome measures across projects."[36]

PROFESSIONALISM IN PHYSICAL THERAPY

In the 2000 House of Delegates, a Vision Statement (Vision 2020) and Vision Sentence (shortened version) were adopted that set the course and strategic plan for transitioning to a doctoring profession (see Box 1-7 for the Vision Statement and Box 4-1 for the Vision Sentence).[1] Vision 2020 included six key elements: Doctor of Physical Therapy, Evidence-Based Practice, Autonomous Practice, Direct Access, Practitioner of Choice, and Professionalism. Most of these tenets have been addressed as separate issues in this chapter. Professionalism, however, underscores all of the elements.

What is professionalism? It is one of the six key elements to transition to a doctoring profession, but do we know how to define it, measure it in new graduates, and recognize it in our collegial interactions? To better understand professionalism, the APTA held a consensus-based conference in July 2002 and invited leading practitioners, researchers, and academicians to define core values of professionalism. The result of this 3-day conference was the document Professionalism in Physical Therapy: Core Values, which was adopted by the APTA Board of Directors in August 2003 (see Table 1-1).[37] Seven core values were defined with sample indicators listed to enable academic programs or other professional organizations to measure when professionalism has been displayed. This document should be reviewed routinely not only by physical therapy students, but also by practitioners to ensure their direction and action in a doctoring profession.

SUMMARY

This chapter reviewed the current issues affecting physical therapy and the profession's continued growth in education, practice, and research. Educational preparation of the PT has evolved to a doctor of physical therapy degree with the development of transitioning DPT programs to enable the full-time clinician to earn a DPT. The role of the PTA has been clarified, and opportunities for recognition of advanced clinical proficiency have been created. Practice settings continue to change with greater autonomy of the practitioner in more diversified settings. PTs and PTAs will continue to work in hospitals, but the role of the PT in that setting has changed with greater demands on clinical decision making. Legislation for direct access continues to grow with introduction of a bill in the U.S. Congress to enable Medicare beneficiaries to have direct access to physical therapy. Physician-owned physical therapy services continue to exist and are proliferating in some parts of the country. The articulated core values of professionalism, specifically altruism, integrity, professional duty, and social responsibility, will cause new graduates of DPT programs to gravitate to practice settings that serve the common good of patients.

Physical therapy is in evolution. We have come a long way, but much remains to be done. In her plenary address at Preview 2020, an APTA conference in November 2004, Colleen Kigin, PT, DPT, MPA, MS, discussed autonomous practice in terms of the profession's current achievements and future responsibilities, the risks inherent in accepting those responsibilities, and the keys to overcoming those risks. While emphasizing that "we've come a long way," Kigin, chief of staff at the Center for Integration of Medicine and Innovative Technology in Cambridge, Massachusetts, pushed for action models that collectively will "create an environment in which we can function as autonomous professionals." Elements of those models, she said, include standardization of data collection systems, "on call" availability to patients, greater community involvement, and an expanded PT role in the shaping of health care policy.[38] As we continue to evolve in education, practice, and research, our physical therapy graduates will serve as the change agents of the future.

REFERENCES

1. APTA Vision Sentence for Physical Therapy 2020 and APTA Vision Statement for Physical Therapy 2020, HOD P06-00-24-35. House of Delegates Standards, Policies, Positions, and Guidelines. Alexandria, VA, American Physical Therapy Association, 2005.
2. Pinkston D: Evolution of the practice of physical therapy in the United States. *In:* Scully RM, Barnes MR (eds): Physical Therapy. Philadelphia, Lippincott, 1989.
3. Report to the House of Delegates Session. Phys Ther 1979;59:1397.
4. Educational Programs for Physical Therapists: Terminology Used to Describe, HOD P06-93-26-51. House of Delegates Standards, Policies, Positions, and Guidelines. Alexandria, VA, American Physical Therapy Association, 2005.

5. A Normative Model of Physical Therapist Professional Education: Version 2004. Alexandria, VA, American Physical Therapy Association, 2004.

6. Evaluative Criteria for Accreditation of Education Programs for the Preparation of Physical Therapists. Alexandria, VA, American Physical Therapy Association. Available at http://www.apta.org/AM/Template.cfm?Section=Home&TEMPLATE=/CM/ContentDisplay.cfm&CONTENTID=25709. Accessed March 20, 2006.

7. The DPT and You: The Future Is Now—Chat transcript, Harris MJ, Jan 15, 2004. Alexandria, VA, American Physical Therapy Association.

8. Threlkeld J, Jensen G, Royeen C: The clinical doctorate: A framework for analysis in physical therapist education. Phys Ther 1999;79:567-581.

9. Coyne C: The DPT: A real world update. PT—Magazine of Physical Therapy 2002;10(2):64-72.

10. Transition DPT Programs. Alexandria, VA, American Physical Therapy Association. Available at http://www.apta.org/AM/Template.cfm?Section=Post_Professional_Degree&CONTENTID=30031&TEMPLATE=/CM/ContentDisplay.cfm. Accessed May 17, 2006.

11. Rothstein J: Education at the crossroads: Which paths for the DPT? Phys Ther 1998;78:454-457.

12. Sahrmann S: Moving precisely? Or taking the path of least resistance? Phys Ther 1998;78:1208-1218.

13. Vector Research, Inc: Executive Summary, Workforce Study. Alexandria, VA, American Physical Therapy Association, 1997.

14. Guide to Physical Therapist Practice, revised ed 2. Alexandria, VA, American Physical Therapy Association, 2003.

15. Education Program Development and Expansion in Physical Therapy, HOD P06-02-32-55. House of Delegates Standards, Policies, Positions, and Guidelines. Alexandria, VA, American Physical Therapy Association, 2005.

16. Bureau of Labor Statistics, US Department of Labor, Occupational Outlook Handbook, 2004-05 Edition, Physical Therapists.

17. A Normative Model of Physical Therapist Assistant Education: Version 1999. Alexandria, VA, American Physical Therapy Association, 1999.

18. Evaluative Criteria for Accreditation of Education Programs for the Preparation of Physical Therapist Assistants. Alexandria, VA, American Physical Therapy Association. Available at http://www.apta.org/AM/Template.cfm?Section=Home&CONTENTID=28816&TEMPLATE=/CM/ContentDisplay.cfm. Accessed March 20, 2006.

19. The Future Role of the Physical Therapist Assistant—Replacement-Packet II, House of Delegates Minutes June 18-20, 2001. Alexandria, VA, American Physical Therapy Association, 2001.

20. Continuing Education for the Physical Therapist Assistant, HOD P06-01-22-23. House of Delegates Standards, Policies, Positions, and Guidelines. Alexandria, VA, American Physical Therapy Association, 2005.

21. Procedural Interventions Exclusively Performed by Physical Therapists, HOD P06-00-30-36. House of Delegates Standards, Policies, Positions, and Guidelines. Alexandria, VA, American Physical Therapy Association, 2005.

22. Guccione A: The effect of changes in the practice environment on employment patterns. PT—Magazine of Physical Therapy 1999;7(5):26-28.

23. PT: Type of Facility. Alexandria, VA, American Physical Therapy Association. Available at http://www.apta.org/AM/Template.cfm?Section=Demographics&TEMPLATE=/CM/ContentDisplay.cfm&CONTENTID=26309. Accessed March 13, 2006.

24. Fosnaught M: Direct access: Exploring new opportunities. PT—Magazine of Physical Therapy 2002;10(2):58-62.

25. Mitchell JM, de Lissovoy G: A comparison of resource use and cost in direct access versus physician episodes of physical therapy. Phys Ther 1997;77:10-18.

26. Joint ventures among health care providers in Florida, State of Florida, conducted by the Florida Health Care Cost Containment Board in conjunction with the Department of Economics and Department of Finance, Florida State University, August 1991.

27. Swedlow A, Johnson G, Smithline N, et al: Increased costs and rates of use in the California worker's compensation system as a result of self-referral by physicians. N Engl J Med 1992;327:1502-1506.

28. HCFA weighs option for wider referral ban. Am Med News 1994;37(23):1.

29. CMS Issues Stark II Final Regulations. Alexandria, VA, American Physical Therapy Association, 2004.

7

30. Opposition to Physician Ownership of Physical Therapy Services, HOD P06-03-27-25. House of Delegates Standards, Policies, Positions, and Guidelines. Alexandria, VA, American Physical Therapy Association, 2005.

31. Webster's New World Dictionary, Second College Edition. New York, Simon & Schuster, 1986.

32. Physical Therapist Education Programs. Alexandria, VA, American Physical Therapy Association, 1992.

33. Woods EN: The restructuring of America's hospitals: What does it mean for physical therapy? PT—Magazine of Physical Therapy 1994;2(6):34-41.

34. Model for Targeting Research Areas in Physical Therapy. Alexandria, VA, American Physical Therapy Association, 1994.

35. Coyne C: Getting hooked on "Hooked on Evidence." PT—Magazine of Physical Therapy. 2002;10(6):34-39.

36. CRN Explores Effects of Muscle Strengthening Exercises. Alexandria, VA, American Physical Therapy Association. Available at http://www.apta.org/AM/Template.cfm?Section=Home&CONTENTID=23342&TEMPLATE=/CM/ContentDisplay.cfm. Accessed April 23, 2006.

37. Professionalism in Physical Therapy: Core Values, BOD 05-04-02-03. House of Delegates Standards, Policies, Positions, and Guidelines. Alexandria, VA, American Physical Therapy Association, 2005.

38. Be change architects and 'embrace the fear,' Preview 2020 speakers urge, PT Bulletin 2004;(5)49.

ADDITIONAL RESOURCES

Castro J: The American Way of Health. New York, Little, Brown, 1994.

An easy-to-read, informative book that details how health care has changed in our country and why we are faced with the issues that we have today. Many stories of different patients are presented to assist the reader in understanding the crisis that has existed.

Depoy E, Gitlin S: Introduction to Research: Multiple Strategies for Health and Human Services. St Louis, Mosby, 1993.

This introductory text was written for members of all allied health professions and teaches the reader how to critically evaluate, implement, and respect a variety of research strategies.

House of Delegates Standards, Policies, Procedures, and Guidelines. Alexandria, VA, American Physical Therapy Association.

Updated annually, including new goals for the APTA.

PT Bulletin. Alexandria, VA, American Physical Therapy Association.

Contains short articles and letters to the editor that address current issues. Published weekly online (http://www.apta.org/Bulletin).

PT—Magazine of Physical Therapy. Alexandria, VA, American Physical Therapy Association.

The May issue of this monthly publication distributed to members of the APTA includes the annual report of the APTA.

REVIEW QUESTIONS

1. Explain the controversy over an experienced PT with a bachelor's degree and a new graduate with a DPT. What issues does this situation raise?

2. Discuss both sides of the debate over PTA attendance at continuing education PT courses.

3. Weigh the objections to direct access against its track record in states that have legislated in its favor.

4. Explain the risks involved in a physician-owned physical therapy service.

5. What is "infringement"? Discuss the issues that it raises and their impact on reimbursement for services.

6. Give a balanced analysis of the advantages and disadvantages of the patient-focused care model.

Approximately 70 percent of Americans are members of at least one association; 25 percent belong to four or more. Although the role of associations varies, these organizational entities offer forums for communication and collaboration, develop ethical standards for the individuals or groups they represent, educate members and the public, and provide a vehicle for change in society.

Environmental Statement, American Physical Therapy Association

8 American Physical Therapy Association

Michael A. Pagliarulo

After reading this chapter, the reader will be able to:

■ Describe the structure and function of the American Physical Therapy Association

■ Distinguish between sections and assemblies within the association
■ Identify and describe organizations that are associated and related to the Association
■ Describe the benefits of belonging to the Association

The definition of physical therapy presented in Chapter 1 demonstrated that this field is a profession because it possesses all the qualities or criteria of a profession. One of these criteria is a representative organization. This chapter focuses on the **American Physical Therapy Association (APTA)**, which is the national organization that represents physical therapy. The organization's mission, structure, and benefits are described here. A historical account of the Association was presented in Chapter 1. Affiliated and related organizations representing physical therapy interests are included at the end of this chapter.

MISSION AND GOALS

The APTA is a national member-driven organization that represents the profession of physical therapy (Figure 8-1). It is composed of more than 66,000 physical therapists (PTs), physical therapist assistants (PTAs), and students throughout the United States and abroad. Membership is strictly voluntary.

In 1993, the House of Delegates (HOD) of the APTA adopted a mission statement and related policy. The statement[1] (Box 8-1) and policy[2] (Box 8-2) demonstrate the profession's interest in serving the public and its members through practice, education, and research.

Goals for the APTA are proposed by the Board of Directors (BOD). They are then reviewed and approved by the HOD. The goals for 2006 were approved by the HOD in June 2005 and are presented in Box 8-3.[3] These goals direct the activities and funding priorities for the new year and reiterate the grounding in education, research, and practice. They are anchored in the Vision 2020 Statement and further promote activities to attain these visions. (See Chapter 1 for further description of Vision 2020.)

ORGANIZATIONAL STRUCTURE

The organizational structure of the APTA is depicted in Figure 8-2. This structure provides a three-tiered approach (local, state, and national) to serve the members and the public. Three units at the state and national levels—chapters, sections, and assemblies—are the **components** of the APTA. Policy-making bodies, with their respective committees and task forces, and staff complete the general plan of this organization. Each level is described in this section, beginning with the primary unit, the membership.

MEMBERSHIP

As stated earlier, membership in the APTA is voluntary; however, it is estimated that approximately two thirds of licensed PTs in the United States are members. This extensive membership provides strength and diversity to the organization.

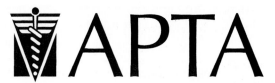

American Physical Therapy Association

Figure 8-1 ■ Logo for the American Physical Therapy Association. (Courtesy of the American Physical Therapy Association.)

BOX 8-1	*Mission of the American Physical Therapy Association*

The mission of the American Physical Therapy Association (APTA), the principal membership organization representing and promoting the profession of physical therapy, is to further the profession's role in the prevention, diagnosis, and treatment of movement dysfunctions and the enhancement of the physical health and functional abilities of members of the public.

From Mission Statement of APTA, HOD P06-93-05-05. House of Delegates Standards, Policies, Positions, and Guidelines. Alexandria, VA, American Physical Therapy Association, 2005.

BOX 8-2	*Mission Statement Fulfillment*

To fulfill the American Physical Therapy Association's (APTA) Mission, to meet the needs and interests of its members, and to promote physical therapy as a vital professional career, the Association shall:

■ Promote physical therapy care and services through the establishment, maintenance, and promotion of ethical principles and quality standards for practice, education, and research.

■ Influence policy in the public and private sectors.

■ Enable physical therapy practitioners to improve their skills, knowledge, and operations in the interest of furthering the profession.

■ Develop and improve the art and science of physical therapy, including practice, education, and research.

■ Facilitate a common understanding and appreciation for the diversity of the profession, the membership, and the communities we serve.

■ Maintain a stable and diverse financial base from which to fund the programs, services, and operations that support this mission.

From Mission Statement Fulfillment, HOD P06-93-06-07. House of Delegates Standards, Policies, Positions, and Guidelines. Alexandria, VA, American Physical Therapy Association, 2005.

8

BOX 8-3	Goals That Represent the Priorities of the American Physical Therapy Association

Goal I: Physical therapists are universally recognized and promoted as the practitioners of choice for persons with conditions that affect movement and function.

Goal II: Physical therapists are universally recognized and promoted as providers of fitness, health promotion, wellness, and risk reduction programs to enhance quality of life for persons across the life-span.

Goal III: Academic and clinical education prepares doctors of physical therapy who are autonomous practitioners.

Goal IV: Physical therapists are autonomous practitioners to whom patients/clients have unrestricted direct access as an entry-point into the health care delivery system, and who are paid for all elements of patient/client management in all practice environments.

Goal V: Research advances the science of physical therapy and furthers the evidence-based practice of the physical therapist.

Goal VI: Physical therapists and physical therapist assistants are committed to meeting the health needs of patients/clients and society through ethical behavior, continued competence, collegial relationships with other health care practitioners, and advocacy for the profession.

Goal VII: Communication throughout the Association enhances participation of and responsiveness to members and promotes and instills the value of belonging to the American Physical Therapy Association (APTA).

Goal VIII: APTA standards, policies, positions, guidelines and the Guide to Physical Therapist Practice, Normative Model of Physical Therapist Education and Evaluative Criteria for Accreditation of Education Programs for the Preparation of Physical Therapists, Normative Model of Physical Therapist Assistant Education and Evaluative Criteria for Accreditation of Education Program for the Preparation of Physical Therapist Assistants, and Professionalism in Physical Therapy: Core Values are recognized and used as the foundation for physical therapist practice, research, and education environments.

These goals are based upon APTA Vision Statement for Physical Therapy 2020 (Vision 2020) developed by the Association in 2000. The goals encompass the Association's major priorities as it moves toward realization of the ideals set forth in Vision 2020. The Board is committed to these goals as the foundation from which to lead the Association. The Association's awareness of cultural diversity, its commitment to expanding minority representation and participation in physical therapy, and its commitment to equal opportunity for all members permeate these goals. These goals are not ranked and do not represent any priority order.

From Goals That Represent the Priorities of the American Physical Therapy Association, HOD P06-05-15-24. House of Delegates Standards, Policies, Positions, and Guidelines. Alexandria, VA, American Physical Therapy Association, 2005.

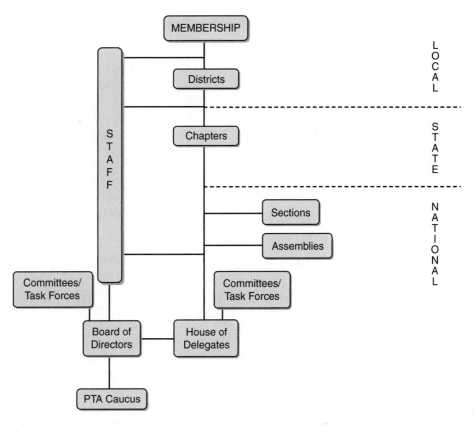

Figure 8-2 ■ Organizational chart of the American Physical Therapy Association. Note how the membership drives this organization. Staff members provide support at all levels, including membership, local, state, and national. Washington, D.C., and Puerto Rico are also chapters.

The primary membership categories of the APTA are physical therapist (formerly active), physical therapist assistant (formerly affiliate), and their respective student categories.[4] Other categories include life, retired, corresponding, honorary (not a member in any other category and has made outstanding contributions to the APTA or health of the public), and Catherine Worthingham Fellow of the APTA (physical therapist member for at least 15 years who has made notable contributions to the profession; may use the initials FAPTA). Requirements for membership include graduation from (or enrollment in) an education program approved (or seeking candidacy) by a recognized accrediting agency. In addition, the applicant must sign a pledge indicating compliance with the Code of Ethics (physical therapist and related categories) or Standards of Ethical Conduct for the Physical Therapist Assistant (physical therapist assistant and related categories) and pay dues.

Service to the membership has always been one of the main purposes of the APTA. Members have had a sense of pride and commitment to the organization. In fact, during the formative years of the profession, membership in this organization was considered the standard for competence. This proud heritage remains today; however, membership is not required to demonstrate competence.

DISTRICTS

As noted in Figure 8-2, a **district** is the most local organizational unit in the structure of the APTA. Districts do not exist in all jurisdictions, such as small states. Membership is automatic where they do exist and may be based on location of residence or employment as provided in the bylaws of the APTA.

Districts are more common in locations with high population densities or large geographical areas and frequently consist of one or more counties. This arrangement provides a mechanism for convenient meetings and participation. It also provides a basis for representation in a body that conducts business at the next level of organization, the chapter.

CHAPTERS

In accordance with the standing rules of the APTA, a **chapter** "must coincide with or be confined within the legally constituted boundaries of a state, territory, or commonwealth of the United States or the District of Columbia."[5] In 2006, the APTA consists of 52 chapters, one for each state, the District of Columbia, and Puerto Rico. Membership in a chapter is automatic and based on location of residence, employment, education, or greatest active participation (in the last case, only in an immediately adjacent chapter). In contrast to districts, which are not permitted to assess dues, each chapter requires dues for PT and PTA members and, in a few cases, student categories.

Chapters are an important component of the APTA. They provide a mechanism for participation at a state level and proportionate representation at the national level (see later discussion of House of Delegates). Participation is facilitated through authorized special interest groups and assemblies to address the needs of recognized subsidiary groups. Chapters also provide an important voice for members at the state level of government. This capacity is essential to maintain statewide legislation and regulations appropriate to the profession and practice of physical therapy.

SECTIONS

A **section** is organized at the national level exclusively. In accordance with the bylaws of the APTA, sections provide an opportunity for members with similar areas of interest to "meet, confer, and promote the interests of the respective sections."[4] Membership in one or more of the 18 sections listed in Table 8-1 is voluntary; however, only a member of the APTA can join a section. Students are permitted and encouraged to join.

In addition to the publications listed in Table 8-1, section members share information at an annual **Combined Sections Meeting** in early February. This meeting provides a mechanism for educational and business sessions. Section leadership can then accurately represent the members at other APTA and government arenas.

A specialty area within a section may form a **special interest group (SIG)**. Bylaws authorize SIGs within a chapter, section, and assembly, but they are most common in sections. This capability provides an opportunity for members

Table 8-1
Sections of the American Physical Therapy Association

Section	Area(s) of Interest	Publication(s)
Acute Care	Physical therapy practitioners working with acutely ill patients	*Acute Care Perspectives*
Aquatic Physical Therapy	Addresses the administrative, research, and clinical needs of members to advance the practice of aquatic physical therapy	*Journal of Aquatic Therapy* *Waterlines Newsletter*
Cardiovascular & Pulmonary	Health, wellness, prevention, and rehabilitation services for individuals with cardiovascular or pulmonary impairments	*Cardiopulmonary Physical Therapy Journal*
Clinical Electrophysiology	Electrotherapy/physical agents, clinical electrophysiological evaluation, and wound management SIG: Wound Management	*Electrophysiology Newsletter*
Education	Developing new practitioners, educators, educational leaders, and administrators SIGs: Academic Administrators, Academic Faculty, PTA Educators, and Clinical Educators	*Journal of Physical Therapy Education* *Bulletin*
Geriatrics	Clinical excellence of PTs and PTAs working with older adults SIGs: International Association of Physical Therapists Working with Older People, Balance and Falls, Health and Wellness, and Osteoporosis	*Issues on Aging* *Gerinotes*
Hand Rehabilitation	Hand and upper extremity rehabilitation	*Hand Prints*
Health Policy & Administration	Administration, leadership, professionalism, health policy, legislation, regulation, and ethical standards affecting the practice of physical therapy SIGs: Cross-Cultural and International, Technology	*The HPA Resource*
Home Health	Practice in home health care and other "out-of-hospital" settings	*Quarterly Report*
Neurology	Neurological injury and disease SIGs: Brain Injury, Degenerative Diseases, Spinal Cord Injury, Stroke, Balance and Falls, and Vestibular Rehabilitation	*Journal of Neurological Physical Therapy*
Oncology	Physical therapy for individuals diagnosed with cancer or HIV/AIDS SIG: HIV/AIDS, Lymphedema	*Rehabilitation Oncology*

8

Continued

Table 8-1
Sections of the American Physical Therapy Association—cont'd

Section	Area(s) of Interest	Publication(s)
Orthopaedic	Management of patients with musculoskeletal disorders SIGs: Occupational Health, Foot and Ankle, Performing Arts, Pain Management, and Animal Physical Therapist	*Journal of Orthopaedic and Sports Physical Therapy Orthopaedic Physical Therapy Practice*
Pediatrics	Highest quality of life for all children, people with developmental disabilities, and their families	*Pediatric Physical Therapy Section on Pediatrics Newsletter*
Private Practice	Growth, economic viability, and business success of PT-owned physical therapy services	*Impact*
Research	Clinical and basic scientific research	*Section on Research Newsletter Michels Research Forum Proceedings*
Sports Physical Therapy	Athletic injury management, including acute care, treatment and rehabilitation, prevention, and education	*The Journal of Orthopaedic and Sports Physical Therapy*
Veterans Affairs	High-quality physical therapy in the Department of Veteran Affairs	*VAntage PoinT*
Women's Health	Women's health across the life span	*Journal of the Section on Women's Health Highlights in Women's Health*

PT, Physical therapist; *PTA*, physical therapist assistant; *SIG*, special interest group.
Data from Component Contacts Online: Sections. Alexandria, VA. American Physical Therapy Association. Available at http://www.apta.org/AM/Template.cfm?Section=Chapters&Template=/aptaapps/componentsonline/componentsonline.cfm. Accessed April 24, 2006.

in one of these components to further organize into smaller areas of common interest. For example, the Section for Education has four SIGs, two for academic administrators (physical therapist and physical therapist assistant education programs) and one each for clinical education and academic faculty. Participation in any SIG is voluntary.

ASSEMBLIES

An **assembly** is similar to a section in that it provides a mechanism for members with common interests to meet, confer, and promote their objectives.

The differences are that assemblies are composed of members of the same class (category) and may exist at the state and national levels. One exception to the class limitation applies to student and student physical therapist assistant members, who may combine into one assembly. In fact, the Student Assembly is the only assembly that currently exists at the national level. This provides an important vehicle for communication and a voice for students.

HOUSE OF DELEGATES

The **House of Delegates** is the highest policymaking body of the APTA. Officers, directors, and members of the Nominating Committee are elected by the HOD. Its general powers, noted in Box 8-4,[4] are derived from the bylaws of the APTA.

The HOD is composed of voting delegates from all chapters and nonvoting delegates (who may speak and make motions) from each section, the Physical Therapist Assistant Caucus, the Student Assembly, and the BOD. Representation is proportionate; however, the complex formula for determining the size of the HOD ensures that the total number of delegates will always be slightly above 400. In addition, each chapter is entitled to at least 2 delegates, each section 1 delegate, the Physical Therapist Assistant Caucus 5 delegates, and the Student Assembly 2 delegates.

In accordance with the bylaws, the annual session of the APTA is the HOD meeting. This session spans 3 days and is held in conjunction with an **annual conference and exposition** in June. The conference (known as "PT XXXX"; the Xs represent the year) continues for another 2 to 3 days and includes an extensive program of presentations and activities. Beginning in 2007, these two events will occur separately every 4 years, with the HOD preceding the annual conference.

Ad hoc committees and task forces, in addition to standing committees, may be created by the HOD to address issues that it deems important. When these groups are created, definite charges and time lines are stipulated in the motion that created the unit.

8

BOX 8-4   *General Powers of the House of Delegates*

The House of Delegates of the American Physical Therapy Association has all legislative and elective powers and authority to determine policies of the Association, including the power to:
- A. Amend and repeal these Bylaws;
- B. Amend, suspend, or rescind the Standing Rules;
- C. Adopt ethical principles and standards to govern the conduct of members of the Association in their roles as physical therapists or physical therapist assistants; and
- D. Modify or reverse a decision of the Board of Directors.

From Bylaws of the American Physical Therapy Association. Phys Ther 2005;85:1254-1263.

BOARD OF DIRECTORS

Six officers of the APTA and nine directors constitute the **Board of Directors**. The officers are the president, vice president, secretary, treasurer, speaker of the HOD, and vice speaker of the HOD. The duty of the BOD is to carry out the mandates and policies established by the HOD. Full meetings generally occur in November and March.

The BOD and HOD must work closely together for effective operation of the APTA. While the HOD establishes the policies and positions of the APTA, the BOD, elected by the HOD, communicates these issues to internal and external personnel or agencies. This communication of issues is an important representative function of the BOD.

Similar to the HOD, the BOD may create ad hoc committees and task forces to carry out its business. These units will also have specific charges and time lines. In addition, the BOD may establish councils to respond to unique service needs of the APTA.

PHYSICAL THERAPIST ASSISTANT CAUCUS

The Physical Therapist Assistant Caucus (PTA Caucus) was created by the HOD at its meeting in 2005. This was part of the major organizational changes that affected the PTAs and replaced the Representative Body of the National Assembly (see Chapter 3 for further details of these changes). The PTA Caucus meets once a year immediately preceding the HOD. This provides a mechanism for representation and discussion of issues and perspectives pertinent to PTAs and presentation to the HOD. Details of its operation were established before its initial meeting in 2006.

STAFF

The organizational chart in Figure 8-2 indicates that APTA staff serves the organization at multiple levels. During any business hour, a member (or non-member) can call the APTA headquarters in Alexandria, Virginia, at its toll-free number, (800) 999-APTA (2782), and speak to any of its more than 160 staff members. Staff may also be contacted through links from the APTA website (www.apta.org). This direct benefit is important to access information and services. Staff also provide support for activities of the chapters, sections, and assemblies and for operation of the HOD, BOD, PTA Caucus, and all national level committees and task forces.

Key staff members also provide important representative functions to outside agencies, similar to duties of the BOD. This role is particularly true for the chief executive officer and senior vice presidents. These individuals are responsible for the following divisions: Executive; Communications; Finance/Administration; Foundation for Physical Therapy; Education; Governance, Components, and Meetings; and Practice and Research.

ASSOCIATED ORGANIZATIONS

In addition to the components identified in Figure 8-2, several other organizations have a mission and set of goals that complement those of the APTA. Some of these agencies function independently of the APTA, whereas for others the link is more than philosophical. In all cases, the association is mutually beneficial. These organizations are briefly described in the following sections and labeled in Figure 8-3.

AMERICAN BOARD OF PHYSICAL THERAPY SPECIALTIES

The **American Board of Physical Therapy Specialties (ABPTS)** was created by the HOD in 1978 to provide a formal mechanism to recognize physical therapists with advanced knowledge, skills, and experience in a special area of practice. A specialization program was established to achieve board certification and enhance the quality of care in the specialty area. Participation in the program is voluntary; however, PTs shall not present themselves as "board-certified clinical specialists" unless they have successfully completed the certification process.

Each specialty area must be approved by the HOD, but criteria for each area are established by the ABPTS. Seven specialty areas have been approved and are listed in Table 8-2.

To be recognized as a "board-certified clinical specialist," a PT must pass a written examination and present the following qualifications: licensure to practice physical therapy in one of the chapters of the APTA and evidence of at least 2000 hours of clinical practice in the specialty area, at least 25% of which must have been done within the 3 years preceding the examination. The first three specialists were recognized in 1985 in the area of cardiopulmonary physical therapy. More than 6000 clinical specialists have been certified. For more information on the ABPTS, visit the APTA website.

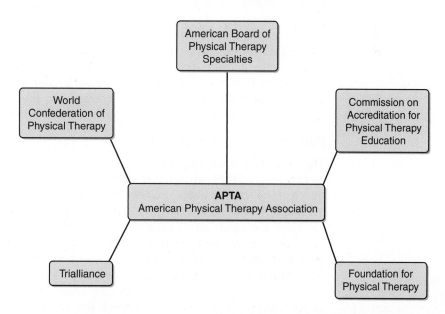

Figure 8-3 ■ Organizations associated with the American Physical Therapy Association.

Table 8-2
Approved Specialty Areas in Physical Therapy

Specialty Area	Year Approved
Cardiopulmonary physical therapy	1981
Clinical electrophysiologic	1982
Geriatrics	1989
Neurology	1982
Orthopaedics	1981
Pediatrics	1981
Sports physical therapy	1981

COMMISSION ON ACCREDITATION IN PHYSICAL THERAPY EDUCATION

The **Commission on Accreditation in Physical Therapy Education (CAPTE)** is responsible for evaluating and accrediting professional (entry level) PT and PTA education programs. It is recognized by the U.S. Department of Education and Council for Higher Education Accreditation. CAPTE is composed of 26 members from the educational community, the physical therapy profession, and the public. (See Chapter 1 for a historical account of accreditation in physical therapy.)

The relationship between the APTA and CAPTE is integrated, yet they are technically independent. A Department of Accreditation within the APTA manages the accreditation program. However, CAPTE reviews the data and determines the accreditation status of each education program. Moreover, CAPTE establishes the evaluative criteria for the accreditation decisions. For more information on CAPTE, visit the APTA website.

FOUNDATION FOR PHYSICAL THERAPY

The **Foundation for Physical Therapy** was established in 1979 by an action of the APTA HOD to promote and provide financial support for research in physical therapy. Its current mission is to fund research in physical therapy that supports evidence-based practice, enhance the quality of physical therapist services, and increase the number of PT researchers.[6] Because it is an independent entity, its governing body is separate from the APTA and consists of clinicians, researchers, and business leaders. The Foundation has awarded more than $10 million in the areas of research grants, scholarships for doctoral degree education, and postdoctoral fellowships. Special projects are also funded. For example, in 2002, the Foundation awarded a $1.5 million, 3-year grant for the Clinical Research Network centered at the University of Southern California. Activities of this network will assess the effects of strengthening exercises in a variety of disabilities. Through these comprehensive programs the Foundation promotes clinically focused research to improve the practice and cost effectiveness of physical therapy. For more information on the Foundation, visit the APTA website or call (800) 875-1378.

TRIALLIANCE

The **Trialliance** was formed in 1988 and consists of the APTA, the American Occupational Therapy Association, and the American Speech-Language-Hearing Association. This organization meets at least three times per year to discuss issues of mutual concern. This unified voice provides greater strength when interacting with government and private agencies.

WORLD CONFEDERATION OF PHYSICAL THERAPY

The **World Confederation of Physical Therapy (WCPT)** represents physical therapy on a global level. This organization promotes health on a worldwide level by fostering high standards in physical therapy research, education, and practice and by providing vehicles to exchange information. Member organizations are from 92 nations around the world, including the APTA. In addition to an annual business meeting, an international congress is held every 4 years to provide a forum to share information and collaborate on mutual goals. For more information, visit the website at www.wcpt.org.

OTHER RELATED ORGANIZATIONS

FEDERATION OF STATE BOARDS OF PHYSICAL THERAPY

The **Federation of State Boards of Physical Therapy (FSBPT)** is an independent agency that has been instrumental in coordinating activity among all of the state boards that regulate physical therapy. It exists to protect the health, safety, and welfare of the public by promoting uniformity in regulations pertaining to physical therapy in each state. Areas of attention include the licensing examination and state practice acts for physical therapy. Regarding the examinations, the FSBPT develops, maintains, and administers the national licensing examination for PTs and PTAs. It has been involved in revising the examination and standardizing passing criteria among the states. Concerning state practice acts, the FSBPT has created a model practice act for physical therapy to be used in these laws. This model is an attempt to standardize language and legal references to the practice of physical therapy. For more information on the FSBPT, visit its website (www.fsbpt.org) or call 703-299-3100.

AMERICAN ACADEMY OF PHYSICAL THERAPISTS

This organization was founded in 1989 to address the unmet needs of the African American physical therapy community. Its mission is to provide relief to poor and disadvantaged African American and other minorities by fostering innovative programs in health care, encouraging minority students to pursue careers in allied health, and conducting clinical research related to conditions that affect the minority communities.[7] For more information, visit its website at www.aaptnet.org/home/ or call 888-313-2278 (AAPT).

8

BENEFITS OF BELONGING

Benefits of belonging to the APTA are both intangible and tangible. The intangible benefits relate to the commitment to high-quality service that the organization provides to its members and public. As the recognized voice for this profession in the United States, it is appropriate for PTs, PTAs, and students to join the APTA. Through the organizational structure described previously, members are represented in a wide variety of public and governmental areas. No other organization will advocate for the best interests of PTs, PTAs, or the patients and clients whom they serve.

The tangible benefits of belonging to the APTA are identified in Table 8-3 and briefly described here. Legislative efforts are provided through lobbying, direct contact with government officials, and a strong infrastructure to represent the members. In this era of rapidly changing health care management and reimbursement, this membership benefit is critical for success of the profession. Information is made available through Internet access to the APTA, phone contact with staff (see the earlier section on staff), and publications. The

Table 8-3
Benefits of Belonging to the American Physical Therapy Association

Benefit	Examples
Legislative efforts	Lobbying for Medicare direct access
Information	*Physical Therapy* *PT—Magazine of Physical Therapy* *PT Bulletin Online* Website (www.apta.org) Staff assistance on issues affecting practice, education, and research
Continuing education	Annual Conference Combined Sections Meeting National Student Conclave Preview 2020 Home study courses
Professional development	Networking and education through districts, chapters, sections, and student assembly
Research	Promote research funding and activities by supporting the efforts of the Foundation of Physical Therapy
Reimbursement	Workshops on reimbursement, coding, and managed care Group rates for insurance and credit card programs Professional liability, auto, health, disability, long-term care insurance plans Mastercard

Data from Extend Your Reach: Benefits of Belonging Checklist. Alexandria, VA, American Physical Therapy Association, 2006.

website contains a great deal of current and reference information; however, some of it is restricted to members. Continuing education offerings, including annual events and home study courses, are available to members at considerable discount from nonmember prices.

Professional development occurs through interaction at the local, state, and national levels, which is available through district, chapter, section, and assembly events. Practice and research activities include promoting clinical competency through guidelines and policies, advising government agencies and insurance companies of practice standards, and defending the need for research funding to appropriate sources. Services in the area of reimbursement, perhaps the most significant issue currently confronting the profession, include input into Current Procedural Terminology (CPT) coding changes, workshops for both members and payers, and coordinated legislative efforts on behalf of PTs, PTAs, and students. Insurance and other financial benefits include low-cost group programs and investment and retirement planning.

Special incentives are provided for student membership. Fees for membership and participation in activities are generally 10% to 25% of the cost for a physical therapist member. In addition, the Career Starter Dues program eases the transition from student to physical therapist/physical therapist assistant membership. Upon graduation, student members automatically convert to the respective physical therapist or physical therapist assistant membership category for the remainder of the membership period. For the next year of membership, dues are 50% of the respective category.

SUMMARY

This chapter described the purposes, infrastructure, benefits, and organizations related to the APTA. Purposes of the APTA include serving the public and its members to enhance the profession and practice of physical therapy. Its governing bodies are organized into three levels: local (districts), state (chapters), and national (HOD and BOD). Opportunities for participation in areas of special interest exist in sections and assemblies. Staff members are readily available to support the organization at all levels and interact with external agencies. Other related organizations in the United States and across the globe further promote physical therapy, and the APTA participates in these organizations through either direct membership or interaction. Benefits of belonging include outcomes that are intangible (professional commitment) and tangible (legislative efforts, information, continuing education, professional development, practice and research support, reimbursement actions, and low-cost insurance). Through its purpose, organization, and activities, the APTA provides widespread opportunities and strong representation for the profession and practice of physical therapy.

REFERENCES

1. Mission Statement of APTA, HOD P06-93-05-05. House of Delegates Standards, Policies, Positions, and Guidelines. Alexandria, VA, American Physical Therapy Association, 2005.
2. Mission Statement Fulfillment, HOD P06-93-06-07. House of Delegates Standards, Policies, Positions, and Guidelines. Alexandria, VA, American Physical Therapy Association, 2005.
3. Goals That Represent the Priorities of the American Physical Therapy Association, HOD P06-05-15-24. House of Delegates Standards, Policies, Positions, and Guidelines. Alexandria, VA, American Physical Therapy Association, 2005.
4. Bylaws of the American Physical Therapy Association. Phys Ther 2005;85:1254-1263.

5. Standing Rules of the American Physical Therapy Association. Phys Ther 2005;85:1251-1253.

6. Annual Report (Foundation News). 2005;13(6).

7. Our Mission. Atlanta, American Academy of Physical Therapists. Available at http://www.aaptnet.org/home/index.php?id=16&sec=home-nav. Accessed April 24, 2006.

REVIEW QUESTIONS

1. Select at least three components of the APTA mission statement and apply them to Figure 8-2 by indicating at what level of APTA each goal should be most logically tackled. (There may be more than one answer.)

2. Apply the goals listed in Box 8-3 to the various levels of the APTA's organizational structure (Fig 8-2) and compare them with your applications in question 1 and with the definitions of the various APTA components given in this chapter.

3. What is the difference between an assembly, section, and SIG? How do they differ in function and membership?

4. Visit a website of one of the organizations associated with the APTA to discern differences in scope and function. What advantage does it offer over membership in the APTA alone?

Part II

Practice

Society needs us so they can follow the path of moving precisely toward optimum health.

Shirley Sahrmann, PT, FAPTA

9

Physical Therapy for Musculoskeletal Conditions

Barbara C. Belyea and Hilary B. Greenberger

hypermobile joint
hypomobile joint
joint mobilization and manipulation
manual muscle testing (MMT)
massage
muscle endurance
muscular strength
myofascial release
nerve entrapment
objective examination
open kinetic chain exercise
paraffin treatment
passive range of motion (PROM)
proprioception
proprioceptor
range of motion (ROM)
range-of-motion exercise
resisted exercise
resisted test
short-wave diathermy
soft tissue mobilization
special tests
sprain
strain
strength

subjective examination
tendinitis
tendinopathies
tendinosis
thermal agent
ultrasound
whirlpool

OBJECTIVES ▬▬▬

After reading this chapter, the reader will be able to:

■ List common conditions seen in musculoskeletal physical therapy
■ Identify the components of an initial musculoskeletal examination
■ Define and give examples of the various tests and measures used in physical therapy for musculoskeletal conditions
■ List the general goals of a therapeutic exercise program
■ Describe the various types of therapeutic exercises
■ Describe various physical agents used to address musculoskeletal problems

Conditions that affect the musculoskeletal system are the primary domain of physical therapists who specialize in orthopaedic physical therapy. One of the largest clinical specialties within the physical therapy profession, orthopaedic physical therapy encompasses a wide array of therapeutic techniques and philosophies of treatment. Physical therapists (PTs) and physical therapist assistants (PTAs) in the field of orthopaedics work in a variety of clinical settings and treat patients of diverse ages with a variety of physical and medical problems. This chapter describes the types of patients with whom an orthopaedic PT would work and presents some commonly used examination techniques and interventions.

GENERAL DESCRIPTION

Although the clinical interests or approaches to treatment may be diverse, the common thread throughout physical therapy for musculoskeletal conditions is the focus on a patient's function. By examining the patient's functional ability, the PT determines the cause and extent of any functional disability, referred to as a **dysfunction,** and works with the patient/client to return the individual to an optimal level of function. A person's function can be affected when a disruption occurs in the musculoskeletal system, either from traumatic injury or from repeated stress to tissue. Dysfunctions may be caused by a structural imbalance of muscle or bone, birth defects, surgery, or degenerative changes in the body.[1] Dysfunctions of the musculoskeletal system often result in symptoms of pain, stiffness, edema (swelling), muscle weakness or fatigue, or loss of **range of motion** (**ROM;** movement at a joint).

To conduct a comprehensive examination, generate an accurate diagnosis, and develop an appropriate plan of care, therapists must have an extensive understanding of anatomy, biomechanics, pathokinesiology, and exercise physiology. They must also be knowledgeable in the application of a variety of intervention techniques and be able to analyze clinical situations and problem solve to determine which approach is the most appropriate for each patient situation. Effective communication skills are also critical for PTs and PTAs so they can establish good rapport with patients and provide the necessary information to gain the patient's adherence to the plan of care.

DEVELOPMENT

Several factors contribute to the continued growth of musculoskeletal physical therapy. New contributions to the scientific literature provide therapists with evidence supporting the effectiveness of various treatment interventions that allow better evidence-based clinical decision making. The development of sophisticated technology and new intervention techniques has also provided new treatment options for PTs who evaluate and treat this patient population. Changes in lifestyle have contributed to the growth of orthopaedic physical therapy. Increasing interest and participation in physical fitness by the general population have resulted in an increase in musculoskeletal dysfunction caused by overuse or traumatic injuries. The increased use of computers and other technical machinery requiring repeated motions has also had an impact on the incidence of overuse injuries in the upper extremity. Individuals who must sustain postures at a computer or operate machinery while performing repeated motions with their hands may be at risk for the development of muscle injury or nerve entrapment requiring intervention by a PT. An increase in life span has also resulted in the growth of this area of physical therapy as people are living longer, more active lives and experiencing symptoms related to degenerative changes in their bodies.

A great deal of similarity exists between orthopaedic physical therapy and sports physical therapy. In both areas the focus of rehabilitation is to regain optimum function and return the patient to the previous level of function and activity. A sports physical therapist must therefore incorporate sport-specific activities into the treatment program to make sure that the patient can meet the physical demands of the sport with respect to strength, endurance, balance, and speed. An orthopaedic physical therapist may work with athletes but may also treat a variety of musculoskeletal conditions that are not related to sports activities.

COMMON CONDITIONS

Within the broad scope of musculoskeletal physical therapy, a variety of patient problems may be treated. These conditions range from injuries sustained through athletic participation, work-related injuries, and dysfunction after orthopaedic surgical procedures to the degenerative changes that accompany the aging process. As previously stated, patients with musculoskeletal conditions referred for physical therapy may have pain, swelling, weakness, or loss of motion resulting from stress to the musculoskeletal system. This stress may include damage to bones or soft tissue such as muscles, tendons, joint capsules, ligaments, bursae, cartilage, and fascia in the extremities or spine.

OVERUSE INJURIES

Repeated stress to the musculoskeletal system can cause overuse injuries that may result in pain, inflammation, and dysfunction. The following examples describe some common conditions caused by overuse injuries.

Bursitis. **Bursitis** is an inflammation of bursae, which are fluid-filled sacs throughout the body that decrease friction between structures. Bursae become irritated and painful when they are repeatedly pinched between two structures. A common example of this mechanism of injury occurs at the shoulder; the subacromial bursa may be pinched during repeated movements when the shoulder is in an overhead position, such as when painting, reaching, or throwing.

Tendinopathy. Tendons are the structures that connect muscle to bone. Repeated use of or rapid overstretching of muscles can overload and injure the tendon. Disorders of tendons **(tendinopathies)** can be the result of inflammation **(tendinitis)** or degenerative changes caused by overuse **(tendinosis).** Tendinopathies usually result in painful movements and are frequently seen in the patellar tendon at the knee in people who perform repeated jumping (e.g., dancers, basketball players) and at the elbow in people who do repeated or sustained gripping activities (e.g., carpenters, tennis players). Excessive overload to a tendon can also result in a complete tear or rupture, which is commonly seen in the ankle (Achilles rupture) or elbow (biceps rupture) and must be surgically repaired.

Nerve Entrapment. Pressure on a nerve, causing **nerve entrapment,** may result from a variety of sources and usually causes symptoms of tingling, pain, weakness, or any combination of these. A common condition of nerve compression at the wrist is referred to as carpal tunnel syndrome. Patients with carpal tunnel syndrome usually complain of numbness and pain in the hand and fingers, which commonly results from repeated activities with the wrist in a flexed position (e.g., musicians, computer keyboard operators).

TRAUMATIC INJURIES

Musculoskeletal injuries may also occur as a result of direct trauma. Bones, muscles, ligaments, and other soft tissue may be injured when they sustain a direct blow or when they are placed under excessive stretch. The following are just a few of the common conditions that can arise from direct trauma to the musculoskeletal system.

Ligament Sprain. Ligaments are supporting structures at joints that serve to stabilize the joint and prevent excess movement. When ligaments are overstretched, their fibers can tear and cause pain and instability at the joint. A common site of **sprain** is at the ankle when the lateral (outside) ligaments are overstretched. This injury occurs when a person lands on the foot in a turned-in position. Another common site of ligament sprain is the anterior cruciate ligament (ACL) at the knee. Injuries to this ligament are usually the result of a twisting movement of the knee when the foot is planted, commonly occurring in sports that require jumping or quick changes in direction, such as soccer or volleyball.

Fracture. Direct trauma to bone can result in a break, or **fracture,** of the bone. Fractures can occur in any bone in the body, but are commonly seen at the wrist or the hip after falls. Elderly individuals are particularly prone to fractures, because of changes in the structure of their bones resulting from inactivity, inadequate nutrition, and degenerative conditions. Fractures are best diagnosed through the use of radiographs.

Muscle Strain. A sudden contraction of a muscle or excessive stretch on a muscle can cause tearing of the muscle fibers, known as a **strain.** Muscle strains can occur in any area of the body and can range in severity. A strain of the rotator cuff muscles at the shoulder can result in shoulder pain and weakness when lifting the arm, and cervical strains may be the result of a sudden movement of the neck, as with a whiplash injury.

Surgical Conditions

Individuals who have had surgery are another group of patients commonly seen by the orthopaedic physical therapist. Injuries resulting from repeated stress, acute trauma, or disease processes may require surgical intervention for appropriate healing. The following are examples of orthopaedic surgery in which patients can benefit from physical therapy intervention to reduce pain and regain motion and strength that will allow optimal movement and function.

Total Joint Arthroplasty. Painful movement caused by degenerative changes at joint surfaces can be alleviated through surgical replacement of the joint surfaces. Joints most commonly replaced are weight-bearing joints, primarily the hips and knees. A variety of plastic and stainless steel implants are used to effectively replace degenerated joint surfaces. Therapeutic intervention is necessary postoperatively to ensure maximum strength and function and to provide patient education to prevent complications such as dislocation.

Amputation. Surgical amputation is the removal of a portion of an extremity because of trauma, inadequate blood flow, or the presence of a malignant growth. Inadequate circulation can be a result of disease processes such as diabetes mellitus or peripheral vascular disease, whereas a growth may indicate the presence of cancer. Postoperative physical therapy often addresses regaining strength in the remaining portion of the limb and functional training with a prosthesis.

9

MEDICAL CONDITIONS

Numerous medical conditions may also affect the musculoskeletal system by causing pain, weakness, or loss of function. Systemic diseases such as rheumatoid arthritis, cancer, or acquired immunodeficiency syndrome may cause impairments that disrupt the musculoskeletal system and result in functional challenges that can be addressed by the orthopaedic PT.

PRINCIPLES OF EXAMINATION

Treating a patient with a musculoskeletal condition requires the PT to have a comprehensive understanding of anatomy, pathology, biomechanics, and pathokinesiology. The first step in understanding the needs of a patient is a thorough examination. Reexaminations are performed throughout the rehabilitative process to monitor patient progress toward established functional goals.

This section describes the following components of an initial examination: patient history, systems review, and tests and measures performed by the PT. The history is part of the **subjective examination,** whereas the remaining parts constitute the **objective examination.**

PATIENT HISTORY

The **history** involves gathering information about the current and past health status of the patient. The information is obtained by interviewing the patient or the patient's family or by accessing the patient's medical record. The history is a qualitative measurement based on the *patient's* perception of the problem and is therefore included in the "S" portion of the "SOAP" note (see Chapter 2).

The role of the therapist during the interview is to guide the patient through pertinent questions. This interaction allows the therapist to develop a rapport with the patient and to understand the patient's insight into and opinion of the problem. The interview also assists the therapist in appropriately directing the remainder of the examination. Often, the patient interview will give the therapist ample information to make a tentative physical therapy diagnosis. Questions asked during the interview include information on the cause of the condition, current symptoms, previous physical therapy treatments, past medical history, and lifestyle as it pertains to work and recreation. Box 9-1 lists typical questions asked during the patient interview.

The patient is commonly asked to draw the location of the pain on a body chart (Figure 9-1). Pain scales are also often used to gauge the amount of pain the patient is experiencing (Figure 9-2). On completion of the history taking, the therapist should have gained information regarding the description and location of symptoms, nature of the disorder (acute versus chronic condition), behavior of the symptoms (what activities make the symptoms either better or worse), and functional difficulties the patient may be experiencing.

SYSTEMS REVIEW

The objective portion of the examination refers to quantitative or qualitative measurements that are taken by the PT. This portion of the examination begins with systems review and is included in the "O" section of the SOAP note (see

BOX 9-1 *Questions Typically Asked During The Subjective Component of an Initial Physical Therapy Evaluation*

1. What brings you to physical therapy today?
2. What do you feel is your primary problem? Is it stiffness? Pain? Weakness? Instability?
3. Was the onset of the problem slow or sudden? Was the problem caused by a specific incident or mechanism of injury?
4. Have you ever had this problem before? If so, were you treated for it? How long did it take to recover?
5. What provokes your symptoms? What relieves your symptoms?
6. Are your symptoms worsening or improving?
7. Are your symptoms constant or intermittent?
8. Can you describe your pain? Does your pain spread to other parts of your body?
9. What is your occupation?
10. What activities are you unable to do because of your symptoms?
11. Have you had any radiographs ("x-rays") taken or diagnostic tests performed?
12. Are you currently taking any medication for this problem?
13. How is your general health?
14. Is there anything else you would like to tell me that I have not asked and that would be pertinent to your problem?

Chapter 2). Systems review provides additional information about the general health and fitness level of the patient separate from the specific reason the patient has sought advice from a PT. The information gathered during the systems review assists the therapist in developing an appropriate plan of care and identifying health problems that may require consultation or referral to another health care provider. In a patient with a musculoskeletal condition, common system reviews may include monitoring of heart rate and blood pressure, assessment of skin integrity, and a gross assessment of joint ROM, strength, and coordinated movements.

TESTS AND MEASURES

During the tests and measures portion of the examination, specific numbers or grades may be assigned (quantitative measurement), as is the case with ROM or strength measurements. Other times, parts of the examination are performed by observing and describing patterns of movement, deformities, or both (qualitative measurement). The purpose of the tests and measures is to establish baseline values and observations that can be used for comparison after a single treatment or a series of treatments. The PT can then make appropriate changes in the plan of care based on the amount of progress or lack of progress found with repeated tests and measures.

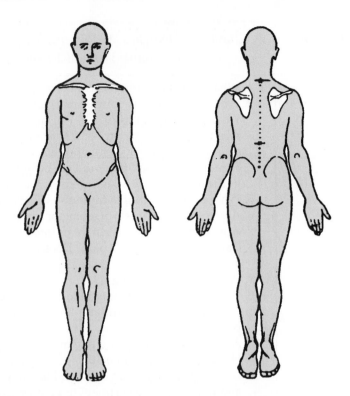

Figure 9-1 ■ Body chart to indicate areas of pain. The patient is asked to indicate areas of pain with Xs, areas of numbness with slashes, and areas of tingling with plus signs.

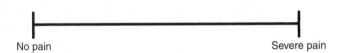

No pain   Severe pain

Figure 9-2 ■ Visual analog scale. On the line provided, the patient is asked to mark the degree of pain experienced.

This section briefly describes some of the tests and measures performed in an orthopaedic physical therapy setting. The purpose is to familiarize introductory level students with common terms used when working with a patient who has a musculoskeletal problem.

Observation. Observation is the "looking" phase of the examination. It may begin in the waiting room, where the therapist can observe the patient's general attitude, posture, and willingness to move. A perfunctory gait assessment may be made as the patient enters the examination area. Once the patient is appropriately undressed, a more detailed inspection can be made, including observation of obvious deformities such as an abnormal curvature of the spine, joint subluxations (a condition in which a joint partially dislocates), asymmetrical body contours, swelling, and color and texture of the skin. Many musculo-skeletal injuries are a result of or are exacerbated by poor sitting and standing postures. Therefore particular attention is paid to the standing and sitting posture of the patient.

Active Range of Motion. **Active range of motion (AROM)** refers to the ability of the *patient* to *voluntarily* move a limb through an arc of movement. AROM provides the therapist with information regarding the quality of the movement (smooth versus rigid movement), the willingness of the patient to move the limb, any pain produced during movement, and whether the patient has any limitations in the motion as compared with the unaffected side. An example of AROM of the shoulder in multiple planes is provided in Figure 9-3.

Passive Range of Motion. **Passive range of motion (PROM)** refers to the amount of movement at a joint that is obtained by the *therapist* moving the segment *without assistance from the patient.* In some instances, because of injury or prolonged immobilization, a joint may have less motion than is considered functional. This condition is referred to as a **hypomobile joint.** In other cases, such as a joint subluxation, the joint may have excessive motion, which is referred to as a **hypermobile joint.** PROM also gives the therapist an indication of the degree and pattern of pain, as well as the "feel" of the movement.

Many methods may be used to measure and document AROM and PROM. The most common measurement technique, **goniometry,** is performed with a **goniometer.** Examples of goniometers are shown in Figure 9-4. The amount of motion available at any joint depends on the structure of the joint. In addition, norm values for joint ROM depend on several factors, including the patient's age and gender.[2] Typically the therapist compares ROM values of the affected joint with those on the unaffected side. Figure 9-5 shows a PT conducting a PROM measurement of a patient's knee flexion.

Strength. **Strength** can be defined as the amount of force produced during a voluntary muscular contraction. This contraction may be performed statically (no motion) or dynamically (through an ROM). When one is assessing the status of the muscles and tendons, a quick **resisted test** is used. This test allows the therapist to determine the general strength of a muscle group and assess whether the muscle contraction produces pain. If the resisted test shows that a muscle or muscle group is weak or painful, further testing may be performed to isolate the specific muscle. To isolate and test specific muscles, **manual muscle testing (MMT)** is performed (Figure 9-6). MMT allows the therapist to assign a specific grade to a muscle. This grade is based on whether the patient can hold the limb against gravity, how much manual resistance can be tolerated, and whether the joint has full ROM. Several systems of grading are widely used. One of the most common grading systems was initially described by Robert Lovett, MD, and later modified by Henry Kendall, PT, and Florence Kendall, PT.[3] This key to muscle grading is outlined in Table 9-1.

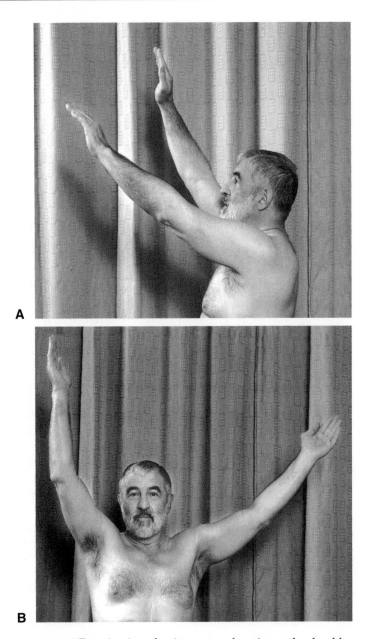

A

B

***Figure* 9-3** ■ Examination of active range of motion at the shoulder; note the decreased ROM in the left shoulder. **A,** Shoulder flexion. **B,** Shoulder abduction. (Courtesy of Dewey Neild.)   *Continued*

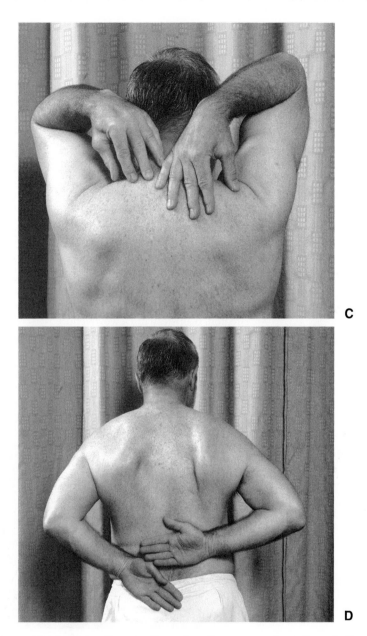

C

D

9

Figure 9-3, cont'd ■ Examination of active range of motion at the shoulder; note the decreased ROM in the left shoulder. **C,** Shoulder external rotation. **D,** Shoulder internal rotation.

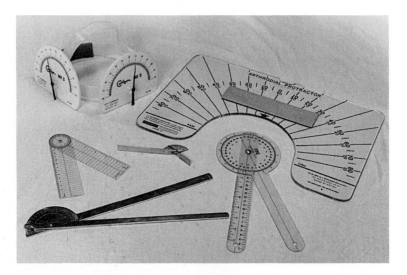

Figure 9-4 ■ Variety of goniometers to measure joint angles. The size and type vary to measure long and short limb segments and the cervical region. (Courtesy of Dewey Neild.)

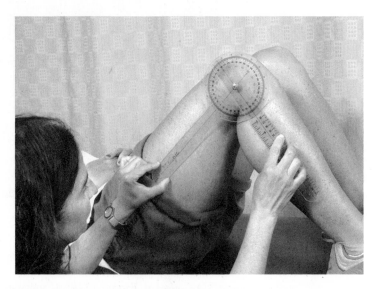

Figure 9-5 ■ Physical therapist conducting a goniometric measurement of knee flexion. (Courtesy of Dewey Neild.)

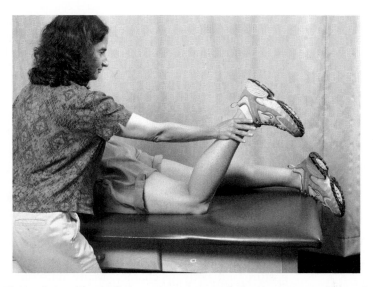

Figure 9-6 ■ Physical therapists commonly perform manual muscle tests to determine muscle strength. Pictured is the manual muscle test for the hamstring musculature. (Courtesy of Dewey Neild.)

Table 9-1
Key to Manual Muscle Testing Grades

	Function of the Muscle	Grade	Symbols	Symbols
No movement	No contraction felt or seen in the muscle	Zero	0	0
	Tendon becomes prominent or feeble; contraction felt in the muscle with no visible movement of the part	Trace	T	1
Supported in horizontal plane	Moves through partial range of motion	Poor –	P –	2 –
	Moves through complete range of motion	Poor	P	2
	Holds against slight pressure in test position	Poor +	P +	2 +
	Moves through partial range of motion against gravity			
	Gradual release from test position	Fair –	F –	3 –
	Holds test position (no added pressure)	Fair	F	3
	Hold test position against slight pressure	Fair +	F +	3 +
Tests in the antigravity position	Holds test position against slight to moderate pressure	Good –	G –	4 –
	Holds test position against moderate pressure	Good	G	4
	Holds test position against moderate to strong pressure	Good +	G +	4 +
	Holds test position against strong pressure	Normal	N	5

Modified from Kendall FP, McCreary EK, Provance PG, et al: Muscle Testing and Function, ed 5. Baltimore, Lippincott Williams & Wilkins, 2005.

With the development of sophisticated technical equipment, many other methods are now available to measure strength, including hand-held dynamometers and computerized instruments such as isokinetic devices. These devices allow the therapist to obtain strength curves of isolated muscles, as well as specific force values.

Flexibility. **Flexibility** refers to the ability to move a limb segment through a specific ROM. The amount of flexibility at a given joint depends on two factors. First, the soft tissue surrounding the joint must be pliable to allow movement between the joint surfaces. This feature is referred to as **accessory motion** of the joint. Accessory motion is the ability of the joint surfaces to glide, roll, and spin on each other. Second, the muscle or muscles crossing the joint must be at an appropriate length to allow motion to occur. For example, the ability to stand up and touch the toes while keeping the knees straight depends on the flexibility of the back and posterior hip muscles, as well as the ability of the spinal vertebrae to move.

Appropriate flexibility or balance of muscles is a key component of proper posture and body mechanics. Many musculoskeletal problems seen in the physical therapy clinic can be linked to muscle imbalances that have caused movement dysfunctions.[4] For example, if the muscles surrounding the shoulder did not act synergistically (because of lack of flexibility), compensation might occur at joints distal and proximal to the shoulder, such as the elbow and cervical spine.

A PT may perform a number of tests to determine flexibility. One common test for the lower extremity is the 90/90 straight leg raise (Figure 9-7). This test objectively measures flexibility of the hamstring muscles on the posterior aspect of the thigh.

Functional Tests. The ultimate goal of therapy is to return the patient to the previous level of activity, which may include anything from the ability to go grocery shopping independently to returning to athletic competition. With some types of injuries a return to the previous level of activity is not feasible. In these cases the ultimate goal would be to return the individual to the highest level of function achievable.

Traditionally, functional assessment has referred to such activities as the patient's bed mobility, transfers between a variety of surfaces (e.g., moving from a sitting position in a wheelchair to a standing position), and ability to perform activities of daily living (ADLs), such as hair combing, dressing, and bathing. PTs may spend a large percentage of their time during the initial examination assessing the patient's ability to perform these ADLs. Box 9-2 lists examples of ADLs.

Individuals who wish to return to activities other than ADLs require more aggressive types of functional testing. Examples of these types of functional tests are hop tests, jump tests, lunge tests, excursion tests, and balance tests. Gary Gray and others have described these and other types of functional tests in detail.[2,5-7]

Special Tests. **Special tests** are used to examine specific joints to indicate the presence or absence of a particular problem. The purpose of these tests is to

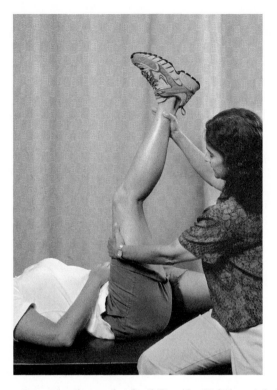

Figure 9-7 ■ Example of a test for flexibility: the 90/90 straight leg raise. (Courtesy of Dewey Neild.)

confirm or reinforce a physical therapy diagnosis. Because so many special tests are available for each joint, only those that appear to be indicated based on the results of tests and measures are performed. Examples of special tests are those that examine nerve compression (Phalen's test; Figure 9-8, *A*), shoulder impingement (Hawkins' test; Figure 9-8, *B*), and ligamentous knee injuries (Lachman's test; Figure 9-8, *C*).

Palpation. A comprehensive understanding of anatomy is essential for any PT. In the clinical situation the therapist uses the sense of touch, known as palpation, to assess what is occurring below the skin and what musculoskeletal structures are involved in an injury. When palpating an area of the body, the therapist is feeling for areas of pain and tenderness, areas of restriction, swelling, and proper orientation of structures.

Other Diagnostic Procedures. Depending on the patient's injury or complaint, other examination procedures may be performed to provide a more complete assessment of the patient. The patient may be referred to other personnel for these procedures. Such complementary procedures may include a variety of imaging techniques, such as radiographs (x-rays), computed tomography (CT) scans, and magnetic resonance imaging (MRI). If the patient has had neuro-

9

BOX 9-2 | *Examples of Activities of Daily Living*

Eating
- Eat with spoon
- Eat with fork
- Cut with knife
- Open milk carton
- Pour liquid
- Drink from cup

Dressing and Undressing
- Reach clothes in closet
- Put on shoe
- Manage zippers
- Remove coat

Bathing and Grooming
- Turn on faucet
- Wash hands
- Dry with towel
- Manage cosmetics
- Brush teeth

Bed and Bathroom
- Get out of bed
- Transfer to toilet
- Reach objects on nightstand
- Sit up in bed

Transfer and Ambulatory Activities
- In and out of bus
- In and out of car
- Safe outdoor ambulation
- Endurance

Other Activities
- Propel wheelchair forward
- Propel wheelchair backward
- Manage elevator
- Hold book
- Dial a telephone
- Use scissors

logical damage, full sensory testing may be indicated. Additional tests for patients with cardiopulmonary conditions may include an assessment of lung capacity. Some of these tests are presented in more detail in Chapters 10 and 11.

PRINCIPLES OF EVALUATION, DIAGNOSIS, AND PROGNOSIS

Based on evaluation of the findings from the comprehensive examination, the physical therapist identifies the patient's impairments, functional limitations, and disability and then determines the diagnosis and prognosis. Once the problems have been identified, the therapist and patient develop goals to address each problem. Common short-term goals are to decrease pain and edema and increase strength and motion. The ultimate long-term goal for patients with musculoskeletal dysfunctions is to achieve an optimal level of function, whether that means returning to work, resuming athletics, or performing daily activities independently. Therapeutic goals should include how each goal is to be measured and the expected time frame to achieve each goal. Once goals have been established, the therapist develops a plan of care designed to achieve these outcomes.

The plan of care is based on determining which interventions will most effectively improve a patient's function. Numerous intervention options and rehabilitation approaches are available to the orthopaedic PT. Some therapists focus their treatment approaches on exercises, whereas others incorporate physical agents or manual techniques. In most instances a combination of techniques is appropriate when designing a comprehensive plan to address the needs of a patient with musculoskeletal dysfunction. When selecting a plan of

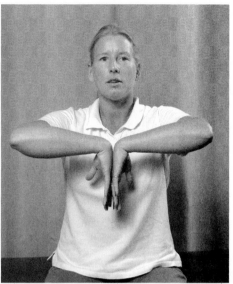

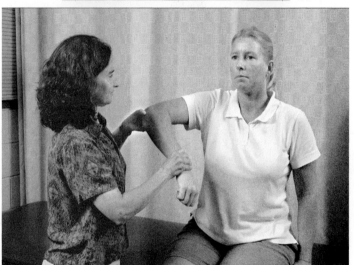

Figure 9-8 ■ Examples of special tests. **A,** Phalen's test for nerve compression. **B,** Hawkins' test for shoulder impingement. (Courtesy of Dewey Neild.)   *Continued*

care, the therapist must consider the goals of the patient and the desired outcome of therapy.

PRINCIPLES OF DIRECT INTERVENTION

The following discussion of intervention options introduces the reader to the typical indications and uses of various techniques. The techniques described include physical agents, manual techniques (including soft tissue and joint mobilization), and therapeutic exercise. The reading list at the end of the

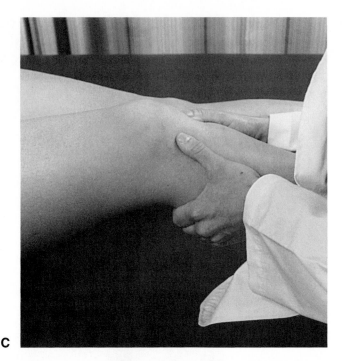

C

Figure 9-8, cont'd ■ Examples of special tests. **C,** Lachman's test for anterior cruciate ligament instability. (Courtesy of Dewey Neild.)

chapter gives sources for in-depth information regarding the application of these and other techniques.

PHYSICAL AGENTS

Many therapeutic agents are available for PTs to incorporate into rehabilitation programs when treating patients with musculoskeletal dysfunction. Based on the intended purpose and method of application, physical agents can be divided into two categories: thermal agents (thermotherapy) and electrical stimulation (electrotherapy). Thermal agents can be subdivided into agents that apply superficial heat, deep heat, and cold. The decision regarding which agent to use is based on a thorough examination of the patient's symptoms, the desired outcomes of therapy, and the therapist's knowledge of the physiological and clinical effects of each physical agent. Table 9-2 lists common physical agents used in physical therapy according to their *physical* effects and includes their *physiological* effects and clinical indications.

Thermal Agents. When a tissue in the body sustains an injury, an automatic response is initiated in an attempt to heal the tissue and return it to its pre-injured state. These naturally occurring processes are referred to as inflammation and repair.[8] The inflammation and repair stages of tissue healing can be altered through the use of thermal agents or electrical stimulation. **Thermal**

Table 9-2
Summary of Common Physical Agents Used in Physical Therapy

Physical Effect	Physical Agents	Physiological Effects	Clinical Indications

Superficial heat	Hot packs
	Paraffin
	Fluidotherapy
	Whirlpool
		Increases blood flow
		Increases metabolism:
		   promotes healing and
		   removal of waste products
		Decreases pain
		Decreases stiffness
			Pain
			Joint stiffness
			Wound care

Deep heat	Ultrasound
	Short-wave
	   diathermy
		Increases blood flow
		Increases metabolism:
		   promotes healing and
		   removal of waste products
		Decreases pain
		Decreases stiffness
			Muscle spasm
			Pain
			Joint stiffness

Cold	Ice packs Ice massage Cold whirlpool Cold compression	Decreases blood flow Decreases metabolism Decreases edema Decreases pain	Acute injury Swelling Pain Muscle spasm After exercise

Electrical
   stimulation
	Transcutaneous
	   electrical nerve
	   stimulation (TENS)
	Iontophoresis
	Electrical stimulation
	   for tissue repair (ESTR)
	Neuromuscular electrical
	   stimulation (NMES)
		Decreases pain
		Decreases edema
		Promotes wound healing
		Reeducates muscles
		Decreases spasticity
			Pain
			Edema
			Wounds
			Nerve regeneration
			Muscle weakness
			   and imbalance

9

agents are used to modify the temperature of surrounding tissue and result in a change in the amount of blood flow to the injured area. Besides vascular changes, temperature changes affect the metabolism of the surrounding tissue, in addition to altering neuromuscular and connective tissue. Through the use of therapeutic changes in temperature, the healing process can be accelerated and the injured tissue restored to optimal strength and integrity.

The extent of the therapeutic changes caused by an alteration in tissue temperature depends on the intensity of the thermal agent applied, the length of time the tissue is exposed to the agent, and characteristics of the tissue being treated. The therapist must continually monitor and reexamine the patient to ensure that the thermal agent selected is appropriate and that the treatment outcomes are being achieved.

Thermal agents can be classified as those that provide superficial heat, deep heat, or cold. Superficial heat modalities create an increase in blood flow to cutaneous tissue close to the surface of the skin and are effective in reducing pain and stiffness, increasing range of motion, and promoting healing.[9] Examples of superficial heat agents include hot packs, paraffin, fluidotherapy, and whirlpools.

A **hot pack** is a pouch available in various shapes that is filled with silica gel and soaked in thermostatically controlled water (Figure 9-9). Hot packs are applied to the affected body part with layers of towels to prevent overheating (see Figure 2-11). **Paraffin treatment** involves dipping a patient's involved extremity (usually hands or feet) into a mixture of melted paraffin wax and mineral oil that is maintained at a temperature of approximately 135° F (Figure 9-10). The heat from the paraffin produces the relaxing and pain-reducing effects of other superficial heat treatments and leaves the skin feeling warm and soft, which increases comfort when ROM exercises are performed.

Fluidotherapy is the use of a self-contained unit filled with corncobs finely chopped into a sawdust-type substance. The particles are heated to the desired temperature and circulated by air pressure around the involved body part. In addition to receiving the effects of heating, the patient can exercise while the treatment is in progress. Use of the therapeutic effects of water is known as **hydrotherapy.** A **whirlpool** can be used when the body part or entire body is immersed in a tank of water. A variety of sizes of tanks are available, ranging from a small tank for the distal ends of extremities to a full-body tank known as a Hubbard tank. In addition to its heating effects, hydrotherapy can assist with wound healing.

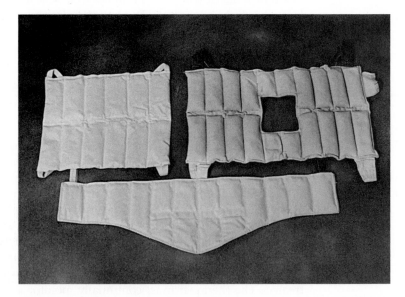

Figure 9-9 ■ Variety of hot packs to apply superficial heat to different body areas. (Courtesy of Dewey Neild.)

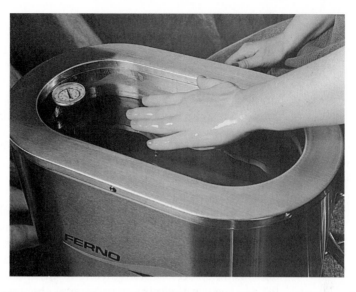

Figure 9-10 ■ Paraffin tank to apply paraffin to a hand. (Courtesy of Dewey Neild.)

Deep heat modalities produce physiological effects similar to those of superficial heat agents, but at a greater tissue depth. Therefore patients with deep muscle or joint dysfunction may receive more therapeutic benefit from the application of deep heat than from a superficial heating agent. Deep heat modalities include ultrasound and short-wave diathermy. Thermal **ultrasound** is the therapeutic application of high-frequency sound waves that penetrate tissue and increase tissue temperature to promote healing and reduce pain (Figure 9-11). Similar results are achieved with **short-wave diathermy,**

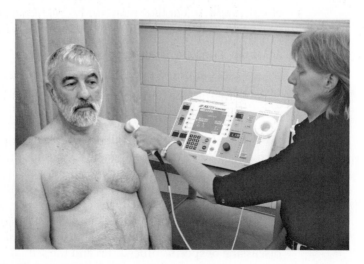

Figure 9-11 ■ Application of ultrasound to produce deep heat in the shoulder region. (Courtesy of Dewey Neild.)

which is the use of electromagnetic energy to produce deep therapeutic heating effects.

In contrast to heating agents, therapeutic cold **(cryotherapy)** may be applied to decrease tissue temperature. Temperature differences produced by the application of cold agents cause a decrease in blood flow and metabolism, which results in a decrease in swelling and pain. Cold is the physical agent of choice for patients who have acute injuries with clinical symptoms of swelling or pain or both (see Figure 2-12). Cold may also be incorporated into a treatment protocol after exercise to help reduce postexercise soreness. Cryotherapy may take the form of commercial cold packs, ice massage, cold whirlpool, or cold used in conjunction with compression.

Electrical Stimulation. PTs and PTAs may use **electrical stimulation** as part of their plan of care to achieve therapeutic results. With the use of electrical stimulation units, electrodes are placed on the skin at specified locations to stimulate nerves, muscles, and other soft tissues in an attempt to reduce pain and swelling, increase strength and ROM, and facilitate wound healing (Figure 9-12).[10] The use of electricity to generate therapeutic benefits is not new, but the numerous electrotherapy devices on the market can make selection of the appropriate device confusing. The therapist must have a clear understanding of the desired effects from the electrical stimulation intervention and have knowledge of the appropriate parameters to use with regard to treatment intensity, voltage, and current type. Common electrotherapy applications are listed in Table 9-2.

Other Physical Agents. Additional physical agents that may be used in the treatment of patients with musculoskeletal dysfunction include mechanical traction, hyperbaric oxygen, biofeedback, laser, and ultraviolet treatment. These modalities achieve therapeutic benefit through mechanisms different from those of thermal or electrical agents, but they may also be used to decrease a patient's pain, promote healing, or improve strength or motion in an attempt to maximize function.

MANUAL THERAPY TECHNIQUES

PTs working with patients who have musculoskeletal dysfunction always have two tools at their ready disposal—their hands. Perhaps in no other patient population is touch so important as it is in the orthopaedic population. Whether palpating a structure during an examination, providing manual force for a patient to resist against when exercising, or performing a mobilization to increase ROM, a therapist's hands are important therapeutic instruments. A variety of manual techniques are currently being used by orthopaedic PTs, and many of these techniques are the subject of clinical research to validate and clarify their purpose and clinical efficacy.

For the purpose of this text, manual techniques are divided into two categories: soft tissue mobilization and joint mobilization and manipulation. A discussion of specific procedures and the schools of thought behind the various techniques is beyond the scope of this text. The reading list at the end of this chapter provides further information regarding this topic.

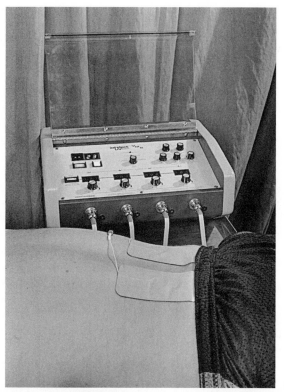

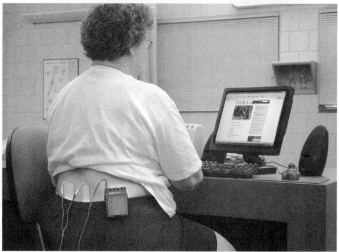

***Figure* 9-12** ■ Use of transcutaneous electrical nerve stimulation (TENS) for the treatment of pain in the low back region. **A,** Clinical unit. **B,** Portable unit. (Courtesy of Dewey Neild.)

Soft Tissue Mobilization. **Soft tissue mobilization** includes a variety of "hands-on" techniques designed to improve movement and function. The techniques are designed to decrease pain or swelling and relax muscle or fascia tension to create proper postural alignment and optimal muscle function.

Two common forms of soft tissue mobilization are massage and myofascial release. **Massage** involves the systematic use of various manual strokes to produce certain physiological, mechanical, and psychological effects. Swedish massage strokes promote relaxation by decreasing pain or swelling, relieving tension, and improving the metabolism of surrounding tissue. More vigorous massage strokes may be used before physical activity to stimulate and prepare the muscles for exertion. Another soft tissue technique known as transverse friction massage is useful for improving the flexibility and function of soft tissues such as muscles, ligaments, and tendons.[11]

Myofascial release involves manual stretching of the layers of the body's fascia, which is connective tissue that surrounds muscle and other soft tissue in the body (see Figure 2-9).[12] Myofascial release techniques are thought to soften and loosen restrictions in muscles and fascia that are limiting normal movement. These techniques are unique in that the stretching force applied by the therapist depends on the response of the patient's tissues to the stretch. The therapist must be able to "feel" fascial tension diminish as stretch is applied and adjust the amount of stretch to the patient's comfort.

Joint Mobilization and Manipulation. In contrast to soft tissue mobilization, which focuses on stretching or relaxing soft tissue, **joint mobilization and manipulation** techniques are used when a patient's dysfunction is the result of joint stiffness or hypomobility (limited motion). Based on knowledge of the anatomy of joint surfaces and the findings from joint examination, the therapist applies specific passive movements to a joint, in either an oscillatory (rapid, repeated movements) or sustained manner. Joint mobilization techniques are intended to reduce the pain and stiffness affecting movement and restore normal joint motion.

THERAPEUTIC EXERCISE

Therapeutic exercise forms the core of most rehabilitation programs.[13] This foundation is based on scientific principles and the knowledge that the human body has the ability to react and respond to physical stresses placed on it. In particular, the muscular and cardiovascular systems are adaptable, depending on the stresses and forces placed on them. When these systems are stressed with a program of progressive exercise, positive changes such as improvement in strength and endurance occur. Similarly, the effects of abnormal stresses, such as prolonged bed rest, can lead to detrimental changes, including osteoporosis and muscle atrophy.[2]

The goals of therapeutic exercise are not only to facilitate and restore normal function in an individual, but also to prevent an initial injury, educate the patient on how to prevent recurrence of an injury, and help maintain normal function. These goals are based on the results of the patient's examination and assessment of needs.

The level of sophistication of an exercise program should not be determined by the type of equipment the clinic has. Some of the most sophisticated exercises can be performed with inexpensive equipment. With creativity, various pieces of equipment can be adapted to incorporate many of the goals of therapeutic exercise. This section describes a variety of therapeutic exercise techniques that may be used with a patient who has a musculoskeletal dysfunction. These techniques include exercises to improve ROM, strength, flexibility, balance and coordination, cardiovascular endurance, and function.

Range-of-Motion Exercise. As mentioned earlier in the chapter, **range-of-motion exercise** can be categorized into two types: passive and active. PROM may be provided manually by the therapist or mechanically by a machine. This type of exercise might be used with (but is not limited to) patients who are restricted to bed rest, have paralysis of one or more limbs, or are in a coma. It may also be used when AROM is contraindicated. AROM can be subdivided into active assisted movement, active free movement, and active resisted movement. When performing **active assisted range of motion,** the patient may be assisted either manually or mechanically if the prime muscle mover is weak (Figure 9-13, *A*). Pendulum exercises in which the patient does not receive any support or resistance are an example of **active free range of motion** (Figure 9-13, *B*). In **active resisted exercises** an external force resists the movement. The last category includes a variety of techniques, several of which are described in the next section.

Resisted Exercise. **Resisted exercise** is a form of active movement in which some form of resistance is provided. The goals of a resisted exercise program are to increase muscular strength and endurance. **Muscular strength** refers to the maximal amount of tension an individual can produce in one repetition. **Muscle endurance** refers to the ability to produce and sustain tension over a prolonged period. If the goal is to increase strength, the program would concentrate on low repetitions with heavy resistance. If the goal is to increase endurance, the exercise program would concentrate on using low resistance for high repetitions. The type of exercise performed depends on the types of activities to which the patient is planning to return. When designing a program, the therapist must consider the type or types of resisted exercise on which the patient should concentrate. Resisted exercise can be categorized into three types: isometric, isotonic, and isokinetic. Definitions and examples of these types are outlined in Table 9-3. Typically, a combination of all three types of exercise is necessary to perform any type of functional activity.

In resisted exercise, resistance can be applied either manually by the therapist or mechanically by the use of equipment. Manual resistance can be applied to isolated muscle groups (as is the case with MMT positions) or to patterns of movement that involve several muscle groups. An example of the latter is a technique called proprioceptive neuromuscular facilitation, which is described in Chapter 10. The use of manual resistance offers many advantages, the primary one being that the therapist can control the amount of resistance provided. This advantage is particularly useful when working with patients in

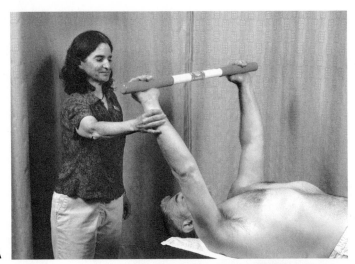

A

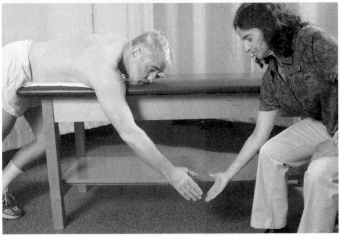

B

Figure 9-13 ■ Range-of-motion exercises are used to maintain or improve joint motion. **A,** Rod can be used to conduct simple active assistive range-of-motion exercises for the shoulder. **B,** Pendulum exercises are effective active free exercises and require no special equipment. (Courtesy of Dewey Neild.)

the early stages of rehabilitation when ROM may need to be limited or the patient can tolerate only mild to moderate resistance. The disadvantage of manual resistance is the difficulty in quantifying the amount of resistance provided. Inability to accurately document the resistance makes it difficult for another therapist to replicate the same force on that patient.

Many pieces of equipment can be used when applying mechanical resistance, from an inexpensive strip of elastic tubing (Figure 9-14, *A*) to expensive and highly technological isokinetic equipment (Figure 9-14, *B*). Other common and frequently used equipment in the clinic includes free weights (Figure 9-14, *C*), exercise machines, and pulley systems.

Table 9-3
Classification of Resisted Exercises

Type of Exercise	Definition	Example
Isometric	Muscle contraction without visible joint movement	Pushing against a wall
Isotonic concentric	Muscle contraction that produces or controls joint motion, resulting in muscle *shortening*	Flexing elbow with dumbbell in hand (biceps brachii muscle)
Isotonic eccentric	Muscle contraction that produces or controls joint motion, resulting in muscle *lengthening*	Extending elbow with dumbbell in hand (biceps brachii muscle)
Isokinetic	A concentric or eccentric muscle contraction that occurs at a constant speed	Knee extensions using an isokinetic device

Flexibility Exercise. Patients recovering from a musculoskeletal injury frequently have decreased flexibility in the muscles crossing the involved joint. Conditions that may produce decreased flexibility include prolonged immobilization and tissue trauma. Many times, prior limitations in flexibility contributed to or were the primary cause of the injury. Therefore **flexibility exercise** is an important component to address with the patient.

Soft tissue, such as muscle, has the ability to change length or adapt over time with stress. Although a variety of techniques can be used to increase flexibility, no consensus has been reached on the most effective way to stretch. Furthermore, a stretching technique that works well for one patient may be ineffective for another.

Stretching techniques can be performed passively with an external force applied either manually or mechanically. Stretching can also be performed by actively inhibiting the shortened muscle. This technique, called contract-relax, requires that the shortened muscle actively contract before a stretching force is applied.

Balance and Coordination Exercise. **Proprioception** is a term used to describe one's awareness of position and movement. The body is made aware of proprioception through various receptors found in the skin and joints. These **proprioceptors** respond to stimuli such as pressure, stretch, and position. After injury, particularly to the knee and ankle, proprioception may be reduced, leading to loss of balance and coordination. Unfortunately, the paucity of well-documented tests to examine balance in patients with orthopaedic dysfunction makes it difficult to monitor changes in balance in a rehabilitation program; however, numerous exercises and equipment can be used to facilitate proper balance. One popular piece of equipment seen in the clinic is a balance board (Figure 9-15). The patient progresses from a sitting to a standing position

9

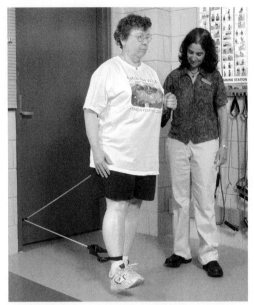

A

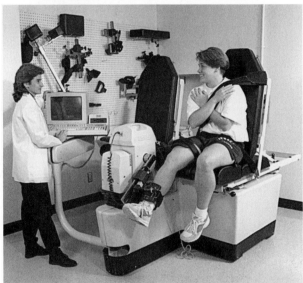

B

Figure 9-14 ■ Different methods of using mechanical resistance for exercise. **A,** Elastic tubing is inexpensive and easy to use. **B,** Isokinetic equipment is generally expensive and sophisticated. (Courtesy of Dewey Neild.)

Continued

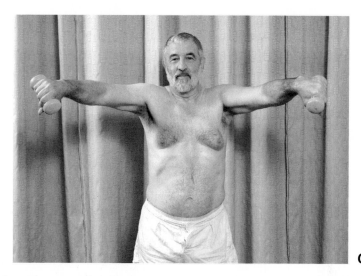

C

Figure **9-14,** *cont'd* ■ Different methods of using mechanical resistance for exercise. **C,** Free weights are readily available to produce mechanical resistance. (Courtesy of Dewey Neild.)

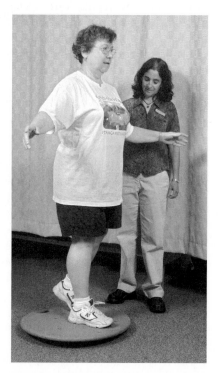

Figure **9-15** ■ Balance board can be used for balance exercises. (Courtesy of Dewey Neild.)

9

while shifting weight from side to side and front to back. This exercise can also be progressed from two-legged weight shift to one-legged weight shift (balancing on one leg). The exercise can be made more challenging by having patients close their eyes and incorporating upper extremity movement with and without weights.

Cardiovascular Endurance Training. Cardiovascular or **aerobics training** refers to exercise performed over a long period at low intensity. Aerobic exercise typically involves large muscle groups used in a rhythmic type of activity. Many modes of exercise are available to improve cardiovascular endurance, including walking, running, stair climbing, cycling, cross-country skiing, and swimming. The PT will choose the most appropriate exercise modality for the patient. For example, a patient who is recovering from a low back injury and has difficulty sitting may participate in a walking program rather than a cycling program. See Chapter 11 for a more detailed description of cardiovascular exercise.

Functional Exercises. As mentioned earlier in this chapter, the ultimate goal in physical therapy is to allow the patient to return to the previous level of function or highest level of function achievable. Therefore exercises mimicking functional movements and activities must be incorporated into the rehabilitation program. A **functional exercise** incorporates strength, flexibility, balance, and coordination. Incorporating all these factors allows patients to return to function with confidence because they know that they performed the same or similar exercises in the clinic.

The use of closed kinetic chain exercises allows the patient to incorporate these functional movements. A **closed kinetic chain exercise** is an exercise in which movement at one joint affects movement at other joints (e.g., a two-legged squat). An **open kinetic chain exercise** is an exercise in which the end limb segment is free (e.g., biceps curl). Many of the exercises traditionally used to strengthen the lower extremity are those in which the foot is off the ground. An example is the use of isokinetic equipment for thigh strengthening; since the lower extremity typically functions with the foot on the ground, however, closed chain exercises are particularly important in the rehabilitation of the lower extremity. Therefore exercises involving the movement of joints while the foot is on the ground facilitate proper proprioceptive feedback that mimics function (Figure 9-16). Closed kinetic chain exercises are also used with patients with upper extremity injuries, particularly those with shoulder dysfunctions.

Aquatic Therapy. The use of water for therapeutic benefit dates back to the ancient Greeks and Romans, who used therapeutic baths for relaxation and pain reduction.[14] "Pool therapy" developed in the 1920s in the United States as part of the rehabilitation program for children with poliomyelitis (see Figure 1-4). As polio declined with the introduction of vaccines, so did the therapeutic use of pools. Recently, however, **aquatic physical therapy** has been shown to be beneficial for a variety of orthopaedic dysfunctions. The

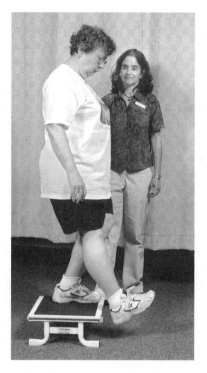

Figure 9-16 ■ Functional exercises, such as descending a step, are designed to mimic daily activities. (Courtesy of Dewey Neild.)

popularity of aquatic therapy has grown significantly, and in 1992, the APTA established the Aquatic Physical Therapy Section.

The Aquatic Physical Therapy Section offers a comprehensive description of this form of therapy (Box 9-3).[15] The description indicates that this form of rehabilitation is effective for a variety of conditions, in addition to maintaining health and fitness in well individuals. As the description indicates, aquatic therapy is a specific intervention that requires the expertise and supervision of a trained specialist to be safe and effective.

Although general exercises and manual techniques may be performed in the water, highly specific techniques have also been developed. In the **Bad Ragaz method**[16] the therapist uses proprioceptive neuromuscular facilitation techniques while the patient is suspended by rings in the water (see Chapter 10 for a description of proprioceptive neuromuscular facilitation). The **Halliwick method**[17] uses a preswim stroke instruction and musculoskeletal rehabilitation. Therapists may also use other exercise techniques or treatment approaches such as Tai Chi or Shiatsu in the water to combine their therapeutic benefits with the effectiveness of the water environment.

The beneficial effects of aquatic therapy depend largely on the fundamental principles of physics, such as the buoyancy, viscosity, and hydrostatic pressure of water. Both physiological and psychological benefits are derived from aquatic physical therapy. The physiological benefits include improved cardiovascular status, increased muscle strength and flexibility, decreased pain, and improved balance without the impact that occurs with exercises on land.

9

BOX 9-3 | Description of Aquatic Therapy

Aquatic physical therapy is the practice of physical therapy by a trained and licensed physical therapist or physical therapy assistant within the environment of a water-filled pool. The buoyancy, support, and accommodating resistance of water enhance exercise and create a safe environment for progressive rehabilitation. The temperature of water (warm or cold) prompts muscle relaxation, facilitates stretching, and generally reduces the sensation of pain.

Treatment sessions conducted by a trained and licensed physical therapist or physical therapy assistant are designed to: improve circulation, strength and endurance, balance and coordination; increase range of motion; decrease tissue swelling; normalize muscle tone; protect joints during exercise; and reduce stress.

Typical problems and conditions that can be treated effectively through aquatic physical therapy techniques are injuries to the neck, shoulder, low back, knee and ankle; chronic pain; arthritis; fibromyalgia; neurological disorders, and conditions limiting the body's ability to bear weight

From APTA Aquatic Physical Therapy Section Purpose Statement. Alexandria, VA, American Physical Therapy Association, 2004.

BOX 9-4 | Precautions and Contraindications to Aquatic Therapy

- Fevers, infections, rashes
- Cardiac history
- Incontinence without protection
- Open wounds without appropriate dressings
- Fear of water
- Limited lung capacity
- Unstable cardiac condition

Modified from Hall CM, Brody LT: Therapeutic Exercise: Movement Towards Function, ed 2. Baltimore, Lippincott Williams & Wilkins, 2005.

Psychological benefits include general relaxation from the warmth of the water, the socialization process that may be associated with group sessions in a pool, and the increased patient confidence and level of satisfaction that accompany patient performance.

Certain contraindications and precautions must be considered when planning and implementing any aquatic therapy session (Box 9-4). These contraindications and precautions must be carefully considered to ensure the safety of the individual.

HOME EXERCISE PROGRAMS

The use of therapeutic exercise in a rehabilitation program is an important component of the physical therapy plan of care. Aside from the physical benefits derived from exercise, it also encourages active participation in the rehabilitative process and allows patients to assume some responsibility for their care. Home exercise programs are an important aspect of patient care. Performing exercises in the clinic two or three times per week is not usually adequate to achieve the desired long-lasting effects of rehabilitation, so home exercises given by the PT become an important component of physical therapy.

PATIENT EDUCATION

As mentioned earlier in the chapter, communication is a critical component of the orthopaedic physical therapy experience. The therapist's depth of knowledge and effectiveness in performing and interpreting the evaluation and the variety of treatment options available are of little value if the therapist does not share this information with patients and inform them of their role in the rehabilitation process. The patient and therapist must work as a team and focus on common goals and sharing of information to achieve optimal results.

The PT and PTA are responsible for educating the patient about exercises to perform at home, postures or positions to avoid during daily activities at work or home, and strategies to prevent the dysfunction from recurring (Figure 9-17).

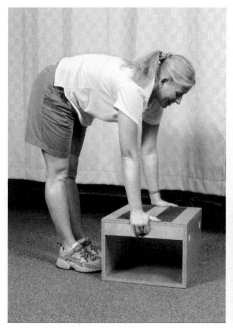
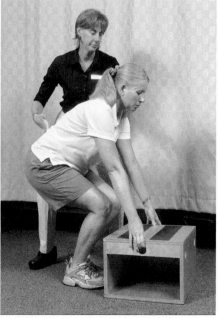

A   B

Figure 9-17 ■ Patient education is essential to rectify improper habits regarding body movement and posture. **A,** Improper lifting can result in straining lower back muscles and ligaments. **B,** Instruction in proper lifting techniques can prevent injuries to the back. (Courtesy of Dewey Neild.)

To communicate effectively, the therapist must create a treatment atmosphere that ensures the patient's comfort and must also provide the necessary information in a clear, easily understood manner.

It is important for the PT and PTA, when working with a patient, to treat the whole person rather than just an injured joint. Each patient comes to physical therapy with a different set of values, expectations, and background. All these factors must be considered to successfully and effectively treat a patient.

SUMMARY

This chapter has presented the role that PTs and PTAs play in physical therapy for musculoskeletal conditions. Common conditions described were overuse and traumatic injuries and surgical and medical conditions. Components of the patient examination were presented. Interventions focused on physical agents, manual techniques, therapeutic exercise, home programs, and patient education. The emphasis in physical therapy for musculoskeletal conditions is on evaluating a patient's function and developing a treatment program that will assist the patient to return to optimal function in the environment, whether that be the athletic field, work site, community, or home.

CASE STUDIES

CASE STUDY ONE

Examination

History: Jack, a 36-year-old English-speaking male, is married and has a 2-year-old child. As an architect, he sits at a computer approximately 5 hours per day and drives 1 hour each way to work. His chief complaint is left-sided lower back pain that spreads into the buttock region and occasionally down the back of the thigh. Symptoms came on suddenly approximately 2 weeks ago after he bent down to pick up house keys; Jack had difficulty standing back up because of pain. He saw a physician, who recommended a course of muscle relaxants and physical therapy. Jack says that the pain has gradually improved since its onset and rates the pain level a "4" on a scale of 1 to 10. The pain worsens when he lifts his daughter from the floor and with prolonged periods of sitting. Symptoms improve with walking. Jack has no complaints of numbness or tingling in the lower extremity but is currently unable to sit for more than 20 minutes without the onset of pain. Radiographs taken 1 week ago were "normal," according to Jack. He has a history of occasional low back discomfort after prolonged sitting, but no previous history of this type of pain. His medical-surgical history and family history are unremarkable. Jack is sedentary but enjoys occasional weekend recreational activities.

Systems Review: Cardiopulmonary examination: blood pressure 136/88 mm Hg and resting heart rate 86 beats per minute. The patient's integumentary system is unremarkable, and he has full ROM of the lower extremity. See below for detailed examination of the lumbar spine. Neuromuscular evaluation shows normal movement patterns of the lower extremities.

Tests and Measures: In tests of gait, locomotion, and balance, gait appears normal with equal weight bearing. In joint integrity and mobility testing, no swelling or temperature changes are noted over the lumbar erectors. Increased tone is seen bilaterally in the spinal muscles. Muscle performance testing finds the lower extremity to be within normal limits; however, the trunk muscles were not tested because of pain. A straight leg raise reproduces the thigh pain at 40 degrees. In standing posture, Jack has a posterior pelvic tilt with a slight lateral shift to the right, a forward head, and rounded shoulders. ROM testing demonstrates lumbar spine movements to be significantly limited in all directions; the chief complaint is exacerbated with flexion movements. Pain centralizes with lumbar extension in the prone position. Regarding sensory integrity, the lower extremity is intact to light touch bilaterally. Testing of reflex integrity reveals deep tendon reflexes (DTRs) of 2 in the left extremity throughout (within a range of 0 to 4) and symmetrical.

Evaluation
The evaluation of Jack's dysfunction is low back pain peripheralizing to the left side with signs and symptoms indicative of low back derangement. Impairments include increased muscle tone of the lumbar erectors, pain with straight leg raise, poor posture, and decreased lumbar ROM. Functional limitations include a decreased ability to sit for prolonged periods. Disabilities include an inability to complete job tasks in a timely fashion because of a decreased ability to sit and inability to participate in recreational activities.

Diagnosis
The patient presents with impairments in joint mobility, motor function, muscle performance, ROM, and reflex integrity secondary to intervertebral disc disorder. (Practice Pattern 4G: Impaired Joint Mobility, Motor Function, Muscle Performance, Range of Motion, Reflex Integrity Secondary to Spinal Disorders)

Prognosis/Expected Range of Visits
Over the course of 4 to 8 weeks, Jack will return to his premorbid level of function with a minimal increase in symptoms. He is to be seen for 8 to 12 visits over the course of 3 months.

Short-Term Goals (2-4 Weeks)
The following short-term goals are set: (1) pain reduced to 1 to 2 (out of 10), (2) abolishment of lateral shift, (3) 50% increase in all lumbar movements, (4) independence in a home exercise program, and (5) ability to demonstrate proper sitting posture throughout the treatment session.

Long-Term Goals/Outcomes (6-8 Weeks)
For the long term, Jack's goals and outcomes are threefold: (1) functional limitations/disabilities—Jack should be able to sit for prolonged periods (up to 6 hours with breaks every hour) without symptoms, as well as return to leisure and recreational activities without symptoms; (2) patient satisfaction—services provided by the PT are deemed acceptable by the patient; and (3) secondary prevention—the risk of impairment, functional limitation, and disability is reduced through adherence to an independent exercise program, and Jack understands and demonstrates strategies to prevent the recurrence of symptoms.

9

Plan of Care/Intervention

Jack's home exercise program will begin with lumbar extension exercises and progress to flexion exercises. He will be educated on proper sitting posture and body mechanics, including lifting techniques. Modalities (ultrasound, hot packs) and manual techniques (joint mobilization, soft tissue massage) are to be used as appropriate for pain relief. As pain resolves, exercises will increase to include functional movements, flexibility exercises, spinal stabilization exercises, and cardiovascular fitness training. The importance of adhering to the home exercise program will be explained. Work site analysis will be performed, followed by recommendations to improve Jack's computer workstation.

Outcomes/Patient Status at Discharge

After 6 weeks of physical therapy, Jack was free of symptoms and all goals had been met. He was discharged with a comprehensive home exercise program. A recommendation was made to initiate a general fitness program at the local health club.

CASE STUDY TWO

Examination

History: Alice, a 72-year-old widow and retired schoolteacher, lives alone. She is right hand dominant. Alice sustained a fractured right radius after slipping on ice 8 weeks ago. She was immobilized in a hand-to-midhumeral cast with her elbow positioned in 90 degrees of flexion and her arm supported in a sling for comfort. The cast was removed yesterday. Her chief complaints are stiffness and weakness throughout the upper extremity and an inability to perform daily activities such as getting dressed and preparing meals. Radiographs taken yesterday reveal "healing without complications." Alice has no past history of the current condition, and her medical and surgical history is unremarkable; she is in generally good health. Her family history is unremarkable. Regarding social habits, Alice walks 1 to 2 miles a day and enjoys cooking, gardening, and the outdoors.

Systems Review: Cardiopulmonary evaluation reveals a blood pressure of 140/90 mm Hg and a resting heart rate of 80 beats per minute. Integumentary examination reveals dry skin over the area covered by the cast. Musculoskeletal assessment discloses full ROM of left upper extremity movements and good range of strength in the left arm. See below for details of the right upper extremity. Neuromuscular evaluation of the left upper extremity reveals normal movement patterns.

Tests and Measures: Joint integrity and mobility testing demonstrates swelling over the dorsal aspect of the right wrist. In muscle performance testing, resisted tests reveal weakness in the following muscle groups: right shoulder abductors and external rotators, elbow flexors and extensors, and wrist flexors and extensors. Manual muscle tests reveal the following (see Table 9-1 for descriptions of grades; grades are based on a scale of 0 to 5):

Right biceps = 4–/5   Left biceps = 5/5
Right triceps = 3+/5   Left triceps = 5/5
Right hand grip = 15 lb   Left hand grip = 25 lb

Testing for pain reveals pain with movement of the right upper extremity. Alice's standing posture is with the head slightly forward and the shoulders rounded, and she holds her arm in a guarded position against her body. Muscle atrophy is noted throughout the upper extremity. ROM testing demonstrates limited and painful active movements of the right shoulder, elbow, and wrist. AROM of the right hand is within normal limits. PROM of the right upper extremity is as follows:

Shoulder: Flexion = 0-160 degrees
Abduction = 0-60 degrees
External rotation = 0-15 degrees
Internal rotation = 0-70 degrees
Elbow: Unable to extend past 60 degrees of flexion
Wrist: Flexion = 0-45 degrees
Extension = 0-45 degrees

Accessory motion is decreased at the right glenohumeral joint. Sensory integrity testing reveals the upper extremity to be intact to light touch bilaterally. In reflex integrity, Alice has upper extremity DTRs of 3 throughout (within a range of 0 to 4) and symmetrical.

Evaluation

Alice has decreased ROM and strength secondary to immobilization after a wrist fracture. Impairments include swelling, decreased upper extremity strength, decreased upper extremity ROM, poor posture, and decreased accessory movement at the shoulder. Her functional limitation is a decreased ability to perform ADLs. Regarding disabilities, Alice is unable to participate in leisure activities, including cooking and gardening.

Diagnosis

The patient presents with impairments in joint mobility, muscle performance, and ROM secondary to immobilization following a Colles fracture (Practice Pattern 4G: Impaired Joint Mobility, Muscle Performance, and Range of Motion Associated with Fracture)

Prognosis/Expected Range of Visits

Over the course of 8 to 12 weeks, Alice will return to her premorbid level of function with minimal limitation. She is to be seen for 6 to 18 visits over the course of 3 months.

Short-Term Goals (2-4 Weeks)

Alice's short-term goals are as follows: (1) decrease swelling by 25%, (2) increase upper extremity strength to the next higher grade, (3) increase right grip strength to 18 lb, (4) increase ROM by 5 to 10 degrees in all limited movements, (5) increase accessory motion to nearly full range, (6) be able to demonstrate proper cervical and shoulder posture, and (7) demonstrate independence in her home exercise program.

Long-Term Goals/Outcomes (10-12 Weeks)

Alice's long-term goals and outcomes are threefold: (1) functional limitations/disabilities—Alice should be able to perform all ADLs independently and to return to all leisure activities; (2) patient satisfaction—services provided by the PT

9

are deemed acceptable by Alice; and (3) secondary prevention—the risk of impairment, functional limitation, and disability is reduced through adherence to an independent exercise program, and Alice should understand the importance of good posture as it relates to the shoulder.

Plan of Care/Intervention

Alice's home exercise program will progressively increase to enhance elbow and wrist ROM and strength. The program will include active assisted, active free, and active resisted exercises such as pendulum, pulley, and cane exercises (Figure 9-13). Alice will be educated on proper sitting posture and the relationship between proper posture and shoulder mechanics. Modalities (superficial heat) and manual techniques (joint mobilization) will be used as appropriate. Proprioceptive neuromuscular facilitation patterns will be incorporated to improve functional movements. As strength and ROM increase, simulated ADLs will be added to the treatment program.

Outcomes/Patient Status at Discharge

After 9 weeks of physical therapy, Alice had functional use of her right upper extremity and was able to return to all activities with minimal limitation. She was discharged with a comprehensive exercise program.

CASE STUDY THREE

Examination

History: Megan is a 20 year-old female college student who presents with (L) anterior knee pain. She states the pain has increased gradually over the past month and is aggravated by prolonged sitting in class, walking/running, and stair climbing. She has had to stop her recreational fitness workout of treadmill running and weight lifting because of the pain. She rates her pain as a "2" (scale of 0-10) during normal activities, but it can be "8" after climbing stairs to her dorm room or excessive walking. She denies any injury to the knee but does report having similar symptoms 3 years ago during high school soccer season. At that time she was referred to physical therapy and was instructed in quad-strengthening exercises that helped manage symptoms somewhat. She has recently been examined by the campus sports medicine physician, who referred her to physical therapy at this time. Her past medical and family history is unremarkable with the exception of a recent 10-pound weight gain.

Systems Review: Blood pressure 115/75 mm Hg, resting heart rate 68; integumentary and neuromuscular examination of uninvolved extremities unremarkable.

Tests and Measures: Standing posture exam reveals internally rotated position of (L) femur, and bilateral pes planus (flat feet). Demonstrates full AROM and PROM of both knees, but limited squat because of pain in (L) knee. Muscle performance testing is WNL at both knees, with slight weakness noted in (L) hip abductors. Flexibility testing reveals + Straight Leg Raise and Ober's tests on (L). Patellar orientation reveals a lateral shift and lateral glide both statically and dynamically on the (L). Functional testing with step-downs reveals poor pelvic control and reproduces pain. Score on Lower Extremity Functional Scale = 66/80.

Evaluation

(L) anterior knee due to muscle imbalances and structural malalignment in the (L) lower extremity. Impairments include (L) knee pain, decreased flexibility of hamstrings and iliotibial band, and excessive foot pronation in standing. Functional impairments include difficulty sitting for prolonged periods of time and negotiating stairs due to pain; disabilities include inability to participate in desired fitness program of running and strength training.

Diagnosis

Patient presents with signs and symptoms consistent with patellofemoral pain syndrome (Practice Pattern 4B: Impaired Posture).

Prognosis/Expected Range of Visits

Over the course of 6-8 weeks, this patient will be able to resume her desired level of activity, including running and strength training, with adequate pain management. She will be seen for 8-12 visits.

Short-Term Goals (2-4 weeks)

(1) Decrease pain with walking and stair climbing to 2-3/10, (2) decrease Lower Extremity Functional Scale score to 70/80, (3) independent with hamstring and iliotibial band stretching exercises, (4) increase strength in hip abductors for improved pelvic control during step-down.

Long-Term Goals (6-8 weeks)

(1) Improve lower extremity alignment, (2) improve score on Lower Extremity Functional Scale to 76/80, (3) resume desired level of fitness, including jogging and lower extremity strength training with manageable knee pain, and (4) prevent further episodes of knee pain by adherence to an exercise program that addresses muscle imbalances.

Plan of Care

Instruction in home exercise program, including cardiovascular training beginning with aquatic therapy and progressing to land-based training as tolerated, flexibility exercises, progressive hip and core strengthening and functional exercises using weights, resisted bands, and involving a variety of surfaces including theraballs and foam rollers. Fit for custom orthotics to address overpronation.

Outcomes/Patient Status at Discharge

After 7 weeks of therapy, patient reports minimal symptoms and goals achieved. She is able to demonstrate good pelvic control while doing repeated step-downs without pain, and she reports tolerating a progressive running program with her orthotics, She has been discharged with instructions to continue the prescribed home exercise program and progress running distance and weight with strength training as tolerated.

REFERENCES

1. Moffroid M, Zimny N: Causes of movement dysfunction and physical disability. *In:* Scully RM, Barnes MR (eds): Physical Therapy. Philadelphia, Lippincott, 1989.
2. Bandy W: Functional rehabilitation of the athlete. Orthop Clin North Am 1992;1:269-281.

3. Kendall FP, McCreary EK, Provance PG, et al: Muscle Testing and Function, ed 5. Baltimore, Lippincott Williams & Wilkins, 2005.

4. Sahrmann SA: Diagnosis and Treatment of Movement Impairment Syndromes. St Louis, Mosby, 2002.

5. Barber SD, Noyes FR, Mangine RE, et al: Quantitative assessment of functional limitations in normal and anterior cruciate ligament–deficient knee. Clin Orthop 1990;255:204-214.

6. Gray GW: Team Reaction: Developing the Lower Extremity Functional Profile. Adrian, MI, Wynn Marketing, 1995.

7. Lephart S, Perrin D, Fu F, et al: Relationship between selected physical characteristics and functional capacity in the anterior cruciate ligament–insufficient athlete. J Orthop Sports Phys Ther 1992;16(4):174-181.

8. Reed B, Zarro V: Inflammation and repair and the use of thermal agents. *In:* Michlovitz SL (ed): Thermal Agents in Rehabilitation, ed 2. Philadelphia, FA Davis, 1990.

9. Michlovitz SL: Biophysical principles of heating and superficial heat agents. *In:* Michlovitz SL (ed): Thermal Agents in Rehabilitation, ed 3. Philadelphia, FA Davis, 1996.

10. Robinson AJ, Snyder-Mackler L: Clinical Electrophysiology, Electrotherapy and Electrophysiologic Testing, ed 2. Baltimore, Williams & Wilkins, 1995.

11. Cyriax J: Textbook of Orthopaedic Medicine, vol 1, Diagnosis of Soft Tissue Lesions, ed 8. London, Bailliere Tindall, 1982.

12. Manheim CJ, Lavett DK: The Myofascial Release Manual. Thorofare, NJ, Slack, 1989.

13. Guide to Physical Therapist Practice, revised ed 2. Alexandria, VA, American Physical Therapy Association, 2003.

14. Wynn KE: Lily ponds, warm springs and fortunate accidents. PT—Magazine of Physical Therapy 1994;2(12):44-45.

15. APTA Aquatic Physical Therapy Section Purpose Statement. Alexandria, VA, American Physical Therapy Association, 2004.

16. Garrett G: Bad Ragaz ring method. *In:* Ruoti RG, Morris DM, Cole AJ (eds): Aquatic Rehabilitation. Philadelphia, Lippincott Williams & Wilkins, 1997.

17. Martin J: The Halliwick method. Physiotherapy 1981;67:288-291.

ADDITIONAL RESOURCES

Andrade CK, Clifford P: Outcome-Based Massage, Baltimore, Lippincott Williams & Wilkins, 2001.

Provides theoretical background and comprehensive descriptions of a variety of manual techniques based on desired outcomes.

Andrews JR, Harrelson GL, Wilk KE: Physical Rehabilitation of the Injured Athlete, ed 3. Philadelphia, Saunders, 2004.

Offers a comprehensive, joint by joint approach to the management of athletic injuries. The book provides hundreds of illustrations of common exercises used in this population.

Bates A, Hanson N: Aquatic Exercise Therapy. Philadelphia, Saunders, 1996.

Provides easy-to-understand aquatic exercises referenced by joint and common musculoskeletal disorders.

Edmond S: Manipulation and Mobilization: Extremity and Spinal Techniques. St Louis, Mosby, 1993.

This is a clinically applicable text that describes manual therapy techniques of the extremities and spine.

Evans RC: Illustrated Orthopedic Physical Assessment, ed 2. St Louis, Mosby, 2001.

Hundreds of tests can be used for making conservative care diagnoses of disorders of the nervous and orthopaedic systems. This manual describes them in a clearly illustrated, sequential fashion. Organization of the text is by region and specifically by initial signs, symptoms, and indications.

Brotzman SB, Wilk KE: Clinical Orthopaedic Rehabilitation, ed 2. Philadelphia, Mosby, 2003.

Thorough text on the examination techniques, differential diagnosis, treatment approaches, and intervention options for a variety of musculoskeletal disorders.

Cameron MH: Physical Agents in Rehabilitation: From Research to Practice, ed 2. St Louis, Saunders, 2003.

A comprehensive text on the clinical decision making and practical application of physical agents.

Edmond S: Manipulation and Mobilization: Extremity and Spinal Techniques, St Louis, Mosby, 1993.

Hall CM, Brody LT: Therapeutic Exercises: Moving Toward Function, ed 2. Philadelphia, Lippincott Williams & Wilkins, 2005.

Offers a comprehensive approach to therapeutic exercise, including separate chapters on aquatic physical therapy, proprioceptive neuromuscular functioning, and closed kinetic chain exercise.

Hecox B, Mehreteab TA, Weisberg J, Sanko J: Integrating Physical Agents in Rehabilitation, ed 2. Upper Saddle River, NJ, Pearson/Prentice Hall, 2006.

Current evidence-based information about the theory and practice related to physical agents.

Kendall FP, McCreary EK, Provance PG, et al: Muscle Testing and Function, ed 5. Baltimore, Lippincott Williams & Wilkins, 2005.

The classic text and "gold standard" on manual muscle testing. Includes an anatomy review provided on CD ROM.

Kolt GS, Snyder-Makler L: Physical Therapies in Sport and Exercise. London, Churchill Livingstone, 2003.

A comprehensive text with an emphasis on the rehabilitation and prevention of injuries seen with exercise and sport. Several chapters devoted to special populations, such as children, female athletes, older adults, and athletes with disabilities.

Magee DJ: Orthopedic Physical Assessment, ed 4. Philadelphia, Saunders, 2002.

An excellent text detailing the evaluation of joints, with good descriptions of special tests.

Robinson AJ, Snyder-Mackler L: Clinical Electrophysiology, Electrotherapy and Electrophysiologic Testing, ed 2. Baltimore, Williams & Wilkins, 1995.

Provides basic theoretical background and clinical applications for electrotherapy based on desired therapeutic outcomes.

REVIEW QUESTIONS

1. What is the difference between active ROM and passive ROM?
2. Without looking at the text, how many questions can you come up with that may be helpful in a patient interview?
3. How would quantitative and qualitative measurements fit into the "SOAP" note?
4. Research some physical therapy books in your school's library to find examples of resisted tests and manual muscle testing. What, in your observation, is the main difference?
5. Try the following study technique: Photocopy Table 9-2 and block out the second column ("Physical Agents") with a folded strip of paper. Can you fill in the applicable agents? Repeat this exercise by filling out column 3 ("Physiological Effects") or column 4 ("Clinical Indications"). Performing this exercise will reinforce the uses and effects of physical agents.
6. Describe the difference in purpose between exercising for muscular strength and exercising for muscular endurance.
7. Explain the difference between open and closed kinetic chain exercises.

9

A *sense of history and an appreciation of why things happened can provide a perspective in understanding the present and in projecting the future.*

Lucy Blair, PT

10 Physical Therapy for Neuromuscular Conditions

Shree Pandya

KEY TERMS

akinesia
amyotrophic lateral sclerosis (ALS)
angiography
bradykinesia
Brunnstrom's approach
computed (axial) tomography (CAT or CT)
electroencephalography (EEG)
electromyography (EMG)
expressive aphasia
hypertonia
hypotonia
lumbar puncture (LP)
magnetic resonance imaging (MRI)
motor control
motor development
motor learning
multiple sclerosis (MS)
nerve conduction velocity (NCV) study

neurodevelopmental treatment (NDT)
paraplegia
Parkinson's disease
perception
proprioceptive neuromuscular facilitation
   (PNF)
quadriplegia
receptive aphasia
rigidity
Rood's approach
sensation
spinal cord injury (SCI)
stroke or cerebrovascular accident (CVA)
tone
traumatic brain injury (TBI)

tremor
vertigo

OBJECTIVES

After reading this chapter, the reader will be able to:

■ Discuss the role of the physical therapist in the management of patients with neuromuscular disorders
■ Describe some of the common neuromuscular conditions in which physical therapists play an essential role
■ Compare the different roles a therapist may play, depending on the patient's condition and problems

GENERAL DESCRIPTION

At the beginning of the last century one could learn about the human nervous system from autopsy tissue samples only. Today, with new technologies, the brain can be seen in action in living human beings. The 1990s were declared the decade of the brain by the U.S. Congress. During this period, tremendous progress was made in the areas of neuroscience, clinical neurology, and genetics. As the function of the brain and nervous system becomes better understood, physical therapists (PTs) are devising effective new techniques and explaining the reasons for the efficacy of previously developed techniques.

Patients with problems related to disorders of the neuromuscular system make up a large proportion of individuals treated by PTs today. Disorders of the neuromuscular system can be inherited or acquired. Acquired disorders may result from trauma or infection, arise secondary to disorders affecting other body systems, or occur as part of the normal aging process. In addition, many disorders whose causes are still unknown (idiopathic) or not well understood affect the neuromuscular system.

Neuromuscular disorders can affect people at any age. For example, inherited disorders such as Friedreich's ataxia or spinal muscular atrophy are present from birth. Traumatic disorders such as spinal cord injuries or brain injuries are most often caused by motor vehicle accidents and most commonly involve the age range from the teens to the thirties. Disorders such as multiple sclerosis (MS), Parkinson's disease, and Lou Gehrig's disease (amyotrophic lateral sclerosis [ALS]) are manifested most often between the thirties and sixties. The two most common neuromuscular disorders encountered with age are stroke (paralysis secondary to disruption of blood flow within the brain) and Alzheimer's disease. When working with patients with neuromuscular problems, therapists are likely to encounter persons of all ages, either sex, and all races.

Depending on the cause of the disorder, the condition may be lifelong or temporary. It may be reversible, static, or progressive. The patient may go through

10

periods of "plateaus" (i.e., relative stability) interspersed with progression. Because of the lengthy course of most neuromuscular disorders, PTs have extended contact with their patients and play a critical role in their care. Depending on the condition, the stage of illness, and the setting of service delivery, the frequency of intervention will vary. For example, patients may be treated as often as twice a day for an hour each session in the rehabilitation or hospital setting, or two or three times a week if the patient is past the acute stage and is being seen in the home or an extended care facility. If the therapist sees the patient on a consultation basis or for education regarding personal care and management, these visits may be as infrequent as monthly, quarterly, or yearly.

From the description just presented, it is apparent that PTs who work with this population encounter diversity in their clients, work settings, and types of services they provide. This situation is a major change from the early days of physical therapy practice and even from 20 years ago, when PTs practiced under physicians' orders only and followed prescriptions for massage, electrotherapy, thermal agents, hydrotherapy, and exercise. Today, the PT is an autonomous member of the health care team and in most states practices under direct access. As described in the patient/client management model, therapists are involved in examination, evaluation, diagnosis, prognosis, intervention, prevention, education, consultation, coordination, and other related activities (see Chapter 2). The next section provides a brief overview of some common neuromuscular disorders and the role of physical therapy in the care and management of patients with these disorders.

COMMON CONDITIONS

STROKE

Stroke or **cerebrovascular accident (CVA)** refers to neurological problems arising from disruption of blood flow in the brain. This disruption may be caused by hemorrhage (bleeding) or blockage from a clot that results in ischemia (decreased oxygen). The type and severity of symptoms will depend on the area of brain tissue involved. The most common symptom is a complete paralysis or partial weakness on the side opposite the site involved. Depending on the site of the lesion, the paralysis may be accompanied by such symptoms as difficulty speaking or understanding the spoken word, visual problems, and neglect of the affected side. Approximately 30% of patients die during the first month. Of the survivors, approximately 30% to 40% have severe disability.[1] A major psychological problem after stroke is depression, which can have a great impact on management. Recovery from stroke occurs most rapidly during the first 6 months, but functional gains can be seen for 2 years or longer. Currently under investigation are several medications that have thrombolytic properties, such as tissue plasminogen activator (tPA), medications that have neuroprotective properties such as glutamate antagonists, and calcium channel blockers, which have the ability to halt or reverse the cascade of events after ischemia. Some (such as tPA) are effective only if given within the first 3 to 6 hours after the stroke. Hence a key issue is to educate the public regarding the symptoms of a stroke and have them seek immediate attention for this "brain attack," just as they would for a "heart attack."

The purpose of physical therapy is to facilitate and enhance the functional recovery occurring in response to the resolution of neurological changes. Once functional recovery plateaus, the therapist and assistant will teach the patient and family to adapt and compensate for the residual deficits in order to function at the optimal level possible within the constraints of the condition.

Figures 10-1 and 10-2 illustrate the preventive and functional training aspects of management of a patient with left-sided paralysis secondary to stroke.

TRAUMATIC BRAIN INJURY

Traumatic brain injury (TBI) is most often caused by motor vehicle accidents or by falls and violence.[2] Because of the nature of the injury, the brain trauma may be associated with fractures, dislocations, lacerations, and the like. The groups most commonly affected are children (from bicycle accidents) and young adults (from car accidents); traumatic brain injury is the most common cause of death and disability in these age groups. Early management is focused on preservation of life and prevention of further damage. The diffuse nature of the brain injury usually results in problems with multiple brain functions and mechanisms. A complex picture is common, with varying deficits in motor and sensory capabilities, intellectual and cognitive functions, and emotional and psychological functions. Because of the complexity and variability of problems that may be encountered with each patient, management and treatment require an individualized plan and a multidisciplinary team approach in which each member plays a specific and significant role. Currently, not enough data are available on long-term outcomes or valid and reliable measures that may help predict out-

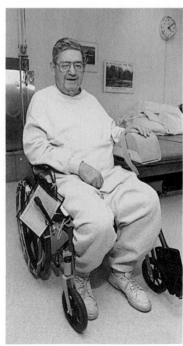

Figure 10-1 ■ Positioning the patient with a stroke to prevent secondary problems in the shoulder and hand on the paralyzed (left) side.

10

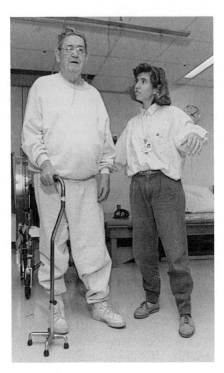

Figure 10-2 ■ Gait training for a patient with left-side paralysis caused by stroke.

comes. This area provides several opportunities for research to answer questions important to patients and their families. TBI is also an area in which prevention through education is crucial. Wearing a helmet when riding a bike and using a seat belt when riding in a car can make the difference between life and death.

SPINAL CORD INJURY

Spinal cord injury (SCI), like TBI, most often results from motor vehicle accidents, falls, violence (especially gunshot wounds), and sports (diving and football). The age group most often affected is between 15 and 25 years of age, and men are affected four times as often as women.[3] Spinal cord damage can also be precipitated by other diseases and conditions, and in these instances older patients are affected more commonly. Depending on the level of injury, all limbs may be affected **(quadriplegia),** or the lower part of the trunk and legs may be affected **(paraplegia).** If the lesion is complete, no residual sensory or motor function can be found below the level of the lesion ("-plegia"). When the cord is partially severed, some distal motor and sensory functions may be preserved ("-paresis").

As with TBI, SCI may be accompanied by multiple injuries, and the early goal of management is preservation of life and prevention of further damage to neural tissue. Further damage is prevented through internal immobilization of the area by fusing the vertebrae with bone grafts, rods, and wires—or externally with devices such as body jackets or casts. Medications are used to prevent further damage to neural tissue and enhance repair and recovery.

While this healing process occurs, it is important to maintain mobility in the joints of the extremities, strength in the unaffected muscles, cardiorespiratory capacity, and endurance. Figure 10-3 illustrates one of the types of body jackets used to provide stability. The patient is working on strengthening the upper extremity and trunk muscles. Once medical and orthopaedic clearance is obtained, more vigorous functional training is begun.

As illustrated in Figures 10-4 and 10-5, the patients are learning mat table–to–wheelchair transfers and wheelchair manipulation skills. Identification of equipment requirements and environmental adaptations is needed for each patient. For example, most patients use a wheelchair as a primary means of

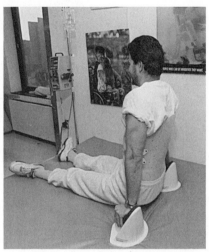

Figure 10-3 ■ Patient with spinal cord injury in a body jacket working on upper body strengthening.

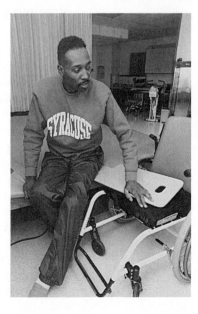

Figure 10-4 ■ Patient with paraplegia working on mat table–to–wheelchair transfers.

10

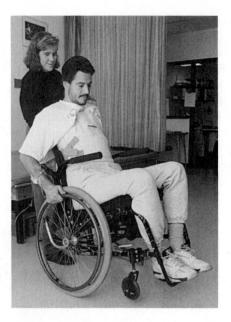

Figure 10-5 ■ Patient with paraplegia working on wheelchair manipulation skills necessary for going up and down curbs.

mobility, and they must be custom ordered for each patient with specific size and adaptation requirements. Figure 10-6 shows a patient with quadriplegia using an electric wheelchair for mobility and a special device that allows him to write. The home will have to be made wheelchair accessible with ramps and other modifications. Thus the therapist plays a major role not only in the treatment, but also in the rehabilitation of patients with SCI by providing family education and consultation on many related issues.

VESTIBULAR DISORDERS

The vestibular system helps detect head position and movement. It consists of two components: (1) the peripheral apparatus, which includes the semicircular canals in the inner ear, and the central component, which includes the vestibular nuclei, and (2) the connections between the peripheral and central components, which include the vestibular nerve, and the central connections between the vestibular nuclei and various brain regions. The vestibular system, in conjunction with other systems, allows us to maintain our orientation in space, control our posture, and maintain our balance. The most common symptoms of vestibular disorders are dizziness, unsteadiness, **vertigo,** and nausea. According to the National Ambulatory Medical Care Survey for 1991,[4] dizziness-vertigo is among the 25 most common reasons Americans visit their doctors. U.S. physicians report a total of more than 5 million dizziness-vertigo visits a year. Vestibular disorders can occur as a result of trauma, infections, toxicity from large doses of antibiotics, and pathological changes underlying other conditions such as multiple sclerosis and stroke.

Over the past two decades, the knowledge and understanding of vestibular function and related disorders have improved tremendously. This has resulted

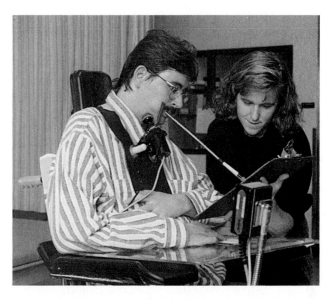

Figure 10-6 ■ Patient with quadriplegia, in a customized electric chair, using a special device that enables him to write.

in better diagnosis based on history, examination, and differential tests to pinpoint the specific disorder and underlying mechanisms. Improved diagnosis allows therapists to better target the treatment, management, and rehabilitation of these patients.

MULTIPLE SCLEROSIS

Multiple sclerosis (MS) is a disease in which patches of demyelination in the nervous system lead to disturbances in the conduction of messages along the nerves. The condition is most often manifested between the ages of 15 and 45 years and affects women more often than men. The specific cause is still unknown. MS can cause a variety of symptoms, depending on the location of the patches of nerve demyelination. Common symptoms include visual problems, sensory problems such as tingling and numbness, weakness, fatigue, problems with balance, and speech disturbances. The course in the early stages is unpredictable. Eventually, the course may take one of four forms[5]: (1) benign, in which the disease seems to go into remission and the patient is relatively symptom free, with no functional disabilities; (2) exacerbating-remitting, in which the patient undergoes periods of worsening followed by periods of improvement; (3) remitting-progressive, which is similar to the exacerbating-remitting form except that improvement after the episode of worsening is not as complete and each occurrence leaves a residual problem or increase in problems that causes general progression of the disease; and (4) progressive, in which the disease progresses unremittingly and causes severe disability.

The role of the therapist with this group of patients is more consultative and educational. Patients may benefit from active treatment during an acute exacer-

10

bation, but otherwise they require periodic evaluation and recommendations because of their changing functional needs.

PARKINSON'S DISEASE

Parkinson's disease is a progressive condition first described by James Parkinson in 1817. It is also referred to as paralysis agitans and idiopathic (cause unknown) parkinsonism and is commonly seen with advancing age. Parkinson's disease is characterized by a classic triad of symptoms.[6] **Tremor** (alternating contractions of opposing muscle groups), usually affecting the hands and feet, tends to occur at rest (i.e., when the part is not being used or moved). **Rigidity,** a disturbance in muscle tone, is manifested as resistance when the limbs are passively moved. **Bradykinesia,** or slowness of movements, or **akinesia,** a poverty of movements, completes the triad.

This condition results from a deficiency in dopamine, a neurotransmitter (chemical messenger) produced in a region of the brain called the substantia nigra. The specific cause of this depletion is unknown. Even though a cure does not yet exist, medications that restore neurochemical balance are available and help alleviate the symptoms. Unfortunately, the effectiveness of the medications diminishes over the years, and the symptoms continue to worsen. Currently, neural cell transplantation is under investigation as an option for a more permanent treatment or cure.

The tremor, rigidity, and bradykinesia have a great impact on the patient's ability to maintain balance and perform such activities as walking, stair climbing, and reaching. Patients tend to have a stooped posture, walk with short, shuffling steps, and lose reciprocal arm movements. The role of the therapist is to educate the patient and family about the secondary problems that result from the basic deficits and teach the patient compensatory strategies to maintain function and prevent or minimize further problems.

AMYOTROPHIC LATERAL SCLEROSIS

Amyotrophic lateral sclerosis (ALS), also known as Lou Gehrig's disease (after the famous baseball player), is a rapidly progressive neurological disorder associated with the degeneration of motor nerve cells. Its cause is unknown. The median age at onset is in the fifties.[7] ALS is characterized by weakness, atrophy (loss of muscle bulk), and fasciculations (muscle twitches). The weakness can be present in limb muscles and cause difficulty in functional activities or can be present in the muscles involved in speech, swallowing, and breathing and cause difficulty in communication, feeding, and respiration. Regardless of where it begins, eventually all muscles are involved. Currently, no cure is available for this disease, and the survival time is about 4 years from diagnosis to death. Riluzole (Rilutek), the only medication that has been shown to slow progression, can extend life by about 3 months.

The role of the therapist is to provide preventive and supportive care for the secondary problems of weakness, recommend appropriate devices and equipment to keep the patient as independent as possible, and educate the family and caregivers regarding handling of the patient. (See also Chapters 13 and 14 for additional neuromuscular conditions common to specific age groups.)

PRINCIPLES OF EXAMINATION

The goal of physical therapy is to improve or maintain functional movements and prevent decline. Functional movements include not only the activities of daily living (dressing, eating, bathing, etc.), but also those necessary for educational, vocational, and recreational purposes. Thus, likely candidates for physical therapy are individuals with disorders of movement or function resulting from involvement of the neuromuscular system.

Assessment of the cause of movement dysfunction requires an examination of the contributing factors, both individually and collectively. Most patients with neurological problems are referred to physical therapy after extensive evaluation by a neurologist, physiatrist, or both. The first step in patient evaluation is to review all the pertinent medical records and data. The therapist will need to make note of not only the current conditions and problems, but also any previous problems or current comorbid conditions that will affect the prognosis. The therapist will also need to note psychological, emotional, and social factors that may have an impact.

Therapists should be familiar with and understand the results and implications of special tests[8] used by physicians to arrive at the medical (etiological or pathological) diagnosis. Some of the tests commonly used include radiography (use of x-rays on photographic film), **computed (axial) tomography (CAT or CT;** computer synthesis of x-rays transmitted through a specific plane of the body), **magnetic resonance imaging (MRI;** creation of computer images by placing the body part in a magnetic field), angiography, lumbar puncture, and electrodiagnostic tests. CT scans and MRIs have become available only during the past two decades as a result of improved (CT) and new (MRI) technologies. They have revolutionized diagnostic capabilities by providing three-dimensional and cross-sectional images of internal structures, including the brain and spinal cord. These tests offer better visualization and differentiation of tissues such as bone, nerve cells, and blood as they relate to the brain and spinal cord. **Angiography** involves injecting radiopaque material into blood vessels to better visualize and identify problems such as occlusion (blockage) of blood vessels, aneurysms, and vascular malformations.

Lumbar puncture (LP) is a procedure used for three main purposes: (1) to measure intracranial pressure, (2) to inject a radiopaque substance for a myelogram, or (3) to obtain a sample of cerebrospinal fluid for examination. The procedure is performed under local anesthesia. A needle is inserted in the space between the L3 and L4 vertebrae until it reaches the subarachnoid space, and then, depending on the purpose of the lumbar puncture, the appropriate procedure is performed. Cerebrospinal fluid is examined for its chemical and cellular content, that is, the specific type and number of cells present. It is also used to identify or obtain bacteriological or viral cultures.

Electrodiagnostic tests are also helpful in identifying the specific neurological disorder. **Electroencephalography (EEG)** involves recording the electrical potential/activity in the brain by placement of electrodes on the scalp. This test is essential in the diagnosis and management of patients with seizure disorders. **Electromyography (EMG)** involves recording the electrical activity in muscle during a state of rest and during voluntary contraction. It helps differentiate

10

disorders primarily related to muscle pathology and those secondary to nerve or neuromuscular junction disorders. A **nerve conduction velocity (NCV) study** involves recording the rate at which electrical signals are transmitted along peripheral nerves. These studies help clarify and differentiate disorders that affect the axons from those that affect the myelin sheath covering the axons. In many cases the PT performs the diagnostic tests, such as EMG or NCV, and provides information directly to the patient.

Knowledge of these tests and the results not only gives the therapist a better understanding of the disorder and its implications and progression, but also enables the therapist to respond appropriately to questions that the patient may have about these procedures.

The next step in the evaluation is an interview with the patient or a family member or caregiver. The interview gives the therapist an opportunity to hear firsthand the sequence of events that brought the patient to therapy. It allows the therapist to ask specific questions that will provide information about the patient's premorbid (predisease) lifestyle and functional level, as well as assess the patient's cognitive and communicative capabilities. The interview also provides the patient and family members with an opportunity to voice concerns and hopes about what the individual wants to achieve through therapy. This interchange between patient and therapist is extremely important in setting realistic short- and long-term goals and expectations. It is a process that will occur periodically as conditions change and goals are met (see also Subjective Examination in Chapter 9).

COGNITION

Functions such as orientation, attentiveness, long- and short-term memory, reasoning, and judgment can be impaired in disorders of the central nervous system and can have a major impact on the patient's ability to function in daily activities and return to school or work. If these impairments are present, they may be more thoroughly evaluated by a neuropsychologist, who can then also act as a resource for other team members regarding strategies to manage the problems. For example, patients with TBI often exhibit behavioral problems. To address these problems successfully, it is important that everyone in contact with the person respond similarly to such behavior and give consistent responses. The specific strategies chosen would be determined by discussion among the team of care providers and the neuropsychologist and would be based on an evaluation and understanding of the underlying phenomena.

COMMUNICATION

Communication is another area that will have a major impact on how the therapist works with the patient. If the patient exhibits a diminished ability to receive and interpret verbal or written communication **(receptive aphasia)** or has an impaired ability to communicate by speech **(expressive aphasia),** the therapist again will have to use specific strategies to work with the patient successfully. For example, when working with patients with receptive aphasia, the therapist may need to physically mime or demonstrate to the patient what is expected or required and to use gestures to augment the words.

The specific components of the physical therapy examination will be determined by various factors such as the current state of the patient, concurrent conditions, mental and emotional status, and age. The examination will include some or all aspects of the components described in the next sections.

FUNCTIONAL ACTIVITIES

The examination may begin with the therapist's asking the patient to demonstrate or describe activities and movements the patient can perform and then describe activities that are difficult or that the patient is unable to perform. The most common activities of daily living involve the ability to move and change positions in bed; to get in and out of bed, a chair, and the like; to stand, walk, and climb stairs; and to get up from the floor in case of a fall. In short, these activities involve the ability to assume and maintain a posture and to function in different positions and environmental conditions. Several components are responsible for the smooth and efficient performance of even the simplest and most routine activities. A problem with even a single component can impair function.

MOTOR CONTROL

The first component to examine in the evaluation of **motor control** is whether the patient is capable of performing voluntary, isolated activity of a specific muscle or whether the patient is capable of performing only movements that are linked together involuntarily. For example, very often in the early stages of recovery after a stroke, a patient is unable to isolate and restrict the activity of bringing the hand to the mouth without the automatic and involuntary activity of raising the shoulder. A second step is to determine whether the patient is able to isolate and *control* specific muscle activity and movements (able to start, stop, reverse, change speed, change direction, regulate force, etc.) and, if so, how well this movement is controlled. A third step is to determine whether the patient exhibits any involuntary movements. Do they occur at rest or with activity? Do the nature and intensity of the involuntary movements change with activity, and are the movements detrimental to the patient's overall functioning? Finally, is the patient exhibiting any reflex reactions caused by damage to specific parts of the nervous system? For example, when damage occurs to the cortex, the patient may exhibit certain reflex reactions that are indicative of control exerted by the brain stem. These automatic reactions will prevent the patient from exerting independent and isolated control and thus affect function (see also Chapter 13).

TONE

Tone is tension exerted or maintained by muscles at rest and during movement. In certain conditions, tone is disturbed and a patient may exhibit **hypotonia** (low tone) or **hypertonia** (high tone). This disturbance in tone may be evident at rest, during activities, or in both conditions. Answers to the following questions are needed before a decision is made regarding interventions: Is the tone disturbance at a level that affects posture and function? What factors seem to increase or decrease it? Does it have a beneficial or detrimental effect on the patient's ability to function?

10

Sensation and Perception

Both sensation and perception are essential for normal movement. **Sensation** is the ability to receive sensory input from within and outside the body and transmit it through the peripheral nerves and tracts in the spinal cord to the brain where it is received and interpreted. Sensory information most essential for movement is visual, vestibular, tactile, and proprioceptive in nature. **Perception** is the ability to both integrate various simultaneous sensory inputs and respond appropriately. It is the ability to respond appropriately that is most often affected in patients with brain lesions, and this has a great impact on movement and function.

Flexibility

Flexibility of the soft tissues, such as muscles and tendons, and alignment and mobility of the joints are important to evaluate. Therapists perform manual tests and use goniometers to help quantify the degree of restriction of movement (see Chapter 9).

Systems Review

The therapist performs a quick check of the other body systems such as the cardiopulmonary system. The purpose of this review is to evaluate the role, if any, that problems in these other systems may be playing in the overall functional limitations of the patient.

PRINCIPLES OF EVALUATION, DIAGNOSIS, AND PROGNOSIS

From the preceding brief descriptions, it is apparent that seemingly simple movements and activities are the result of complex and interconnected mechanisms. Sometimes therapists need several sessions to diagnose the movement disorders and functional limitations and identify the responsible components. Based on the findings of this detailed evaluation, a plan of care can be drawn up to meet the goal of enhancing movement and function.

PRINCIPLES OF DIRECT INTERVENTION

The human nervous system is an incredible system that, because of its plasticity and redundancy, is capable of adaptation and modification after injury or disease. The peripheral nervous system also has the additional capacity of regeneration. Creative treatment approaches are necessary to accommodate these characteristics of the nervous system. This is the challenge and reward of working with patients with neuromuscular disorders.

Early approaches to neurological physical therapy focused on poliomyelitis. This disease causes paralysis of muscles from damage to motor nerve cells. It was one of the conditions responsible for the growth and development of physical therapy in the 1920s and 1930s.[9] As the poliomyelitis epidemics subsided, therapists started working with patients having other neurological conditions, such as stroke and cerebral palsy. As therapists worked with these patients, they found that such treatments as hot packs, massage, stretching, and strengthening exercises—which had worked so well with the patients with polio—were not appropriate or sufficient for patients with other neurological problems. Between the 1940s and 1970s several therapists developed a variety of treatment and handling approaches based on their observations of motor behavior in their patients. They also found that they could influence motor behavior with a variety of sensory inputs (e.g., visual, auditory, thermal, tactile, proprioceptive). To understand and explain the phenomena they were observing, they turned to the literature available at the time. The work of such neurophysiologists as Jackson, Sherrington, and Magnus provided some explanations and influenced treatment philosophies. These early approaches are briefly described here. Techniques based on all these approaches continue to be used to improve motor control. Their efficacy is still being established and researched. No specific technique has proved more effective than others, and therapists continue to mix and match them depending on patient needs.

PROPRIOCEPTIVE NEUROMUSCULAR FACILITATION

Proprioceptive neuromuscular facilitation (PNF), one of the earliest techniques, was developed by Dr. Kabat, a neurologist associated with the physical therapists Margaret Knott and Dorothy Voss.[10] Working with patients who had MS or cerebral palsy, Dr. Kabat observed that the "one muscle–one joint" approach used in the treatment of patients with polio was not applicable to this group. From his observations of normal human movement, he emphasized that most human activities require multidimensional movements; that is, various muscles at various joints complement and enhance one another's activities. Hence, this approach emphasizes specific patterns of movement in the retraining process. Dr. Kabat also observed that motor performance could be facilitated and enhanced by providing the patient with sensory stimuli—specifically, proprioceptive stimuli at specific locations and times within a movement. These techniques, as their name implies, emphasize proprioceptive (joint and position sense) stimuli, but they also use tactile, visual, and auditory stimuli. They are currently used to enhance movement and motor control not only in patients with neuromuscular problems, but also in patients with musculoskeletal problems.

ROOD'S APPROACH

Margaret Rood also recognized and recommended the use of sensory stimuli as part of her handling and treatment regimens. She emphasized the importance of sensory stimuli in arousing, calming, and modulating motor responses.[11] She used a variety of stimuli to influence motor behavior. In addition, she recognized the importance of the autonomic nervous system and in her treatments used such stimuli as neutral warmth to calm a child before proceeding to other interventions. Based on her observations of motor development, she also recommended a skeletal function sequence that required progression through four basic stages of control: mobility, stability, controlled mobility, and skill.

BRUNNSTROM'S APPROACH

Signe Brunnstrom worked with patients who had suffered damage to the nervous system from a CVA.[12] She made detailed observations regarding the movement patterns these patients exhibited as they recovered and was thus able to precisely describe the natural history of recovery of movement and function after a stroke. Her descriptions of the patterns of recovery have been replicated

10

and remain as valid today as when she first wrote about them. Based on her observations, as well as her extensive research and interpretation of the literature available, she made specific recommendations regarding the sequence of movements and activities that would facilitate recovery and function. Her training procedures and treatment sequences progressed from appropriate positioning and activities in bed to training trunk control in sitting and activities to facilitate recovery of motion in the upper and lower extremities. Her recommendations regarding treatment continue to be used as part of the intervention repertoire for patients recovering from a stroke.

NEURODEVELOPMENTAL TREATMENT

Neurodevelopmental treatment (NDT) was developed by Berta Bobath, a physiotherapist, and her husband Karel Bobath.[13] Berta Bobath worked extensively with children with cerebral palsy and adult patients with stroke. Her theories and treatment approach are based on observations of these patient populations and her interpretation of the works of Jackson, Sherrington, and others. Her hypothesis, especially in regard to adult patients with stroke, asserts that because of the damage caused by the stroke, the patient is unable to direct the nerve impulses appropriately. This defect results in abnormal patterns of coordination in posture and movement and abnormal qualities of tone. The aim of treatment is to inhibit the abnormal patterns of movement and facilitate integrated, automatic reactions and voluntary functional activity. The inhibition of abnormal postures is achieved by passively maintaining the patient in corrective postures. Facilitation of automatic reactions and voluntary activity is achieved by handling techniques that require specific placement of hands to support and stimulate the desired reactions.

CURRENT APPROACHES

Over the past 20 years, the understanding of life span **motor development**[14] (age-related processes of change in motor behavior), motor control (neural control of posture and movement), and **motor learning**[15] (process of acquisition or modification of movement) has increased tremendously. This increased understanding has led to a review and reevaluation of the earlier techniques—those that emphasized inhibitory and facilitatory input and modifying motor behavior through handling.[16] Because they are based on principles of motor learning and skill acquisition, current approaches put less emphasis on passive handling of the patient. They recommend more active involvement by the patient, especially in terms of problem solving and finding appropriate solutions.[17] These approaches emphasize the need for the therapist to create the appropriate environment for learning and the appropriate use of feedback to facilitate learning. Shumway-Cook and Woollacott[3,18] recommend that assessment and treatment of clinical problems be based on a systems model of motor control in which a more task-oriented approach is used. They suggest that movement results from a dynamic interplay between perceptual, cognitive, and action systems. They also believe that it is critical to recognize that movement emerges from an interaction between the individual and the task and the environment in which the task is being carried out.

Besides the techniques mentioned above, therapists may choose options specifically targeted to the impairment and dysfunction. These techniques may include stretching or strengthening exercises to improve flexibility and strength. They may also include physical agents such as electromyographic (EMG) biofeedback, neuromuscular electrical stimulation (NMES), or functional electrical stimulation (FES) as adjuncts to improve or facilitate motor control and muscle strength and to reduce spasticity. Other options may be more compensatory or adaptive. For instance, a therapist may teach a patient with impaired sensation in the soles of the feet to rely more on the eyes and visual system for maintenance of balance. Another may initiate the use of braces to improve walking in the case of irreversible paralysis of leg muscles. The therapist may also recommend environmental modifications to help the patient function better. Thus a therapist is constantly challenged to be as creative as possible in treating and managing movement-related problems of function caused by disorders of the nervous system.

SUMMARY

The goal of neuromuscular physical therapy is to treat problems of movement and function that result from damage to the nervous system. If the problems are untreatable and progressive, the goal is to teach the patient and caregivers to accommodate and compensate for the problems and prevent secondary complications. To achieve these goals, therapists need to examine the components necessary for movement and evaluate their role in the dysfunction. Based on the findings, the therapist—in conjunction with the patient, family, and other caregivers—will draw up a plan of care with appropriate short- and long-term goals and specific strategies, which may include hands-on intervention using some of the approaches described above, as well as education of the patient and family members regarding exercises and activities the patient or family can perform to meet these goals. This process of evaluation, assessment, and treatment will occur periodically as goals are met. If goals become unachievable because of physical, psychological, or social factors, reevaluation of goals and strategies becomes necessary. The ultimate objective is to help rehabilitate the patient to function at the highest level attainable within the constraints of the condition.

CASE STUDY

10

CASE STUDY ONE

Jim is an 18-year-old man who sustained a gunshot wound to his thoracic spine. The shot ruptured his spine and caused damage to the spinal cord that resulted in paralysis below the waist. He also sustained abdominal injuries that required surgery. Jim is now medically stable and has been referred to therapy to begin the long process of rehabilitation.

The first task of the team members (which include a physiatrist, nurse, psychologist, social worker, and physical and occupational therapists) is to complete detailed evaluations. This process may take several days because each team member is working within the constraints imposed by the patient's physical and emotional condition. When all the information is gathered, a team meeting is scheduled to discuss the information with the patient and his family and to start setting some short- and long-term goals. At this stage it is too early to tell how extensive and permanent the neurological damage is—it usually takes several months to make a definitive prognosis and hence these goals will probably need periodic review and adjustment.

Even as team members were conducting their evaluations, the PT had already started treatment and management to maintain mobility, increase strength in the uninvolved muscles, and educate the patient about problems arising from loss of sensation. The nurses had initiated a program to manage bowel and bladder function. The psychologist had begun helping Jim cope with the trauma of this unexpected event and the loss of body image and body functions. The social worker was starting to determine Jim's needs on discharge and whether these needs could be met by his family and in the current home environment.

During the next several weeks the team will continue to check Jim thoroughly for any change in or return of sensory or motor activity, which will determine the final prognosis. The team members will start making discharge and placement plans based on Jim's recovery, his functional abilities, the family's needs in being able to care for him at home, their insurance coverage for necessary services, and so on. Team members will continue to work with Jim to teach the new skills necessary to function within the new reality. The PT will play a major role in teaching and training him in these new skills. The therapist will also be involved in ordering equipment, such as the appropriate wheelchair and cushion, to meet the needs of his lifestyle. The therapist will make recommendations to the family for a ramp to gain access to the house. The family may need to widen doorways and remove carpeting to make wheelchair mobility and access easier. They may need to adapt or build a bathroom and bedroom on the main floor level to meet Jim's needs. They may be able to get some financial help or may end up bearing the complete financial burden themselves.

Not only is Jim dealing with many physical and psychological challenges, but also the family is dealing with many emotional issues. As the therapist trains the family to assist Jim, family members will frequently be very open during these sessions and voice their fears and concerns. The therapist's role is to provide not only technical support for the physical needs, but also psychological and emotional support for both the patient and the family.

REFERENCES

1. O'Sullivan SB: Stroke. *In:* O'Sullivan SB, Schmitz TJ (eds): Physical Rehabilitation Assessment and Treatment. Philadelphia, FA Davis, 2001.
2. Fulk GD, Geller AS: Traumatic head injury. *In:* O'Sullivan SB, Schmitz TJ (eds): Physical Rehabilitation Assessment and Treatment. Philadelphia, FA Davis, 2001.
3. Schmitz TJ: Traumatic spinal cord injury. *In:* O'Sullivan SB, Schmitz TJ (eds): Physical Rehabilitation Assessment and Treatment. Philadelphia, FA Davis, 2001.
4. Schubert MC, Herdman SJ: Vestibular Rehabilitation. *In:* O'Sullivan SB, Schmitz TJ (eds): Physical Rehabilitation Assessment and Treatment. Philadelphia, FA Davis, 2001.
5. Brooke M: Diseases of the motor neurons. *In:* Brooke M (ed): A Clinician's View of Neuromuscular Diseases. Baltimore, Williams & Wilkins, 1986.
6. O'Sullivan SB: Multiple sclerosis. *In:* O'Sullivan SB, Schmitz TJ (eds): Physical Rehabilitation Assessment and Treatment. Philadelphia, FA Davis, 2001.
7. O'Sullivan SB: Parkinson's disease. *In:* O'Sullivan SB, Schmitz TJ (eds): Physical Rehabilitation Assessment and Treatment. Philadelphia, FA Davis, 2001.
8. Hallum A: Neuromuscular Diseases. *In:* Umphred DA (ed): Neurological Rehabilitation. St Louis, Mosby, 2001.

9. Bleck TP: Clinical use of neurologic diagnostic tests. *In:* Weiner WJ, Goetz CG (eds): Neurology for the Non-Neurologist. Baltimore, Lippincott Williams & Wilkins, 2004.

10. Pinkston D: Evolution of the practice of physical therapy in the United States. *In:* Scully RM, Barnes MR (eds): Physical Therapy. Philadelphia, Lippincott, 1989.

11. Voss DE, Ionta MK, Myers BJ, et al: Proprioceptive Neuromuscular Facilitation, ed 3. Philadelphia, Harper & Row, 1985.

12. Stockmeyer SA: An interpretation of the approach of Rood to the treatment of neuromuscular dysfunction. Am J Phys Med 1967;46:900-961.

13. Sawner K, Lavigne J: Brunnstrom's Movement Therapy in Hemiplegia. Philadelphia, Lippincott, 1992.

14. Bobath B: Adult Hemiplegia: Evaluation and Treatment. Oxford, Butterworth-Heinemann, 1990.

15. VanSant AF: Life span motor development. *In:* Lister MJ (ed): Contemporary Management of Motor Control Problems. Alexandria, VA, Foundation for Physical Therapy, 1991.

16. Carr JH, Shepherd RB: Movement Science, Foundation for Physical Therapy in Rehabilitation. Rockville, MD, Aspen, 2000.

17. Umphred DN: Merging neurophysiologic approaches with contemporary theories. *In:* Lister MJ (ed): Contemporary Management of Motor Control Problems. Alexandria, VA, Foundation for Physical Therapy, 1991.

18. Carr JH, Shepherd RB: A Motor Relearning Program for Stroke. Rockville, MD, Aspen, 1987.

19. Shumway-Cook A, Woollacott MH: Motor Control: Theory and Practical Applications. Baltimore, Williams & Wilkins, 2001.

ADDITIONAL RESOURCES

The following is a list of Websites for the most up-to-date information regarding the cause, prevention, treatment, and management of various neuromuscular conditions. Several of the lay organizations provide a wealth of educational materials for patients and families, and some also provide links to support groups.

www.ninds.gov : National Institute of Neurological Disorders and Stroke (NINDS)

www.cdc.gov : Centers for Disease Control (CDC) and Prevention

www.neuropt.org : Neurology Section of the American Physical Therapy Association

www.strokeassociation.org : American Stroke Association

www.spinalcord.org : National Spinal Cord Injury Association

www.apda.parkinson.org : American Parkinson Disease Association

www.nmss.org : National Multiple Sclerosis Society

www.vestibular.org : Vestibular Disorders Association

www.mdausa.org : Muscular Dystrophy Association

REVIEW QUESTIONS

1. Why might the physical therapy plan of care change several times for a patient recovering from a stroke?

2. List the kinds of information you might hope to gain from interviewing the patient and family. What other insights does the interview provide?

3. Contrast the differing roles that the physical therapist and physical therapist assistant may assume, depending on the nature of the patient's neurological condition (e.g., contrast the physical therapist's roles in the care of patients with the following: spinal cord injury, stroke, Parkinson's disease, and amyotrophic lateral sclerosis).

4. Describe the purposes of at least three diagnostic tests in neuromuscular disorders. How do they differ in procedure as well?

5. What purpose do body jackets, braces, assistive devices, and environmental modifications serve in neuromuscular rehabilitation?

10

Those aspects of physical therapy commonly referred to as cardiovascular/pulmonary physical therapy are fully recognized as fundamental components of the knowledge and practice base for all entry-level physical therapists.

E.A. Hillegass, PT, and H.S. Sadowsky, PT

11 Physical Therapy in Cardiovascular and Pulmonary Conditions

Ray A. Boone

myocardial infarction
obstructive lung disease
postural drainage
pulmonary function test
respiration
restrictive lung disease
spirometer
target heart rate (THR)
training zone
ventilation

■ Define and describe the effects of common diseases that alter normal function of the cardiovascular and pulmonary systems
■ Outline how the functions of the cardiovascular and pulmonary systems are evaluated both normally and when disease is present
■ Discuss how physical therapists examine, evaluate, and provide interventions to individuals who have cardiovascular or pulmonary disease

OBJECTIVES

After reading this chapter, the reader will be able to:
■ Describe the normal anatomy and physiology of the cardiovascular and pulmonary systems

GENERAL DESCRIPTION

PREVALENCE

Less than 30 years ago, people with cardiovascular and pulmonary conditions had little hope of leading normal lives. In fact, in certain instances exercise was considered deleterious to people with such conditions. Today, the physical therapist (PT) and physical therapist assistant (PTA) play major roles as team members for these patients to enhance their function and improve the quality of their daily lives.

Cardiovascular disease (CVD) remains the number one killer in the United States, claiming over 910,000 lives in 2003 (last full data set available). This represents 38% of the more than 2.4 million people who died that year (Figure 11-1). The economic impact and prevalence of this disease are extensive. Estimated direct and indirect costs for 2006 are $403.1 billion for the 71.3 million American adults who have CVD. The prevalence of two or more risk factors for adults 18 years of age or older varies with ethnicity, education, income, and employment status. These factors were highest among blacks (48.7%) and American Indians/Alaska Natives (46.7%) and lowest among Asians (25.9%). Multiple risk factors ranged from 25.9% for college graduates to 52.5% for those with less than a high school diploma (or equivalent). Individuals with household income of $10,000 or less had the highest prevalence (52.5%), whereas those with $50,000 or more had the lowest prevalence (28.8%). Adults who were unable to work had the highest prevalence (69.3%), followed by retired persons (45.1%), unemployed adults (43.4%), homemakers (34.3%), and employed persons (34.0%).

Coronary heart disease (CHD), disease specifically of the heart and its vascular supply, is responsible for 53% of all deaths caused by CVD (Figure 11-2).[1] This represents 1 of every 5 deaths in the United States in 2003. About every 26 seconds an American suffers a coronary event, and about every minute someone

11

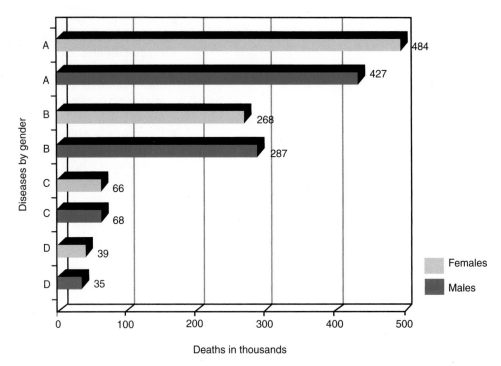

Figure 11-1 ■ Leading causes of death in the United States, 2003. *A*, Total cardiovascular disease. *B*, Cancer. *C*, Chronic lower respiratory pulmonary diseases. *D*, Diabetes. (Modified from Heart Disease and Stroke Statistics—2006 Update. Dallas, American Heart Association.)

dies of a cardiac event. For 2006, an estimated 700,000 Americans will have a new heart attack (myocardial infarction [MI]) and 500,000 will have recurrent attacks. Besides attempts to alter the lifestyle of a person who is at risk for heart disease to decrease the risk factors, direct intervention is commonly used to manage heart disease. In 2003, an estimated 1,244,000 angioplasties were performed. This procedure requires inserting a tube into a coronary vessel and blowing up a balloon on the end of the tube to open up a blockage in the vessel. Nearly half a million bypass procedures were performed and 197,000 pacemaker procedures were completed in 2003.[1]

Chronic obstructive pulmonary disease (COPD) comprises a group of lung diseases that are characterized by obstruction of airflow through the bronchial system and in some cases destruction of lung parenchyma. Emphysema and chronic bronchitis are the two most common COPD conditions and are often found together in the same patient. Asthma is not included in this definition of COPD.

In 2002, an estimated 24 million U.S. adults had some evidence of impaired lung function.[2] In 2003 (last full data set available), 10.7 million people aged 18 or over had a physician-reported diagnosis of COPD. These data indicate that

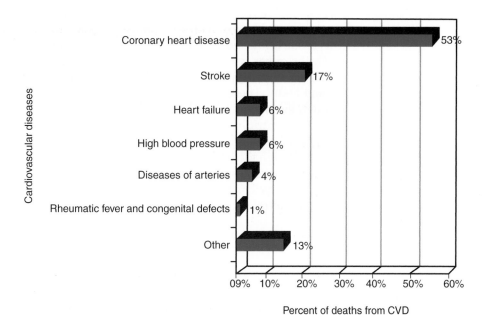

Figure 11-2 ■ Deaths from cardiovascular diseases in the United States, 2003. (Modified from Heart Disease and Stroke Statistics—2006 Update. Dallas, American Heart Association.)

lung disease in the United States is underreported. COPD is the fourth leading cause of death in the United States, and for the last 3 years more women than men were reported to have the disease. As in cardiovascular disease, gender, race, and age affect the population in which COPD develops. In 2003, the highest percentage of individuals suffering from chronic bronchitis was non-Hispanic white females from the South, ranging from 45 to 64 years of age, whereas the greatest percentage of individuals with emphysema was non-Hispanic white males, also from the South but over the age of 65. In 2004, the cost of COPD to the nation was 37.2 billion dollars. This included $20.9 billion in direct health care costs, $7.4 billion in indirect morbidity costs, and $8.9 billion in indirect mortality costs.

Both heart and lung diseases are chronic diseases. Various types of medically trained personnel become involved in caring for people with these problems. PTs and PTAs who work with patients who have cardiovascular and pulmonary diseases must have a thorough understanding of the normal anatomy and physiology of these systems. With this knowledge, appropriate treatment programs can be developed.

CARDIOVASCULAR SYSTEM

Heart. In an adult the heart is in the center of the chest (mediastinum), with the base located superiorly and the apex inferiorly and left of center. The major portion of the heart is made up of muscle tissue referred to as the myocardium. This tissue is layered with muscle fibers running in multiple directions.[3]

The heart has two pairs of matched chambers. The two atria are thin-walled chambers, whereas the two ventricles have much thicker muscular walls (Figure 11-3).[4] These chambers are separated by valves that direct the blood through the chambers in a specific pattern.

The right atrium receives venous blood from the body through the superior and inferior venae cavae. With atrial contraction (atrial systole) the blood then passes through the tricuspid valve into the right ventricle (Figure 11-4, *A*).[4] The left atrium receives oxygenated blood through the pulmonary veins coming from the lungs. During atrial systole, this oxygenated blood passes through the bicuspid (mitral) valve into the left ventricle (Figure 11-4, *B*).

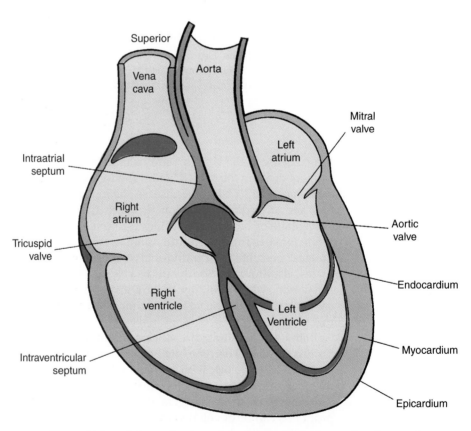

Figure 11-3 ■ Schematic view of the heart and the heart chambers and valves. (From Phillips RE, Feeney MK: The Cardiac Rhythms: A Systematic Approach to Interpretation, ed 3. Philadelphia, Saunders, 1990.)

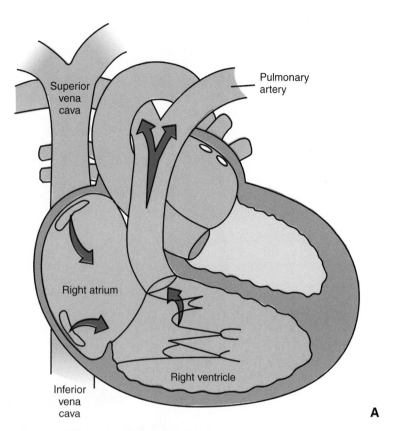

Figure 11-4 ■ **A**, Blood flow through the heart chambers: deoxygenated blood flow from the right atrium to the right ventricle to the lung through the pulmonary artery. *Continued*

Once the right and left ventricles have received blood from their respective atria, ventricular contraction (ventricular systole) occurs. This contraction results in an increase in pressure in the ventricular chambers, which causes the tricuspid and bicuspid valves to close tightly and prevents blood from passing back into the atria. As ventricular contraction continues, venous blood leaves the right ventricle through the pulmonic or semilunar valve and flows into the lungs to be reoxygenated. Oxygenated blood leaves the left ventricle through the aortic valve into the aorta to be transported to the body through the systemic circulation.

It is significant that the ventricles have thicker muscular walls than the atria. This greater muscle mass, especially in the left ventricle, must provide enough force to overcome the resistance to flow that blood encounters as it moves through the peripheral arteries.[5]

Conduction. The myocardium contains special types of tissue responsible for conducting the electrical impulse that causes the myocardium to contract in a synchronized pattern. The synchronized depolarization and repolarization of

11

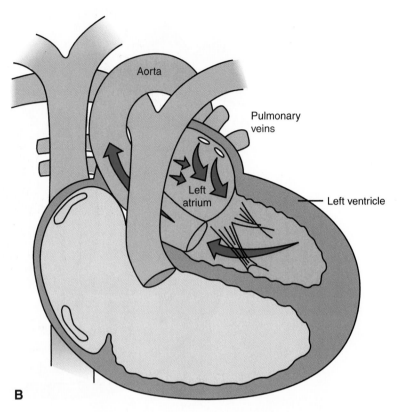

B

Figure 11-4, *cont'd* ■ **B**, Blood flow through the heart chambers: oxygenated blood returning to the left atrium from the lungs via the pulmonary veins, moving into the left ventricle, and exiting through the aorta. (From Phillips RE, Feeny MK: The Cardiac Rhythms: A Systematic Approach to Interpretation, ed 3. Philadelphia, Saunders, 1990.)

cardiac muscle result in efficient movement of blood through the chambers of the heart and through the coronary and peripheral vessels.

The specialized tissues are called nodal and Purkinje fibers (Figure 11-5).[6] The sinoatrial node (SA node) initiates the impulse (sinus rhythm) and is sometimes called the pacemaker of the heart. Once a signal is initiated by the SA node, it travels quickly through the walls of the atria on special tracts to the atrioventricular node (AV node). The impulse also travels to the muscle fibers of the atria and causes them to contract. The AV node transports the signal to the bundle of His, which is where the Purkinje fibers start to spread out into the muscle fibers of the ventricles. For every heartbeat or contraction, the depolarization signal that causes the myocardium to contract must travel through this conduction system.

Both the SA and AV nodes receive autonomic nerve fibers via the sympathetic and parasympathetic systems. These nerve fibers release special neurotransmitters that influence the rate of contraction and myocardial contractility. The ability to

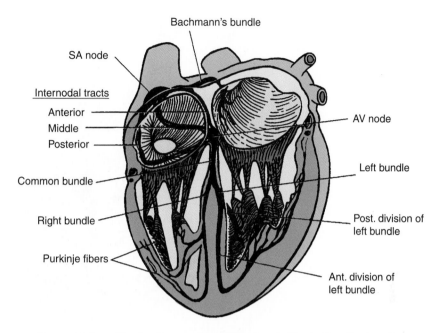

Bachmann's bundle

SA node

Internodal tracts
Anterior
Middle
Posterior

Common bundle

Right bundle

Purkinje fibers

AV node

Left bundle

Post. division of left bundle

Ant. division of left bundle

Figure 11-5 ■ Conduction system of the heart, illustrating the location of the sinoatrial (SA) and atrioventricular (AV) nodes. (From Sanderson RG, Kurth CL: The Cardiac Patient: A Comprehensive Approach, ed 2. Philadelphia, Saunders, 1983.)

influence the heart's rate and contractility is extremely important because this mechanism allows the central nervous system to tell the heart how to respond to increases in demand, such as those made during exercise.[5]

Coronary Arteries. The myocardium receives its blood supply from two major vessels, the right and left coronary arteries (Figure 11-6).[7] These arteries arise from the ascending aorta, which is the major artery leaving the left ventricle and carrying blood to the body (Figure 11-3). In general, the right and left coronary vessels supply the right and left sides of the heart, respectively; however, this arrangement can vary a great deal among individuals. If something occurs that causes blockage of a coronary vessel, it is important to determine exactly how that blockage alters blood flow to the individual's myocardium. When blockage occurs, the person has had a heart attack (MI).

Peripheral Circulation. The blood vessels that make up the peripheral circulation are arteries, capillaries, and veins, and disorders in these vessels can result in cardiovascular and pulmonary dysfunction. PTs and PTAs work with a variety of patients who have disabilities caused by pathological changes in the peripheral circulation.

The arteries, of which the aorta has the largest diameter, and the arterioles have elastic fibers and smooth muscle in their walls. If the smooth muscle

11

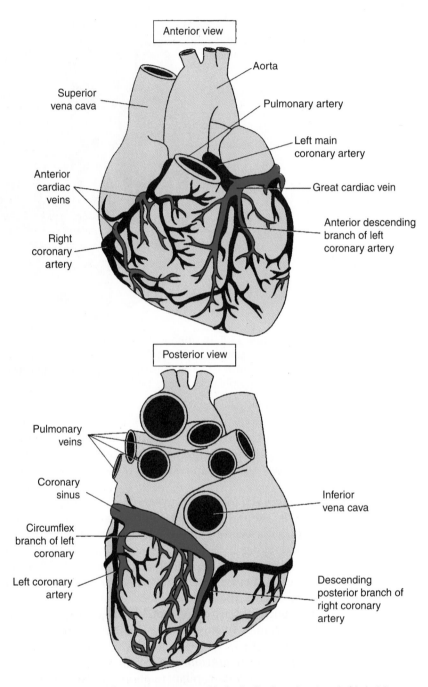

Figure 11-6 ■ Coronary arteries (*dark shading*) and veins (*white*). Note the origin of the arteries from the aorta. (From McArdle WD, Katch FI: Exercise Physiology: Energy, Nutrition and Human Performance, ed 5. Philadelphia, Lippincott Williams & Wilkins, 2001.)

contracts, the diameter of the vessel is decreased, which causes an increase in the resistance to blood flow through the vessels. Arterioles are often referred to as "resistance vessels." Changes in resistance to blood flow in the peripheral circulation directly affect how hard the heart has to work to pump blood through the body. A disease called arteriosclerosis, which is often referred to as "hardening of the arteries," causes plaque to build up on the inner wall and decreases the elasticity of the vessel, with subsequently higher resistance to blood flow.

Capillaries are the smallest vessels in the peripheral circulation. They connect arteries to veins and can be so small that they allow only one red blood cell to pass through at a time. Their walls are only one cell thick, which permits efficient exchange of oxygen and carbon dioxide. Nutrients and waste products also pass through the wall. Capillaries are often referred to as "exchange vessels."

The veins, which return blood to the heart from the body, have much less elastic fiber and smooth muscle in their walls. The larger veins can act as a blood reservoir and are often called "capacitance vessels."

PULMONARY SYSTEM

Respiration. **Respiration** is the process of exchanging oxygen and carbon dioxide between the air we breathe and blood cells that pass through the lungs. **Ventilation** is the process of exchanging air between the atmosphere and the lungs through inspiration and expiration.[8] The mechanics of inspiration and expiration depend on many factors, including the structure of the lungs, chest, and muscles. **Inspiration** occurs when the muscles of ventilation, the most important being the diaphragm, contract to cause an increase in the space within the thoracic cavity. This expansion causes air pressure to drop inside the lungs, which causes air to move into the lungs. **Expiration** is the reverse of this process.

If the body needs increased amounts of oxygen, such as during exercise, the amount of air that must flow into and out of the lungs must markedly increase. When this situation occurs, the muscles of ventilation must work extensively. When disease affects the lungs, the results can be the same. In this case, however, the body is not requiring more oxygen. The ability of air to move normally into and out of the lungs is compromised because of blockage of the tubes that conduct the air. This obstruction results in high resistance to airflow and increased work for the muscles of ventilation.[9]

Conducting Airways and Lungs. **Conducting airways** are the passageways and tubes that transport air into and out of the lungs. The upper conducting airway includes the nose, pharynx, and larynx. This component of the air transport system cleans and humidifies the air and terminates at the beginning of the trachea. The lower conducting airway is made up of the trachea and bronchiole system (Figure 11-7).[9] The bronchiole system consists of tubes branching from the main bronchus out to the terminal bronchioles. It is here that the conduction system ends and air enters into the alveolus, where gas exchange takes place. The alveolus is surrounded by capillaries that contain deoxygenated blood coming from the right ventricle of the heart. It is at this junction that oxygen

11

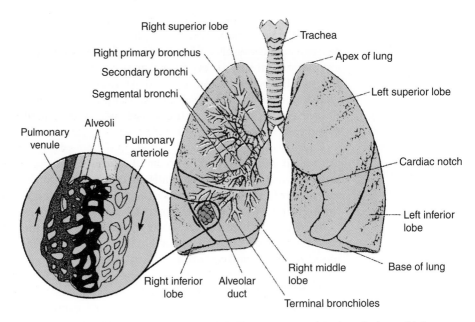

Right superior lobe

Right primary bronchus

Secondary bronchi

Segmental bronchi

Trachea

Apex of lung

Left superior lobe

Cardiac notch

Left inferior lobe

Base of lung

Alveoli

Pulmonary venule

Pulmonary arteriole

Right inferior lobe

Alveolar duct

Right middle lobe

Terminal bronchioles

Figure 11-7 ■ Anterior view of the lower airway showing the bronchial tree, alveoli, and pulmonary circulation. (From Van De Graaff KM, Fox SI: Concepts of Human Anatomy and Physiology, ed 5. Dubuque, IA, WC Brown, 1998.)

and carbon dioxide are exchanged, with the reoxygenated blood returning to the left atrium. The lungs are compartmentalized into a system of lobes, which are present because of the structure of the bronchial airway system (Figure 11-7). A special membrane, the pleura, covers the outer surface of the lungs and the inner surface of the chest wall. The pleura is extremely important to the process of ventilation and maintenance of the continuity of the lungs.[3]

CARDIOVASCULAR AND PULMONARY SYSTEM INTEGRATION

The importance of interaction between the cardiovascular and pulmonary systems is clear: when disease affects one system, eventually the other system will also be affected. For example, if arteriosclerosis develops in the coronary vessels, the amount of oxygen going to the heart muscle will be decreased. With time the heart muscle begins to fail and will not pump blood to the lungs and body efficiently. Eventually, this insufficiency results in an increase in blood volume and pressure in the lungs, which in turn causes a decrease in lung efficiency and, finally, permanent damage.

The degree of success that PTs or PTAs have in establishing appropriate examination or intervention procedures for individuals with cardiovascular or pulmonary disease depends in part on how well they understand how each system functions and interacts. The following section briefly describes common cardiovascular and lung diseases that are treated by physical therapy.

COMMON CONDITIONS

CARDIOVASCULAR DISEASES

Two major categories of disease processes influence the myocardium: ischemic conditions and cardiac muscle dysfunction.[10]

Ischemic Conditions. **Ischemia** occurs in the presence of insufficient blood flow and results in inadequate oxygenation of tissues because of a blocked blood vessel. In CVD, **arteriosclerosis** (hardening of the arteries) affects the coronary vessels and is commonly called **coronary heart disease (CHD).** **Angina** is the condition in which chest pain occurs from ischemia of the heart muscle.

The etiology of arteriosclerosis, which can affect all vessels of the body, is not completely understood. It is clear, however, that the severity of the arteriosclerotic process can be influenced by many risk factors (Box 11-1).[11] Some of these factors cannot be changed, such as having a family history of CHD. However, most of these risk factors can be altered or eliminated completely by changes in behavior. PTs and PTAs help patients with cardiac dysfunction try to alter their behavior as they progress through the rehabilitation process.

Cardiac Muscle Dysfunction. **Cardiac muscle dysfunction** refers to various pathological conditions associated with heart failure.[10] **Heart failure** occurs when a disease process or congenital defect either directly or indirectly causes a decrease in the pumping capability of the heart muscle. These disease processes can occur either acutely or gradually. An example of an acute change in the heart's pumping capability is the occurrence of a **myocardial infarction** (heart attack). In this case one of the coronary arteries suddenly becomes blocked by an **embolus** (clot). When embolism occurs, blood flow to heart muscle beyond the embolus stops, and the part of the heart muscle no longer receiving blood

BOX 11-1 | *Risk Factors That Promote the Development of Coronary Heart Disease*

Major Risk Factors
- Cigarette smoking
- Hypertension (high blood pressure)
- Elevated cholesterol

Minor Risk Factors
- Family history
- Diabetes
- Age
- Gender
- Stress
- Obesity
- Sedentary lifestyle

Data from Heart and Stroke Statistical Update. Dallas, American Heart Association, 1998.

11

dies. If this embolus causes an interruption in blood flow to a large amount of heart muscle, death can result.

If an individual survives a heart attack, other symptoms may develop that further complicate the condition. One of the major complications after infarction is an abnormal rhythm in the sequence of heart muscle contraction (abnormal conduction). This problem makes the heart contraction inefficient. If the left ventricle is seriously damaged from the infarct, it may not contract strongly enough to move the blood through the body appropriately. This deficiency can cause the blood to back up into the lungs, or it may seriously limit function, such as the heart's ability to respond to an increase in physical activity.

When the heart muscle is compromised to the point that it cannot move blood volume effectively, **congestive heart failure (CHF)** will develop. This disorder can occur acutely or chronically. When CHF is present, the ventricles are not adequately pumping the appropriate volume from their chambers. When the right ventricle is not contracting efficiently, blood volume backs into the venous system and fluid collects in the liver, abdominal cavity, and legs. If the left ventricle does not contract appropriately, an abnormal amount of blood volume remains in the lungs and results in fluid collection. The right ventricle then has to work harder because it must try to push blood into the lungs against increased resistance. This increased workload eventually leads to compromised function of the right ventricle (Figure 11-4, *A*).

A person with CHF has many clinical problems. If fluid collects in the lungs, breathing becomes more difficult and the blood is not oxygenated appropriately. If fluid has collected in the legs, walking becomes more difficult. Because of increasing difficulty in performing activities, the patient would have to expend more energy to accomplish simple tasks. With increased energy expenditure, the heart would have to work harder to support simple functional activities. To develop an appropriate treatment program for a patient with problems of this type, a PT must have a thorough understanding of how these disease processes compromise function.

LUNG DISEASES

Diseases of the lung are generally classified as being obstructive or restrictive. If pathological changes in the lung cause an abnormality in airflow through the bronchial tubes, the process is defined as **obstructive lung disease**, whereas if pathological changes cause the volume of air in the lungs to be reduced, the process is defined as **restrictive lung disease.**[10] How lung diseases are classified is a controversial subject. What is most important is that the common diseases that change lung function eventually demonstrate both obstructive and restrictive characteristics.[12]

Chronic Obstructive Pulmonary Disease. **Chronic obstructive pulmonary disease (COPD)** is a group of disorders that produce certain specific physical symptoms. These symptoms include chronic productive cough, excessive mucus production, changes in the sound produced when air passes through the bronchial tubes, and shortness of breath **(dyspnea)**. The specific disorders that can produce these changes include chronic bronchitis (inflammation of the bronchi), emphysema (trapping of air in the alveoli), and peripheral airway disease (collapse of terminal bronchioles). Other disorders sometimes included in this disease group include bronchial asthma (spasmlike contraction of bronchi, resulting in air trapping) and cystic fibrosis (dysfunction of mucous glands, causing blockage of bronchi).[12] Differences between these obstructive diseases include their etiology (cause), pathology (what tissues are affected and how they are changed), and management. However, all of them cause similar symptoms in varying degrees.

The signs and symptoms that develop as COPD progresses include bronchial wall abnormalities causing a decrease in lumen size and alveolar destruction. This process results in trapping of air in the lungs, which causes the lungs to become hyperinflated, and in a decrease in gas exchange in the alveoli, which results in hypoxemia (below-normal oxygenation of blood). Hypoxemia occurs when the lungs cannot adequately supply oxygen to or retrieve carbon dioxide from the red blood cells as the cells pass by the alveoli.

As resistance to airflow increases because of the decreasing lumen size of the bronchioles, the thorax enlarges as a result of air trapping. This enlargement of the thorax causes the respiratory muscles to work harder. With time, the effectiveness of the respiratory muscles decreases. With chronic hypoxemia, changes begin to occur in the function of the heart, in blood pressure, and in the thickness of the blood. All these changes can lead to respiratory failure.[10,12]

Restrictive Lung Diseases. Restrictive lung diseases cause a decrease in the ability of the lungs to expand, which results in a decrease in the volume of air that can move into and out of the lungs. This disease process that affects lung tissue directly is most commonly of idiopathic, or unknown, origin. Known causes include chronic inhalation of air pollutants such as coal dust, silicon, or asbestos. Infections such as pneumonia, cancer of the lung, and changes in heart function (causing chronic fluid collection in the lungs) can also result in restrictive changes. Diseases or trauma to the nerve supply to the muscles of ventilation or disease of the muscles themselves can also result in decreased movement of the chest wall. Thus many disease groups and structural changes in the chest wall can cause restrictive changes.

The signs and symptoms that develop as restrictive disease progresses include some of the same changes seen in COPD, such as shortness of breath and chronic cough. In the case of restrictive lung disease, however, the cough is nonproductive (does not bring mucus out of the lungs). Other changes include tachypnea, or an increase in the rate of breathing, which results in a marked increase in the amount of energy expended on breathing. This increased energy cost can be so severe that it results in weight loss and an emaciated appearance. Patients with restrictive lung disease are also subject to the problems associated with hypoxemia.[10,12]

11

PRINCIPLES OF EXAMINATION

The examination performed by PTs and PTAs is an inclusive process that involves not only the patient, but also the family and other caregivers who are participating in the overall care of the patient. It includes a review of the patient's past medical and social history, review of the body systems, and tests and measures to gather data about the patient's condition. Areas reviewed include not only physical parameters, but also functional, psychological, social, and employment conditions. The tests and measures that are selected to examine a patient/client depend on various parameters, including the age of the patient/client; severity of the problem; stage of recovery (acute, subacute, chronic); phase of rehabilitation (early, intermediate, late, return to activity); and home, community, and work status.[13] Table 11-1 describes tests and measures

Table 11-1
Description of Common Tests and Measures for Patients with Cardiovascular and Pulmonary Conditions

Function or Characteristic	Description
Home, work, and community (job/play/school)	Analysis of the home and work environments to determine the level of functional capacity needed to perform safely within these environments. Examination of the patient's capacity to function at an appropriate level of social interaction with various populations, e.g., family, peers, strangers.
Ergonomics and body mechanics	Determination of the dynamic capabilities required of the patient to safely perform within various environments, e.g., home, work, school, leisure.
Aerobic capacity and endurance	Assessment of cardiovascular and pulmonary performance during controlled exercise and functional activities. Can include measuring oxygen consumption, heart and respiratory rates, blood pressure, dyspnea, and blood gases; electrocardiogram; and heart and lung auscultation.
Ventilation and respiration	Assessment of pulmonary function, arterial blood gases, airway clearance efficiency, and perceived exertion and dyspnea during and after exercise; measurements of strength and endurance of muscles of ventilation and of chest wall mobility and expansion.
Anthropometric characteristics	Determination of body fat composition.
Muscle strength and endurance	Assessment of functional muscle strength and endurance as they relate to exercise protocols.
Posture	Assessment of posture abnormalities and their effect on energy cost during movement.
Range of motion	Assessment of limitations in joint range of motion and impact on energy cost during movement.

Data from Guide to Physical Therapist Practice, revised ed 2. Alexandria, VA, American Physical Therapy Association, 2003.

commonly performed in the examination of patients with cardiovascular and pulmonary conditions.[13]

Other diagnostic tests of the cardiovascular and pulmonary systems beyond the scope of the PT often require invasive techniques and generally place the patient at a certain amount of risk. It is essential that PTs understand the results of these tests to comprehend the severity of the disease and establish an appropriate plan of care.

CARDIOVASCULAR DIAGNOSTIC TESTS AND PROCEDURES

Invasive Procedures. Various pieces of equipment can be used to assess how the heart is functioning or how adequately blood is flowing through an artery. Invasive procedures used to evaluate heart function require that some type of instrument be placed in the body or dye be injected into the blood. One of the most common invasive procedures used to assess heart function is **cardiac catheterization.** The procedure requires passing a catheter (a flexible tube) into an artery in the leg until it reaches the heart. The catheter can then be placed in the left chambers of the heart or in the coronary arteries or pulmonary veins. The catheter can have a special sensory device on the tip to measure pressure; thus its use allows assessment of how much pressure is being generated in chambers of the heart. This measure in turn evaluates the strength of myocardial contraction. Dye can be released directly into the coronary arteries from the catheter, and a special type of imaging technique can then record how well blood flows through the vessels and demonstrate where blockage has occurred. The catheter could also have a small camera in the tip to allow viewing of the heart chamber valves and the inside of the coronary vessels. Other types of invasive procedures may also be performed, all of which require highly trained personnel and sophisticated equipment. These procedures are expensive and generally involve some risk to the patient.[6]

Noninvasive Procedures. Noninvasive procedures are also used to assess heart function. Some of the more common procedures include echocardiography, electrocardiography, and exercise testing. **Echocardiography** is the use of high-frequency ultrasound to assess the size of the heart chambers, the thickness of the chamber walls, and the motion of the chamber walls and heart valves. Generally, the transducer (device that produces the ultrasound and records the returning echo) is placed on the chest wall. In some cases, however, the transducer is placed in the esophagus to improve the accuracy of its recording and allow assessment of the posterior aspect of the heart.[6]

One of the most common and inexpensive methods of noninvasive evaluation of heart function is the **electrocardiogram (ECG).** PTs who work with individuals being monitored by ECG must be able to interpret normal and abnormal ECG readings. This ability requires a basic understanding of the anatomy and conduction system of the heart (see Figure 11-5).

As previously discussed, the conduction system is responsible for initiating depolarization or contraction of the heart muscle. When the conduction and muscle tissues depolarize, a change in electrical potential occurs across the individual cell membranes. This minute electrical change is detected by special

11

electrodes placed on the skin of the anterior chest wall, and the "signal" can be recorded by an ECG machine (Figure 11-8).[10]

The ECG assesses the heart's rate and rhythm (Figure 11-9).[14] When the heart is functioning normally, it produces a consistent ECG pattern. As seen in Figure 11-9, different components of the waveform are assigned names and represent specific events in the heart cycle. For example, the P wave represents

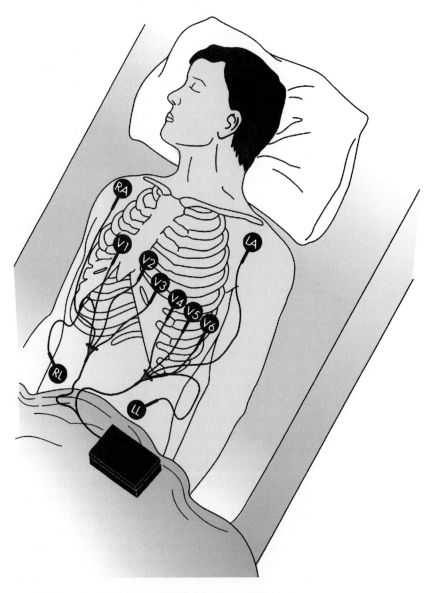

Figure 11-8 ■ Electrode placement for electrocardiographic monitoring. (From Hillegass EA, Sadowsky, HS: Essentials of Cardiopulmonary Physical Therapy, ed 2. Philadelphia, Saunders, 2001.)

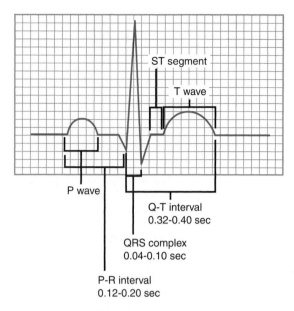

Figure 11-9 ■ Normal electrocardiogram tracing during a single heart cycle. (From Hillegass EA, Sadowsky, HS: Essentials of Cardiopulmonary Physical Therapy, ed 2. Philadelphia, Saunders, 2001.)

atrial depolarization, and the QRS complex represents ventricular depolarization (contraction). If the heart does not depolarize in a normal way or if part of the heart muscle is not functioning correctly, characteristic changes would be seen in the ECG. Other heart problems that can be assessed by ECG include heart muscle hypertrophy and the presence of MI.[15]

Exercise stress testing is a noninvasive method of determining how the cardiovascular and pulmonary systems respond to controlled increases in activity. This technique of assessment is most frequently used to diagnose suspected or established CVD. However, it is also valuable in other applications, such as assessing a patient's performance after coronary artery bypass surgery or heart valve replacement. Often, the exercise stress test is used to assess someone's functional status or help prescribe limitations for occupational activities.[15]

A PT can be involved in administering an exercise stress test. Generally, the therapist is required to have special training in the techniques of testing, especially if the testing protocol requires the patient to exercise at maximum capability. At a minimum, the PT must be able to interpret the data recorded during a stress test to establish a patient's appropriate level of exercise prescription, which should include a specific description of exercise intensity, duration, frequency, and mode.

Several methods can be used to administer an exercise stress test, the most common including walking on a treadmill and riding a bicycle ergometer. Generally, the actual testing procedure includes the following:

■ Continuous ECG monitoring
■ Heart rate monitoring (from the ECG)

11

- Blood pressure monitoring
- Heart and lung sounds
- Feedback from the patient by reporting symptoms

In many stress test laboratories, analysis of expired gas (air) from the lungs is accomplished by having the subject breathe into a collection device. This technique permits a determination of the amount of oxygen the patient used during the test.[10,15]

When an exercise test is performed on a treadmill or bicycle ergometer, the exercise intensity or "protocol" used is very specific and has been tested in many laboratories (Table 11-2).[16] The advantage of following a protocol is that the results of the test can be compared with the results of thousands of other patients on whom the same test has been performed. This comparison helps determine the status of the patient.

PULMONARY DIAGNOSTIC TESTS AND PROCEDURES

As with cardiovascular diagnostic testing, both invasive and noninvasive procedures have been developed to assess lung function and the severity of pulmonary disease. PTs are not generally involved in performing these assessments; however, the information that is provided must be used by PTs so that appropriate evaluation and treatment procedures are established.

Chest Imaging. Chest imaging is the most common noninvasive method of assessing abnormalities of the lungs. Within the last decade, new technology has enhanced the use of what are commonly called x-rays (radiographs). For example, computed tomography (CT scan) is a technique that uses x-rays to take pictures of small slices of the chest and lungs and then a computer to put these individual images into a single picture.

Magnetic Resonance Imaging. Magnetic resonance imaging (MRI) uses the same principle as the CT scan except that the energy source used to take the picture is not x-rays, but magnetic waves.[17]

Table 11-2
Bruce Treadmill Protocol

Stage of Exercise	Time of Each Stage (min)	Speed of Treadmill (mph)	Grade of Treadmill (%)
I	3	1.7	10
II	3	2.5	12
III	3	3.4	14
IV	3	4.2	16

Modified from Ellestad MH, Myrvin H: Stress Testing Principles and Practice. Philadelphia, FA Davis, 1986.

Even though highly technical equipment can provide a great deal of information concerning the condition of the lungs, the standard chest radiograph is often the first diagnostic test used. A PT must be competent in interpreting a standard chest radiograph. To assess this common diagnostic procedure, the therapist must have a thorough understanding of normal anatomy and disease processes that affect the lungs.

Pulmonary Function Tests. A **pulmonary function test** is an assessment of the effectiveness of the respiratory musculature and the integrity of the airways and lung tissue. The testing procedure can help classify the lung disease pattern into obstructive or restrictive by assessing the following:

- Lung volumes
- Lung capacities
- Gas distribution
- Gas diffusion
- Gas flow rate

Generally, in a pulmonary function test the patient blows as hard as possible with the biggest breath into a machine called a **spirometer.** This device measures the various volumes and airflow rates, which are then compared with a normal scale. The degree of change from normal helps assess the seriousness of the obstructive or restrictive disease.[18]

Blood Gas Analysis. **Blood gas analysis** involves assessing arterial blood to determine the concentration of oxygen and carbon dioxide. This measure helps determine how well the lungs are being ventilated or whether the patient has any deficits in respiration. Another parameter that is assessed is the acid balance of the blood. If the lungs are having difficulty maintaining appropriate levels of oxygen and carbon dioxide, the blood generally becomes more acidic. In humans, blood must be maintained at a very specific acid level. Small changes in this acid level can result in severe reactions, possibly even death.[19]

PRINCIPLES OF EVALUATION, DIAGNOSIS, AND PROGNOSIS

The evaluation process results in establishment of a diagnosis and prognosis. A diagnosis is a description of a specific disease obtained by assessing the clinical signs, symptoms, or syndromes resulting from various pathological conditions. Prognosis estimates the maximum level of improvement the patient will experience while progressing through the treatment process.[8] During the process of establishing a diagnosis and prognosis the PT also develops a plan of care. This plan establishes the specific outcomes the patient should be able to demonstrate at the end of the treatment process. It also includes an estimate of how long and how frequently the treatment process will have to be administered to reach the established goals and outcomes, as well as the criteria for discharge.

11

PRINCIPLES OF PROCEDURAL INTERVENTION

As a team member, the PT will be treating a patient in conjunction with several other personnel (e.g., doctors, nurses, nutritionists, psychologists, occupational therapists, social workers, and exercise physiologists). Each of these specialists will be applying specific management procedures. Therefore the PT must be aware of all the treatments the patient is receiving and develop the treatment plan accordingly.

MEDICAL MANAGEMENT

One of the major forms of treating heart and lung disease is medical or pharmacological management. Each year new pharmacological agents become available to treat specific components of the complex symptoms that develop in individuals with cardiovascular and pulmonary disease. Generally, drugs used to treat cardiovascular and pulmonary disease relieve or improve symptoms but do not eradicate the disease.

Understanding the effects of drugs used to treat specific heart diseases is extremely important. Many of these drugs can alter the heart's ability to respond to exercise. For example, drugs that alter how the sympathetic nervous system influences the heart can result in a decreased heart rate and prevent the rate from increasing in response to exercise. Other drugs used to treat the heart can help control the rhythm of contraction, increase or decrease the rate, and increase or decrease the strength of myocardial contraction. They can also improve coronary blood flow or help decrease the resistance to blood flow, thereby decreasing the work the heart must perform.[20]

Medical management of symptoms caused by pulmonary disease focuses primarily on promoting bronchodilation and decreasing inflammation. Drugs producing bronchodilation improve airflow through the bronchial tubes, which helps oxygen reach the alveolus and thereby decreases the work of breathing. Antiinflammatory agents help control the results of infection or inflammation. As in the case of cardiac drugs, pulmonary drugs can have adverse effects, including alteration of heart function, gastrointestinal distress, nervousness, muscle tremor, headache, anxiety, sweating, and insomnia.[20]

SURGICAL MANAGEMENT

Like drug management, surgical management of cardiovascular and pulmonary disease does not generally alter the disease process but does improve the quality of life by relieving symptoms. In the case of CHD the arteriosclerotic process is not stopped, but coronary artery blood flow can be improved through surgery, which in turn enhances heart performance.

Two methods are commonly used to improve coronary blood flow to the heart, angioplasty and bypass surgery. **Angioplasty,** which is the process of mechanically dilating the coronary artery, does not require surgically opening the chest. A catheter is placed through an artery in the leg and then positioned in the coronary vessel blocked by arteriosclerotic plaque. A balloon is then inflated or laser light is used to destroy the plaque.[21]

Coronary artery bypass grafting (CABG) requires surgically opening the chest wall and grafting a small artery or a leg vein from the aorta to a point beyond the blockage or plaque. This technique bypasses the blockage and thereby reestablishes blood flow to the heart through the previously blocked vessel. Several vessels may be bypassed during the same surgery.[21]

Another major surgical intervention is heart transplantation, which is performed only when the heart has failed and all other therapies have been tried. A patient selected for heart transplantation is screened carefully. The patient is generally younger than 60 years, free of other diseases or infection, and emotionally stable with strong family support. The two major problems that a heart transplant patient faces are infection and rejection. If the patient overcomes these problems, the survival rate at the end of 1 year is greater than 80% and after 5 years it is greater than 50%.[22,23]

Surgical intervention is also required for inserting a pacemaker. A **cardiac pacemaker** is an electronic device that produces a pulse to control heart depolarization. In other words, it replaces the function of the SA node. This intervention is generally done to control severe cardiac arrhythmias. The electrodes can be inserted through a vein in the arm up to the heart and placed on the inner surface of the heart. The generator is then placed below the skin on the anterior chest wall and sutured in place. When a pacemaker is present in a patient, the PT and PTA must monitor the patient closely during exercise. Most pacemakers used today can produce variable rates in response to exercise; however, if maximum-intensity exercise is performed, careful monitoring is mandatory.[24] Surgical management is not as frequently used for common lung diseases as it is in the management of cardiac diseases. Resection of lung disease generally applies to removal of malignant and benign tumors, fungal infections, cysts, tuberculosis, fistulas, or bronchiectasis. Pathological changes that occur from obstructive or restrictive diseases generally do not require surgery. When surgery on the heart or lungs is performed, however, the PT and PTA play a major role in preoperative and postoperative care.

When the chest wall is opened, the patient must generally be connected to a machine that breathes for the patient and, in the case of heart surgery, a machine that pumps the blood because the heart is stopped. This very serious interruption of the normal function of the heart and lungs results in certain changes that will have to be managed no matter what surgical procedure is performed.[25] Box 11-2 identifies some of the problems a patient will have preoperatively and postoperatively that must be managed by a PT.[26]

PHYSICAL THERAPY CARDIAC REHABILITATION PROCEDURES

The PT is responsible for establishing an appropriate level of intensity, duration, frequency, and mode of exercise for an individual with cardiac disease, which means monitoring the patient's cardiovascular response to the exercise to ensure the patient's safety. In addition, the therapist must review all the medical data obtained from invasive and noninvasive testing procedures to select an appropriate level of activity for the patient's program.

To help the PT accomplish this activity, individuals with cardiac disease are generally classified according to the severity of the condition. Table 11-3 presents two classification systems that use functional and therapeutic terms to determine the patient's basic condition and the type of activity in which the individual might engage.[27]

Other guidelines used by the PT to help establish appropriate cardiac rehabilitation activities include phases of recovery. Cardiac rehabilitation is typically divided into inpatient and outpatient stages. The inpatient stage is often referred to as phase I (acute), whereas the outpatient stage is generally

11

BOX 11-2	*Factors Influencing Recovery Following Chest Surgery*

Preoperative Factors
- Risk factor profile
- Underlying pulmonary or heart disease
- Other medical problems

Factors During Operation
- Pulmonary collapse and hypoxemia
- Direct trauma to heart or lungs
- Heart arrhythmias
- Danger of emboli (clots) in lungs
- Damage to the mucous membrane of the lungs
- Poor humidity to lungs
- Reaction of lungs to anesthesia
- Drying of pleura

Postoperative Factors
- Atelectasis (collapse of alveoli)
- Narcotics to suppress pain
- Incisional pain preventing deep breathing
- Inactivity promoting shallow breathing
- Inability to clear lung secretions because of decreased coughing
- Pain
- Weakness

Modified from Howell S, Hill J: Acute respiratory care in open heart surgery. Phys Ther 1972;52:253-260.

broken down into phase II (subacute), phase III (intensive rehabilitation), and phase IV (ongoing rehabilitation).[10,21,28] This classification system varies a great deal and often remains specific to a program. For instance, phase IV is frequently combined with phase III.

The person would participate in phase I of the cardiac rehabilitation program as an inpatient. Table 11-4 lists the kinds of exercises and activities of daily living that a PT or PTA would supervise or monitor.[21] The therapist or assistant must monitor the ECG, heart rate, blood pressure, and other physiological parameters to ensure that the patient stays within the predetermined safety range. It is important to note that the patient is involved in educational activities, including risk factor modification, understanding the medications being taken, and discharge planning. This education program could also include flexibility exercises and learning how to take one's own pulse.

After discharge, the individual participates in the outpatient phases of the cardiac rehabilitation program. These phases focus on exercises that will gradually and safely increase the individual's functional capacity. The early stages of outpatient rehabilitation (phase II) are performed under supervision and monitored closely. Generally, patients attend outpatient cardiac rehabilitation

Table 11-3
Functional and Therapeutic Classifications of Patients with Diseases of the Heart

Functional Classification		Therapeutic Classification	
Level	Description	Level	Description
I	Patients with cardiac disease, but without resulting limitations of physical activity. Ordinary physical capacity does not cause undue fatigue, palpitation, dyspnea, or anginal pain.	A	Patients with cardiac disease whose physical activity need not be restricted in any way
II	Patients with cardiac disease resulting in slight limitation of physical activity. Patients are comfortable at rest. Ordinary physical activity results in fatigue, palpitation, dyspnea, or pain.	B	Patients with cardiac disease whose ordinary physical activity need not be restricted but who should be advised against severe or competitive effort
III	Patients with cardiac disease resulting in marked limitation of physical activity. Patients are comfortable at rest. Less than ordinary physical activity causes fatigue, palpitation, dyspnea, or anginal pain.	C	Patients with cardiac disease whose ordinary physical activity should be moderately restricted and whose more strenuous efforts should be discontinued
IV	Patients with cardiac disease resulting in an inability to carry out any physical activity without discomfort. Symptoms of cardiac insufficiency or anginal syndrome may be present even at rest. If any physical activity is undertaken, discomfort is increased.	D	Patients with cardiac disease whose ordinary physical activity should be markedly restricted
		E	Patients with cardiac disease who should be at complete rest or confined to bed or chair

Data from Functional and Therapeutic Classifications of Patients with Diseases of the Heart. Dallas, American Heart Association, 1999.

11

programs that have representatives of the entire rehabilitation team (e.g., occupational therapy, physical therapy, nutrition). During phase II, close physician management is always available. Depending on the severity of the problem, the patient will attend supervised training sessions three or four times a week for 10 to 12 weeks. If recovery has continued well, a stress test will be performed to help determine whether the patient has improved or responded to the exercise program.

Table 11-4
Seven-Step Inpatient Rehabilitation Program for Myocardial Infarction

Step	Supervised Exercises	Activities of Daily Living	Educational Activities
1	Active and passive ROM of all extremities, in bed; teach patients ankle plantar flexion and dorsiflexion, repeat hourly when awake	Partial self-care, feed self, dangle legs on side of bed, use bedside commode	Orientation to CCU, personal emergencies, social service aid as needed
2	Active ROM of all extremities, sitting on side of bed	Sit in chair 15-30 min 2-3 times/day; complete self-care in bed	Orientation to rehabilitation team, program; smoking cessation, if needed; educational literature, if requested; planning transfer from CCU
3	Warm-up exercises, stretching, calisthenics; walk 50 ft and back at slow pace	Sit in chair, go to ward class in wheelchair, walk in room	Normal cardiac anatomy and function, what happens with myocardial infarction
4	ROM and calisthenics; walk length of hall (75 ft) and back, average pace; teach pulse counting	Out of bed as tolerated, walk to bathroom, walk to ward class with supervision	Coronary risk factors and their control
5	ROM and calisthenics, check pulse counting, practice walking few stair steps, walk 300 ft twice daily	Walk to waiting room or telephone, walk in ward corridor	Diet, energy conservation, work simplification techniques (as needed)
6	Continue above activities; walk down flight of stairs (return by elevator), walk 500 ft; instruct on home exercises	Tepid shower or tub bath with supervision, go to occupational therapy, cardiac clinic teaching room, with supervision	Heart attack management; medications; exercise; family, community adjustments on return home
7	Continue above activities; walk up flight of steps, walk 500 ft; continue home exercise instruction, present information regarding outpatient exercise program	Continue all previous ward activities	Discharge planning: medications, diet; return to work; community resources; educational literature; medication cards

CCU, Cardiac care unit; *ROM,* range of motion.
Data from Functional and Therapeutic Classifications of Patients with Diseases of the Heart. Dallas, American Heart Association, 1999.

Progression to phases III and IV involves more independent and aggressive activities. To proceed to these levels, the individual must (1) be able to self-monitor the exercise program, (2) have no contraindications to exercise, and (3) be emotionally stable.[19] These phases include a gradual increase in exercise intensity. Periodic checkups by the professional team occur most frequently in phase III. Once phase IV has been attained, the patient should be functioning at the maximum safe capacity.

During the outpatient phases of the cardiac rehabilitation program, the exercises emphasize aerobic training that includes rhythmic activity of large muscle masses. Appropriate aerobic training involves a warm-up period, a peak period, and a cool-down period. The length of time for these periods may vary with the status of the patient, but generally the warm-up and cool-down phases should be at least 8 to 10 minutes each. The peak period should last 20 to 60 minutes. It is during the peak period that the patient must reach and maintain a target heart rate. [10,12]

A **target heart rate (THR)** is calculated as a percentage of the individual's maximum heart rate. The maximum heart rate can be accurately determined only by a maximum stress test. However, it is commonly *estimated* by subtracting one's age from 220. The THR is then determined to establish a person's **"training zone,"** or the minimum and maximum heart rates that must be achieved to produce an aerobic training effect. The percentage of the maximum heart rate that is selected depends on the individual's level of fitness, symptoms, and ECG findings. If the person has cardiac disease and is very deconditioned, the training zone levels will be small, perhaps only a maximum of 120 beats per minute or 20 to 30 beats per minute above resting levels.[10] By contrast, a training zone for a young athlete may fall between THRs of 60% to 85% of that person's maximum heart rate capacity. To produce a "training effect" or a change in aerobic capacity, this individual would have to reach a heart rate in the established "training zone." The important thing to remember is that as aerobic capacity improves, the amount of work the heart has to perform at a specific exercise intensity decreases. This improvement in aerobic capacity in turn improves the patient's functional capacity without causing the heart to be overworked.

Besides the intensity of exercise (how hard a patient works during a single exercise period) and the duration of exercise (how long each exercise period should last), factors to consider in the planning of an aerobic training program include the mode of exercise (what the patient does, such as walking, jogging, bicycle riding) and the frequency of exercise (how many times a day or week the patient exercises).[15] The mode of exercise must allow for aerobic performance, which includes rhythmic contraction of large muscle groups over several minutes (20 to 60 minutes). Running, swimming, walking, and bicycle riding all promote this type of activity. An individual with cardiac disease, however, may not be able to sustain 20 minutes of exercise at one time; therefore several periods of exercise throughout the day would be more appropriate. The frequency of exercise may also be determined by the patient's condition. Normally, in the latter phases of their program, individuals with cardiac disease must generally perform a minimum of 20 minutes of exercise three to five times per week to promote or maintain aerobic training.[7]

11

The PT and PTA must continuously monitor the patient during all phases of the exercise program. Appropriate monitoring includes assessing heart rate, blood pressure, and respiratory rate responses to the specific exercise intensity. This monitoring is quite important, especially in the early phases of rehabilitation, to ensure that the patient does not exercise at an unsafe level. As the patient progresses, the therapist must teach self-monitoring for safe participation in activities, thus moving the patient one step closer to independent activity. When the patient can function independently at maximum functional capability, the therapist's responsibilities have been met.

PHYSICAL THERAPY PULMONARY REHABILITATION PROCEDURES

As with patients who have cardiac dysfunction, the PT is responsible for establishing an appropriate level of exercise programming for individuals with pulmonary disease. The intensity and duration of the program must be at an appropriate level to promote a training effort that will enhance the patient's ability to perform daily functions aerobically. Aerobic performance occurs when the active muscles receive all the oxygen they need to perform their task. To select the appropriate intensity and duration of exercise, the PT must review the results of all examination procedures performed on the patient. From these data and the physical therapy evaluation, the appropriate exercise program can be established. It is important to remember that during aerobic exercise the PT and PTA must monitor the patient's cardiovascular response to the exercise, such as the heart rate, blood pressure, and breathing rate and depth, as well as elicit feedback on how the patient feels. In this way, excessive exercise that could put the patient at risk is prevented.

Other components of physical therapy treatment for patients with pulmonary disease include techniques for secretion removal, respiratory muscle training and breathing, and saving energy.

Secretion removal techniques are performed in patients who produce excessive mucus in the bronchi of the lungs as occurs in obstructive pulmonary disease. The technique applied to promote mucus removal is called **postural drainage**. The patient is placed in a certain position ("posture") to passively drain fluid from a specific portion of the lung. The therapist applies percussion (or clapping), vibration, and shaking to specific areas of the chest wall overlying specific lobes of the lung (Figure 11-10).[29] Percussion promotes movement of mucus through the bronchial tubes. Having the patient assume Trendelenburg's (inverted) position and cough immediately after the percussion or vibration procedure also helps move mucus out of the different sections of the lungs.

Producing a good cough is essential for maintaining normal lung function in everyone. If the respiratory muscles are weakened or do not work properly, the efficiency of the cough mechanism is reduced. This reduced cough efficiency can occur in both the obstructive and restrictive disease patterns. It also occurs in patients who have experienced trauma, such as an individual with quadriplegia after spinal cord injury or patients who have had thoracic surgery.

The PT can help the patient enhance coughing in three ways: by strengthening both the primary and secondary muscles of ventilation, by changing

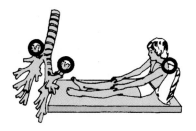
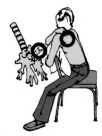

UPPER LOBES Apical Segments

Bed or drainage table flat.
Patient leans back on pillow at 30° angle
against therapist.
Therapist claps with markedly cupped hand
over area between clavicle and top of
scapula on each side.

UPPER LOBES Posterior Segments

Bed or drainage table flat.
Patient leans over folded pillow at 30° angle.
Therapist stands behind and claps over upper
back on both sides

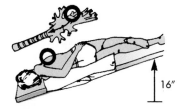
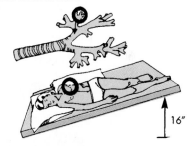

RIGHT MIDDLE LOBE

Foot of table or bed elevated 16 inches.
Patient lies head down on left side and rotates
1/4 turn backward.
Pillow may be placed behind from shoulder to
hip. Knees should be flexed.
Therapist claps over right nipple area. In
females with breast development or tenderness,
use cupped hand with heel of hand under
armpit and fingers extending forward beneath
the breast.

LEFT UPPER LOBE Lingular Segments

Foot of table or bed elevated 16 inches.
Patient lies head down on right side and rotates
1/4 turn backward. Pilow may be placed behind
from shoulder to hip. Knees should be flexed.
Therapist claps with moderately cupped hand
over left nipple area.
In females with breast development or
tenderness, use cupped hand with heel of hand
under armpit and fingers extending forward
beneath the breast.

Figure 11-10 ■ Positions and guidelines for performing postural drain-
age to remove fluid from the lungs. See also Figure 2-11. (From Rothstein
JM, Roy SH, Wolf SL, Scalzitti D: The Rehabilitation Specialist's
Handbook, ed 3. Philadelphia, FA Davis, 2005.)   *Continued*

11

the breathing pattern, and by teaching the patient how to use different devices
to support the chest wall so that the expiration force generated during coughing
is enhanced.[25]

Patients are taught energy-saving techniques so they can perform their daily
activities more efficiently, thereby decreasing the demand on the pulmonary
system. The PT determines the activity needs for the patient in the home or
work environment and then helps select assistive devices that can be used to
perform certain tasks. Examples of such devices include a bathtub seat for

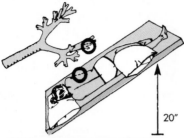

LOWER LOBES Lateral Basal Segments

Foot of table or bed elevated 20 inches.
Patient lies on abdomen, head down, then rotates
1/4 turn upward. Upper leg is flexed over a pillow
for support. Therapist claps over uppermost portion
of lower ribs. (Position shown is for drainage of right
lateral basal segment. To drain the left lateral basal
segment, patient should lie on his right side in the
same posture.)

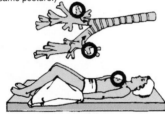

LOWER LOBES Anterior Segments

Bed or drainage table flat.
Patient lies on back with pillow under knees.
Therapist claps between clavicle and nipple on
each side.

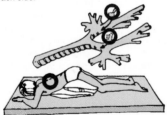

LOWER LOBES Superior Segments

Bed or table flat.
Patient lies on abdomen with two pillows under hips.
Therapist claps over middle of back at tip of scapula
on either side of spine.

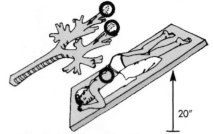

LOWER LOBES Posterior Basal Segments

Foot of table or bed elevated 20 inches.
Patient lies on abdomen, head down, with pillow under
hips. Therapist claps over lower ribs close to spine on
each side.

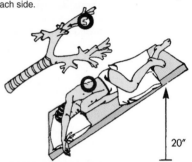

LOWER LOBES Anterior Basal Segments

Foot of table or bed elevated 20 inches.
Patient lies on side, head down, pillow under knees.
Therapist claps with slightly cupped hand over lower
ribs. (Position shown is for drainage of left anterior basal
segment. To drain the right anterior basal segment,
patient should lie on his left side in same posture.)

Figure 11-10, *cont'd* ■ Positions and guidelines for performing postural
drainage to remove fluid from the lungs. See also Figure 2-11. (From
Rothstein JM, Roy SH, Wolf SL, Scalzitti D: The Rehabilitation
Specialist's Handbook, ed 3. Philadelphia, FA Davis, 2005.)

showering in a seated position or a long shoehorn to make putting on shoes easier. The therapist also teaches these patients how to divide an activity into components so that each part of an activity is performed in stages. This technique is sometimes referred to as pacing.[10,12,25]

The PT and PTA engage in direct intervention during pulmonary rehabilitation. They also participate in helping to modify the patient's risk factor profile, such as promoting weight management, good nutrition, smoking cessation, and a positive psychological state. They must be prepared to monitor the activities of other health care professionals and ensure that their treatment program is integrated into a comprehensive care plan. The primary goal for pulmonary rehabilitation is to help the patient achieve the highest functional level allowed by the pulmonary impairment.

THE "WELL" INDIVIDUAL

A discussion of cardiovascular and pulmonary physical therapy would not be complete without reviewing the concept of the "well" individual (person without a diagnosis of any cardiovascular or pulmonary disease). These individuals may be candidates for fitness programs aimed at improving their functional work capacity. A PT or PTA needs to be prepared to offer guidance to such persons. Generally, these exercise programs focus on a specific purpose for starting exercise. Such purposes may include stress reduction, weight management, improvement in physique and body image, alteration of cardiac risk factors, or enhancement of functional capacity.[10]

The aging population represents a large group of "well" individuals who can benefit from exercise but have a tendency to be sedentary. Specific cardiovascular and pulmonary changes occur with aging, one of the most specific being a decrease in the safe maximum heart rate. It is well established that the heart rate is inversely related to age. As a person grows older, the maximum heart rate declines. At the same time the pulmonary system demonstrates a decline in both static and dynamic measurements. Although endurance training in the elderly cannot reduce cardiac changes, it can reduce pulmonary changes.[7]

Just as an individual with cardiac or pulmonary disease needs an examination, so does the "well" individual. This examination should include reviewing the risk factor profile, including smoking and family history. The PT should examine the functional status of the musculoskeletal system. The performance results of an exercise stress test, body composition (percentage of body fat), strength, and flexibility should also be reviewed. Any preexisting conditions, such as orthopaedic abnormalities, must also be considered. An important aspect of the examination is to determine the individual's specific interests. Does he or she like to swim, run, or ride a bicycle? Understanding the person's interests could help the therapist design a program more likely to induce compliance with the exercise routine.

Box 11-3 presents a summary of benefits gained from aerobic and strength-training programs.[10] This type of information can be used to encourage a sedentary person to engage in a regular exercise program. Appropriate assessment and monitoring, however, must accompany any regular exercise.

BOX 11-3   *Benefits of Aerobic Exercise and Strength-Training Programs*

Benefits of an Aerobic Exercise Program
- Improvement in aerobic capacity
- Increased efficiency to extract oxygen in trained muscles
- Increase in stroke volume
- Decrease in resting heart rate
- Decrease in submaximal heart rates
- Change in body composition (loss of fat)
- Decreased clotting factors in blood
- Decrease in resting blood pressure in hypertensive individuals
- Altered method of cholesterol transport
- Increase in high-density lipoproteins (HDLs)
- Slight decrease in low-density lipoproteins (LDLs)
- Decrease in various fats produced by the body
- Increase in using carbohydrates as an energy source
- Improvement in psychological well-being
- Improved response to stress
- Decrease in physiological responsiveness to stimuli
- Improved self-image
- Decrease in risk for developing heart disease owing to elimination of a number of the risk factors

Benefits of a Strength-Training Program
- Increase in strength of trained muscles
- Increase in use of anaerobic metabolism
- Improved ease in performing many activities of daily living, especially with upper body strength training
- Increase in bone mass
- Increase in size, endurance, or both, of trained muscles
- Improvement of body image and self-esteem

Modified from Hillegass EA, Sadowsky HS: Essentials of Cardiopulmonary Physical Therapy, ed 2. Philadelphia, Saunders, 2001.

SUMMARY

Cardiovascular and pulmonary physical therapy has, over the past three decades, become an inherent part of the knowledge and practice base of the PT. This chapter presented the prevalence of the cardiovascular and pulmonary impairments, a fundamental review of the structure and function of the related systems, common conditions, a description of invasive and noninvasive diagnostic tests, principles of medical and rehabilitation procedures, and the physical therapy approach to the "well" individual. A thorough understanding of the anatomy, physiology, and function of the cardiovascular and pulmonary system is essential to develop the skills necessary to make appropriate clinical decisions for proper examination, management, and progression of patients with cardiovascular/pulmonary diseases. It is also essential for PTs and PTAs to remember that no matter what the diagnosis, when exercise is applied as an intervention, the cardiovascular and pulmonary response to that exercise must always be monitored.

PTs working with individuals who have cardiovascular or pulmonary disease must also be acutely aware of their role as team members. Whether guiding a PTA in applying appropriate exercise intensity or discussing maximum exercise intensity levels with a cardiologist, the PT must take into account the total management program the patient with cardiovascular or pulmonary disease is experiencing.

CASE STUDIES

CASE STUDY ONE

Clinical History

Joe is a 60-year-old man who retired after 30 years as a high school math teacher. He had not experienced any previous symptoms of heart disease, such as chest pain or shortness of breath, but had been taking medicine over the past 3 years for mild high blood pressure, which was well controlled. His risk factor profile included the following:

Family history—mother and older brother died of heart disease

Smoking—between the ages of 16 and 40, one pack per day

Sedentary—has not engaged in any regular exercise program since the age of 50

Obesity—has "been carrying" an extra 30 lb since his mid forties

One week ago he was admitted to the emergency room after 1 hour of severe chest pain. The ECG demonstrated severe abnormalities indicating a change in the function of the anterolateral part of his heart. He was rushed to the operating room, where cardiac catheterization revealed major blockage in different sections of his left coronary artery. Angioplasty was performed on two areas of artery blockage, and it improved blood flow through the left coronary artery by 90%.

Cardiac Rehabilitation

After surgery, Joe was admitted to the cardiac care unit. He was prescribed medications that helped control his heart rate, improve the strength of the heart's contractions, and prevent arrhythmias. The PT assessed the patient's status and, after conferring with the cardiologist and ward nurse, initiated the activities outlined in Table 11-4. The PT reported the following results at the end of the exercise period:

1. Resting heart rate (beats per minute): 86 while lying in bed, 98 while sitting, 105 while standing, 135 while performing activities of daily living such as brushing teeth at the bedside.
2. Blood pressure: 130/90 while lying in bed, 110/80 while sitting, 110/65 while standing, 100/60 while performing daily activities.
3. ECG: no indication of any change in pattern except when performing daily activities. This change demonstrated possible mild ischemia.

After 2 days in the cardiac care unit, Joe was transferred to the ward. Following appropriate examination, the PT initiated the exercise and education programs

11

for ward activities listed in Table 11-4. After the first 2 days of this exercise routine, the patient demonstrated appropriate physiological responses to the exercises. The PTA assumed the responsibility for the ambulation and range-of-motion exercises. The patient was discharged after 1 week of hospitalization. He had an understanding that the medicine he took was to help prevent arrhythmias. He had learned how to take his own pulse and was instructed to not engage in any activities that caused his heart rate to exceed 135 beats per minute. At the time of discharge, he was instructed to move his bed to the first floor of his home to avoid a flight of stairs.

Outpatient Program

Joe returned to the outpatient cardiac rehabilitation program conducted in the physical therapy department 3 days after discharge. He reported that he had not had any difficulty at home; however, further inquiry revealed that he did not engage in any activity other than activities of daily living and walking around the house.

The PT initiated phase II of cardiac rehabilitation by determining how long Joe could walk on a treadmill at his preferred rate before reaching the THR of 135 beats per minute. This rate was established by the cardiologist at the time of discharge as the maximum exercise heart rate that Joe could reach. Over the next three outpatient visits (1 week), the PT established the following exercise routine to be performed at home twice daily:

1. 15 minutes of warm-up and stretching
2. 20 minutes of stationary bicycle riding
3. 15 minutes of cool-down exercises

Joe remained on this exercise program for 3 more weeks. During that time he came to the cardiac rehabilitation program to meet with a nutritionist and a psychologist. He then underwent an exercise stress test on a treadmill, which revealed that he could safely reach a maximum heart rate of 146 beats per minute before incurring serious changes in heart function. Phase III cardiac rehabilitation was then initiated and included bicycle riding and fast walking with increasing intensity, duration, and frequency. At the end of 6 weeks of monitored phase III activities, another stress test revealed that Joe could reach a safe maximum heart rate of 160 beats per minute. His resting heart rate and blood pressure were now within normal limits, he lost 20 lb, and his diet was cholesterol free. He was no longer taking any cardiac medication. The cardiologist approved Joe's transfer into phase IV cardiac rehabilitation with 3-month checkups by the PT and another stress test in 1 year.

CASE STUDY TWO

Clinical History

Martha is a 58-year-old homemaker with a history of shortness of breath on exertion. She admits to a 25-year history of smoking but stopped 5 years ago. She states that she has a productive cough in the morning. Recently, she was admitted to the hospital with a temperature of 102° F and a productive cough. Severe upper respiratory tract infection was the diagnosis. This was Martha's third such admission in the past year. After discharge the physician requested a full pulmonary examination and initiation of rehabilitation to reduce the frequency of hospitalization.

The results of pulmonary testing revealed that her ability to forcefully expire a normal volume of air in 1 second was markedly decreased even though the total volume of air in her lungs remained near normal. The carbon dioxide concentration in her blood was elevated, and the amount of oxygen was below normal. A chest radiograph demonstrated mild inflammation of the bronchial tubes.

Examination

Physical therapy examination of her chest revealed that her breathing pattern depended mostly on the diaphragm with little chest wall motion. The angle between her ribs and sternum has increased, which indicates that her lower chest wall has permanently expanded beyond normal. There is evidence that her accessory muscles of ventilation around the neck and shoulders contract during quiet inspiration. When Martha was placed on a treadmill and asked to walk at 3 mph with no grade, she demonstrated a further drop in the oxygen saturation of her blood, shortness of breath, and mild wheezing.

Pulmonary Rehabilitation

The results of the examination led to a diagnosis of moderate obstructive lung disease accompanied by physical deconditioning. The primary goals for Martha's rehabilitation program would be to achieve a daily walk or jog of 30 continuous minutes without shortness of breath, improve her functional capacity, and perform pulmonary hygiene to assist with clearing of her lungs each morning.

The PT instructed Martha in the appropriate postural drainage positions that she will use for 10 minutes on each side of the chest before getting out of bed in the morning. She was taught breathing exercises that will help mobilize her lower chest wall, increase the strength of her diaphragm and intercostal muscles, and improve her ability to perform a forceful cough. Martha must also learn specific diet modifications and how to monitor for symptoms that might occur if her blood oxygen concentration drops too severely.

Martha's exercise program includes progressive walking. The heart rate achieved when shortness of breath requires her to stop will be used as the maximum heart rate. Warm-up and cool-down periods will occur before and after the continuous walking period. The duration, intensity, and frequency of the exercise program will be increased until she can achieve 30 continuous minutes of walking without shortness of breath. In conjunction with the exercise program, the PT must educate the patient on how she will monitor herself safely and perform the exercise routine independently.

11

REFERENCES

1. Heart Disease and Stroke Statistics—2006 Update. Dallas, American Heart Association. Available at http://circ.ahajournals.org/cgi/content/short/113/6/e85. Accessed May 11, 2006.
2. Trends in Chronic Bronchitis and Emphysema: Morbidity and Mortality. New York, American Lung Association. Available at http://www.lungusa.org/atf/cf/{7A8D42C2-FCCA-4604-8ADE-7F5D5E762256}/COPD1.pdf. Accessed May 11, 2006.
3. Williams PL: Gray's Anatomy, ed 38. Philadelphia, Saunders, 1995.
4. Phillips RE, Feeney MK: The Cardiac Rhythm: A Systematic Approach to Interpretation, ed 2. Philadelphia, Saunders, 1990.

5. Moore KL, Dalley AF: Clinically Oriented Anatomy, ed 5. Philadephia, Lippincott Williams & Wilkins, 2005.

6. Sanderson RG, Kurth CL: The Cardiac Patient: A Comprehensive Approach, ed 2. Philadelphia, Saunders, 1983.

7. McArdle WD, Katch FI, Katch VL: Exercise Physiology—Energy, Nutrition, and Human Performance, ed 5. Philadelphia, Lippincott Williams & Wilkins, 2001.

8. Dorland's Medical Dictionary, ed 30. Philadelphia, Saunders, 2003.

9. Van De Graaff KM, Fox SI: Concepts of Human Anatomy and Physiology, ed 5. Dubuque, IA, WC Brown, 1998.

10. Hillegass EA, Sadowsky HS: Essentials of Cardiopulmonary Physical Therapy, ed 2. Philadelphia, Saunders, 2001.

11. Heart and Stroke Statistical Update. Dallas, American Heart Association, 1998.

12. Brannon FJ, Foley MW, Starr JA, et al: Cardiopulmonary Rehabilitation: Basic Theory and Application, ed 3. Philadelphia, FA Davis, 1998.

13. Guide to Physical Therapist Practice, revised ed 2. Alexandria, VA, American Physical Therapy Association, 2003.

14. Dubin D: Rapid Interpretation of EKG, ed 6. Tampa, FL, Cover Publishing, 2000.

15. American College of Sports Medicine: Guidelines for Exercise Testing and Prescription, ed 6. Philadelphia, Lippincott Williams & Wilkins, 2000.

16. Ellestad MH, Myrvin H: Stress Testing Principles and Practice. Philadelphia, FA Davis, 1986.

17. Minter RA: Chest Imaging: An Integrated Approach. Baltimore, Williams & Wilkins, 1981.

18. Cohen S (ed): Pulmonary Function Tests in Patient Care. New York, American Journal of Nursing Company, 1980.

19. Cohen S (ed): Blood Gas and Acid Base Concepts in Respiratory Care. New York, American Journal of Nursing Company, 1976.

20. Ciccone CD: Pharmacology in Rehabilitation, ed 3. Philadelphia, FA Davis, 2002.

21. Wenger NK, Hellerstein HK: Rehabilitation of the Coronary Patient, ed 3. New York, Churchill Livingstone, 1992.

22. Hills LD: Manual of Clinical Problems in Cardiology, ed 3. Philadelphia, Little, Brown, 1989.

23. Wuff KS: Management of the cardiovascular surgery patient. *In:* Brunner LS, Suddarth DS (eds): Textbook of Medical-Surgical Nursing, ed 10. Philadelphia, Lippincott Williams & Wilkins, 2003.

24. Reul GJ: Implantation of a permanent cardiac pacemaker. *In:* Cooley DA (ed): Techniques in Cardiac Surgery, ed 2. Philadelphia, Saunders, 1984.

25. Frownfelter DL: Chest Physical Therapy and Pulmonary Rehabilitation: An Interdisciplinary Approach, ed 2. Chicago, Year Book, 1987.

26. Howell S, Hill J: Acute respiratory care in open heart surgery. Phys Ther 1972;52:253-260.

27. Functional and Therapeutic Classifications of Patients with Diseases of the Heart. Dallas, American Heart Association, 1999.

28. Irwin S, Tecklin JS: Cardiopulmonary Physical Therapy, ed 4. St Louis, Mosby, 2005.

29. Rothstein JM, Roy SH, Wolf SL, Scalzitti D: The Rehabilitation Specialist's Handbook, ed 3. Philadelphia, FA Davis, 2005.

ADDITIONAL RESOURCE

Frownfelter D, Dean E: Principles and Practice of Cardiopulmonary Physical Therapy, ed 3. St Louis, Mosby, 1996.

Practical and readable, this text covers the basics of cardiopulmonary physical therapy. Throughout the text the theme of oxygen transport is stressed. Features include key terms, review questions, and a glossary. A case studies workbook is also available.

REVIEW QUESTIONS

1. Create a diagram that illustrates the processes of respiration and ventilation.
2. Explain why we look at the cardiovascular and respiratory systems together. Don't they have distinctly different functions?
3. Generate and label a diagram that helps you identify events associated with different components of the heart cycle.
4. Research the use of at least one of the cardiovascular or pulmonary diagnostic tools discussed in this chapter. Prepare a demonstration, especially if you are able to include a visit to a treatment facility as part of your research.
5. Make up a simple description of a patient in need of cardiac rehabilitation. (A paragraph is long enough.) Then create a flow chart of the typical therapy process and the changes made as the patient progresses.
6. Repeat the steps assigned in question 5, but this time apply it to a patient in pulmonary rehabilitation.

11

Problems cannot be solved at the same level of awareness that created them.
Albert Einstein

12

Physical Therapy for Integumentary Conditions

R. Scott Ward

KEY TERMS

arterial insufficiency
chronic inflammation
collagen
dermatitis
dermis
epidermis
ground substance
hypertrophic scar
inflammatory phase
inflammatory skin diseases
integument
keloid scar
maturation phase
neoplastic skin diseases
neuropathic (neurotropic) ulcer
pressure ulcer
proliferative phase
scar contraction
scar contracture
total body surface area (TBSA)
Vancouver Burn Scar Scale
venous insufficiency

OBJECTIVES ▮▬▬▬

After reading this chapter, the reader will be able to:

- Discuss the structure and function of the skin
- Discuss the process of wound healing, including the three major phases—inflammation, proliferation, and maturation

- Describe common problems associated with the integument (including vascular compromise, trauma, and disease) and the basic examination principles related to those conditions
- Describe basic intervention principles and strategies necessary in complete patient care (including prevention, management, and education)

Various types of integumentary (skin) wounds or impairments in skin integrity, the consequences of these wounds, and any associated effects of the wound such as inflammation, pain, edema, and scar formation can lead to significant functional limitations and disability. Physical therapists (PTs) and physical therapist assistants (PTAs) must be aware of the importance of the integumentary system in normal human function. They should be able to provide programs or interventions to prevent loss of skin integrity. Appropriate management of patients with various impairments of the skin is a critical part of physical therapy practice.

GENERAL DESCRIPTION

INTEGUMENT

The **integument**, the largest organ of the body, ranges from about 1 to 4 mm in thickness and consists of two layers—the epidermis and the dermis. Beneath the dermis lies a layer of subcutaneous tissue. The integument is basically a protective organ, but it also serves a role in temperature control and provides important sensory information regarding the environment. Figure 12-1 illustrates the structure of the skin and its appendages.

Epidermis. The **epidermis** is very thin in comparison to the overall thickness of the skin. The thickness of the epidermis generally ranges from about 0.06 to 0.1 mm. It is thicker only on the soles of the feet and the palms of the hand, where the most superficial layer of the epidermis, the stratum corneum, may increase the thickness to 0.6 mm. This thicker stratum corneum is often referred to as callus. The preponderant cells in the epidermis are keratinocytes produced in the basal cell layer. The basal cell layer is also where the epidermis is anchored to the dermis. Keratinocytes take a minimum of 28 days to differentiate through their epidermal phases until they are finally sloughed off the most external surface of the stratum corneum. It is the stratum corneum that restricts the loss of fluids from internal tissue and separates this same internal tissue from the external environment.

Other cells that make up the epithelium are Langerhans cells, Merkel cells, and melanocytes. Langerhans cells play a role in the immune response in skin. Merkel cells are acknowledged as sensory receptor cells that provide information about tactile stimuli. Melanocytes (located in the basal cell layer) synthesize

12

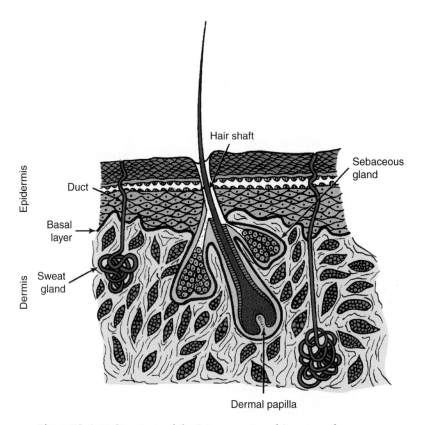

Figure 12-1 ■ Structure of the integument and its appendages.

melanin, which is a pigment that principally serves as primary protection against harmful ultraviolet radiation. Once produced, melanin is transferred from melanocytes to keratinocytes. Melanocytes are also present in the dermis and hair follicles (as well as other sites, such as the retina).

Other components of the epidermis that penetrate into the dermis are hair follicles, sebaceous glands, apocrine glands, and sweat (eccrine) glands. The basal cell layer surrounds each of these structures because of their connection with the epidermis. Hair is formed at the follicle by a process of keratinization that produces three layers of cells. The hair follicle is an invagination of the epidermis. Hair type and amount depend on several factors, including hormonal influence, age, and heredity. Sebaceous glands produce a fatty secretion and are found in association with every hair follicle (pilosebaceous glands). Some sebaceous glands not associated with hair follicles are also found in a general distribution over the body with the exception of the soles of the feet, the palms of the hands, and the lower lip. The main function of the sebaceous glands is to keep the skin "moisturized" and pliant and to prevent it from drying and cracking. The apocrine glands begin to secrete a commonly colorless and odorless oily sweat at the onset of puberty. These glands are localized in the anogenital and axillary areas. The odor associated with perspiration in these areas results from bacterial decomposition of the secretions. Sweat is a hypotonic solution that is delivered to the skin surface by sweat glands. Normal function of the sweat glands is critical in temperature regulation.

Dermis. The **dermis** consists of fibrous and elastic connective tissue encompassed by a ground substance. The dermis varies from 1 to 4 mm in thickness and has two subdivisions—the papillary dermis and the reticular dermis. The papillary dermis, which is composed of a loosely organized collagen matrix and is highly vascular, forms in reflection to the basal cell layer of the epidermis. The junction between these two layers of skin is far from flat. The ridges formed at the dermal-epidermal junction (epidermal ridges and dermal papillae, respectively) provide protection against potentially damaging perturbations such as shearing and deepen the dispersion of the epidermal basal cell layer. The reticular dermis is composed of more densely bundled collagen fibers and less ground substance than the papillary dermis. The ground substance of the dermis is made up of various proteoglycans, glycoproteins, hyaluronic acid, and water. This "gel" forms the interstitial environment that accommodates the composite of dermal elements—fibroelastic collagen, blood vessels, and nerves—along with the epidermal appendages. The fibrous collagen supplies fortification against mechanical stresses on the skin while still allowing the deformation necessary for movement. The elastic connective tissue restores the collagen network to its "resting" arrangement, and the ground substance acts as a "cushion" to protect against many detrimental compression forces.

Blood vessels and nerves are also found within the dermis. The vascular structure in the dermis is vast and allows typically efficient diffusion of gases and nutrients to promote healthy cell function. The vascular system of the dermis additionally participates in the inflammatory response, an important component of wound healing. Along with the sweat glands, the capillaries in the skin also contribute to human thermal regulation. An equally expansive and efficient lymphatic system is associated with the vascular system in the dermis. The dermal nervous network provides the central nervous system with essential sensory information about temperature, pain, and various tactile stimuli (light touch, deep touch, and vibration) singly or in combination to allow for recognition of objects and textures. Efferent nerves innervate the vessels, sweat glands, and arrector pili muscles of the hair follicles.

Subcutaneous Tissue. This layer of tissue consists of loose connective tissue, often containing various amounts of adipose tissue. The loose connective tissue binds the skin to the organ immediately below it in a fashion that allows a reasonable amount of movement of the skin over the underlying organ without displacement or damage.

WOUND HEALING

12

Wound healing is commonly described in three phases: the inflammatory phase, the proliferative phase, and the remodeling phase. Each of the phases, along with applicable interventions for each phase, will be discussed briefly in this section. It is important that all the phases of wound repair occur simultaneously to some extent. For example, inflammation can occur while the proliferative process is in progress.

Inflammatory Phase. With any injury comes an **inflammatory phase** that initiates repair of the damaged tissue.[1] Local cellular and vascular reactions are included in this wound-healing phase.[2] Initial blood loss is decreased by the immediate vasoconstriction of vessels. The vasoconstrictive response may last about 5 to 10 minutes. This time frame also allows the accumulation of platelets and the formation of temporary "platelet clots" along the damaged endothelial lining of the vessels. Activation of the clotting cascade leading to the eventual formation of fibrin clots begins at this time.

The period of vasoconstriction is followed by an episode of vasodilatation and increased capillary permeability. Leukocytes, which are chemotactically recruited to the wound site, are delivered by the increased flow of blood with vasodilatation. Early battles against infection are waged at this point by neutrophils.[3,4] Macrophages also migrate to the wound site to phagocytose wound debris and spent cells. Macrophages release factors important in wound repair, such as cytokines, growth factors, and collagenases.[5,6] Lymphocytes also follow neutrophils into the wound site. They play an important role in the immune response because they release factors that stimulate macrophages and fibroblasts.[7-9] The increased capillary permeability during inflammation can lead to the formation of local edema. Edema hinders healing by reducing the local arterial, venous, and lymphatic circulation and increases the chance of infection for the same reasons. Edema may also restrict motion, which increases the possibility of tissue fibrosis.

Exposure of injured nerves and release of chemical mediators at the wound site can produce pain. Pain often causes a patient to restrict activity because the activity may increase the pain. Decreases in appropriate activity can lead to a reduction in motion and mobility.

The inflammatory phase of healing may normally last about 2 weeks. Longer periods of inflammation are referred to as **chronic inflammation**.

During this phase, appropriate physical therapy interventions might include wound care, edema management, positioning, splinting, cautious passive range-of-motion exercises, active range-of-motion exercises, ambulation, and functional activities such as activities of daily living.

Proliferative Phase. Fibroblasts start converging on the wound site during inflammation, and the **proliferative phase** of wound healing commences with the production of collagen by these cells. Fibroblasts produce a connective tissue scaffold made up of elastin, collagen, and glycosaminoglycans. This process contributes to one of the major events during the proliferative phase of healing—rebuilding and strengthening of the wound site. Elastin is an elastic fibrous protein that provides flexibility to the wound, but it makes up only a small percentage in comparison to collagen.

Collagen is the chief protein produced by fibroblasts.[10] Collagen fibrils formed by fibroblasts combine and form collagen fibers. Collagen fibers supply the preponderance of strength to the wound. The strength lies in the collagen fiber, not in the amount of collagen at the wound site,[11,12] so a patient does not need a big scar to have a strong and well-healed wound.

Ground substance (glycosaminoglycans, water, and salts) occupies the space in between the elastin, collagen, vascular structures, and other cells in the healing wound. The ground substance allows cell proliferation and migration and provides some cushion for the healing tissue.

Angiogenesis (the formation of new blood vessels) begins during the inflammatory phase of healing, but the majority of regrowth occurs during the proliferative healing phase. Vascular genesis is important for the distribution of nutrients and oxygen to cells at the site of healing.

Wounds that are not deep enough to destroy the epidermal basal cell layer can heal through real epidermal regeneration. In epidermal regeneration, proliferation of both epithelial cells at the margin of a wound and epidermal cells from any existing basal cell (such as those in the dermis that encompass hair follicles or sweat glands) ultimately leads to wound coverage. Deeper wounds that do not have basal cells available may still achieve wound closure with epithelium that migrates from adjacent uninjured skin. This process generally occurs only in smaller wounds.

One other concern associated with the proliferative phase of healing is wound contraction. Wounds begin to contract slightly during inflammation; however, aggressive contraction at the wound commences during the proliferative phase. Fibroblasts, particularly myofibroblasts, have contractile capability.[13-16] It appears that the physiological function of wound contraction is to decrease the surface area of the wound, but contraction takes place in wounds of all sizes. Although potentially beneficial in small wounds, contraction is more frequently the cause of decreased mobility and cosmetic change, particularly in wounds associated with joints.

Physical therapy interventions for the proliferative phase of healing may include wound care, edema management, positioning, splinting, cautious passive range-of-motion exercises, active range-of-motion exercises, ambulation, and functional activities such as activities of daily living, similar to interventions during the inflammatory phase. In addition, active assisted range-of-motion exercises, stretching, strengthening exercises, and endurance exercises may be appropriate. During this phase wounds must be handled carefully because a wound may be at only 15% to 80% of its normal strength.[17,18]

Maturation Phase. The **maturation phase** of healing is also often referred to as the remodeling phase. During the maturation phase, collagen continues to be actively deposited while it is also going through active lysis. The balance between the amount of collagen deposition by fibroblasts and the magnitude of collagen lysis influences the ultimate appearance of the scar (if scar formation occurs). If deposition exceeds lysis, either a **hypertrophic scar** or a **keloid scar** forms.[19,20] Keloid scars differ from hypertrophic scars in that they extend beyond the original boundaries of the wound.

During the maturation phase, collagen fibers are deposited in an unorganized fashion. The arrangement of these fibers, however, is influenced by stresses placed on them. For example, stretching an actively forming scar will cause

12

the collagen fibers to align themselves along the length of the stretch and therefore become oriented in an alignment that favors mobility over restriction of movement.

The maturation phase of wound healing may last for several months. While the phase is active, that is, while collagen is being produced, the wound continues to contract with varying degrees of vitality. As the phase nears its end, wound contraction tends to diminish. Contraction during this phase is often referred to as **scar contraction.** If scar contraction leads to either a permanent or a semifixed positional fault at a joint, it is referred to as a **scar contracture.** Race, family history, depth of the wound, size of the wound, patient age, and location of the wound all appear to be factors affecting scar formation.[21-24]

All therapeutic interventions listed for the previous two phases may be applied to the maturation phase of healing. However, the PT or PTA can generally be more aggressive with manipulation of the wound site. Depending on circumstances, the maturation phase may also be the phase when work-hardening and work-conditioning exercises are energetically pursued. Moreover, depending on the size and location of the scar, techniques to control scar formation should be instituted.

Additional Considerations. The variables of repair and patient response to skin wounds include depth of the damage, location of the injury, size of the wound, healing time, and etiology of the disruption. The depth of injury probably has the greatest impact on repair and eventual healing of a wound. For example, superficial wounds that leave a majority of the epidermal basal cells intact often heal without complication. Deeper skin damage that destroys much if not all the epidermal basal cell layer may take weeks to heal or require surgical intervention to hasten repair. Generally, the deeper the wound, the longer it takes to heal. Figure 12-2 illustrates depths of wounds and the integumentary structures involved at the varying depths.

The location of the injury can affect rehabilitation in many ways. For example, wounds on the feet can affect gait, wounds on hands can affect activities that require hand function, and wounds over any joint can lead to impairment in motion and therefore also lead to changes in strength and activities of daily living. Furthermore, wounds at cosmetic sites such as the face and hands may offer psychological challenges for a patient to overcome.

The size of a wound, often measured as the percentage of **total body surface area (TBSA)** affected, has an effect on the extent of the physiological response. A few of the physiological responses that should be considered include the local inflammatory response, the basal metabolic rate, temperature control, cardiopulmonary stresses, hematopoietic reactions, and pain. For example, a large skin wound (such as an extensive burn injury) may dangerously decrease the ability of a patient to control body temperature. Also, a big wound will lead to an increased basal metabolic rate and impose extra nutritional demands on a patient that must be met to avert the protein catabolism that could lead to muscle loss. Infection is a potential problem with any open wound, and increased wound size may increase the risk of infection. As wound size increases, so does the magnitude of the physiological response.

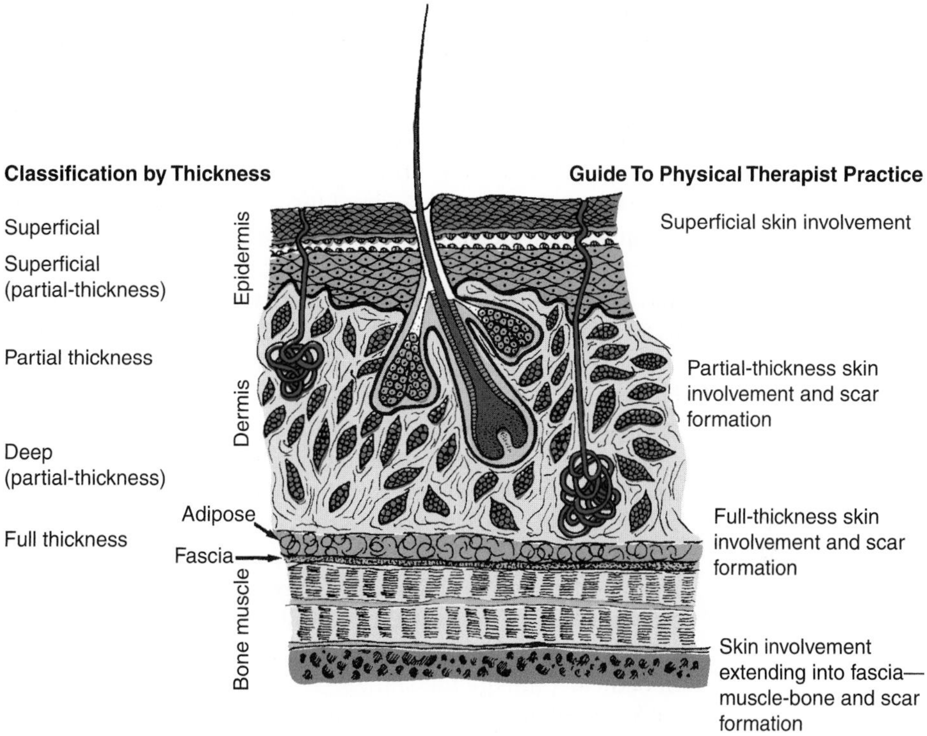

Figure 12-2 ■ Structures involved in varying depths of skin injury.

Wounds that require a long time to heal are associated with two primary problems. First, the risk of infection increases the longer that the wound is open. Second, a wound that takes longer than 2 to 3 weeks to heal is more likely to scar.

COMMON CONDITIONS

Damage to the integument most commonly results from vascular compromise or trauma. Vascular deficiencies such as local tissue ischemia (pressure ulcers and arterial disease) and venous insufficiency can create an unhealthy tissue environment that leads to skin breakdown. Wounds from various types of trauma may include cuts, abrasions, and burns.

The etiology of a wound can provide insight into its prognosis. For example, patients with wounds caused by arterial disease usually require surgical intervention to improve arterial function and eventually improve healing of the associated skin wound. Electrical injuries should lead to the suspicion that tissue deeper than the skin has been damaged.

VASCULAR COMPROMISE

Wounds caused by **arterial insufficiency** are most commonly situated on the foot or ankle, but they also occur at other locations. These wounds are caused by primary loss of vascular flow to an anatomical site, which leads to tissue death.

12

Venous insufficiency (venous stasis) can also lead to ulceration of the skin and generally occurs on the lower part of the legs.[25] Venous stasis may result from venous hypertension, venous thrombosis, varicose (dilated) veins, or obstruction of a portion of the venous system. The precise cause of ulcers caused by venous stasis has not been determined. One theory to explain venous stasis ulceration includes the notion of "fibrin cuff formation" caused by increased capillary leakage of fibrinogen (as well as other large molecules) as a result of venous hypertension.[26] Fibrin then accumulates in the interstitial space and around capillaries and produces an obstacle to the transportation of oxygen and nutrients to tissue. Another theory regarding venous stasis ulcers is referred to as "white cell trapping." Venous hypertension decreases capillary flow and the subsequent removal of leukocytes. The trapped cells then occlude capillaries, which leads to ischemic damage, and may also release substances that bring about direct local tissue damage.[27]

Pressure on tissue causes ischemia, producing damage, tissue hypoxia and death, and a wound referred to as a **pressure ulcer.**[28,29] Only a few hours of pressure can cause severe tissue injury.[30,31] Pressure occurs most commonly over areas of bony prominence, such as the sacral/coccygeal area, ischial tuberosity, heel, lateral malleolus, and greater trochanter. Pressure may increase or decrease, depending on the patient's position.[32] Table 12-1 lists sites at risk for pressure ulcers by position. For example, simply being positioned incorrectly in bed can damage the skin.

Although most pressure ulcers occur at sites of bony prominence, they can develop at any location in which enough pressure is generated to cause ischemia. Inactivity and immobility increase the chance of development of pressure sores.[33] Shearing of the tissue at the site of pressure can further increase the tissue damage. Shearing may occur when a patient is moved from

Table 12-1
Body Areas Commonly at Risk for Pressure Ulcer Development

Position	Areas at Risk
Supine	Occiput, elbows, scapulae, spinous processes, sacrum, coccyx, heels
Seated	Elbows, spinous processes, sacrum, coccyx, ischial tuberosities, greater trochanters, heels
Side-lying	Ear, shoulder, elbow, greater trochanters, medial and lateral aspects of knees, medial and lateral malleoli, heels
Prone	Forehead, nose, chin, anterior of shoulder, iliac crest, patella, dorsal surface of foot or toes

Data from Kosiak M: Etiology and pathology of ischemic ulcers. Arch Phys Med Rehabil 1981; 62:492-498.

one surface to another or moves (slides) on the same surface. This activity causes friction damage to the skin. Friction can denude the epidermal covering and increase the likelihood for pressure ulcer formation. If the skin is exposed to moisture for a certain period, it may become macerated and more liable to break down. Common sources of moisture may include sweat, urine, and feces. Poor nutrition increases the risk for pressure ulcers. Several age-related changes, such as a decrease in overall soft tissue mass that increases the protuberance of bony prominences, atrophy of the dermis, decreased vascularization, and impaired sensory perception, amplify the risk that pressure ulcers will develop.

Ischemic injury can take place as a result of loss of sensory feedback. An ulcer secondary to insensitivity is called a **neuropathic (neurotropic) ulcer.** Decreased sensation limits a person from making appropriate adjustments to potentially damaging situations. For example, a patient with sensory loss in the soles of the feet caused by diabetes mellitus may not notice a tiny pebble in the shoe. Blood flow to the tissue compressed by the pebble decreases as the person continues to bear weight on the stone. Pressure ulcers may also occur with loss of sensory feedback, such as in the case of a patient with a spinal cord injury. If the patient does not perform frequent weight shifts, ischemia resulting from pressure will cause damage to the integument. Neuropathic ulcers may also form as a result of motor neuropathy, leading to anatomical deformity that causes pressure points that would not normally be present.

TRAUMA

Abrasions are integumentary wounds caused by scraping away skin through contact with a rough object or surface. Lacerations are cuts or tears of the integument and may be caused by sharp objects or surfaces. Injuries in which much if not all the skin and generally the subcutaneous tissue are separated from the underlying tissue are referred to as avulsion injuries. When an avulsion injury occurs in a hand or a foot, it may be called a degloving injury. A puncture wound is a hole in the skin created by a pointed, generally sharp object. Burn injuries include damage to skin from many possible causes, such as flame, chemicals, scalding, radiation, and electrical current.

As with some cases of ischemic skin damage, trauma can arise from loss of sensory feedback. Decreased sensation prevents a person from making appropriate adjustments to potentially damaging situations. For example, a patient with decreased sensation in the upper extremities because of edema resulting from surgical removal of axillary lymph nodes may not perceive the hazardous temperature of a dish when removing it from the oven or dangerously hot water, either of which could lead to a burn injury.

DISEASE

The skin can be affected by a number of disorders that may be either benign or life threatening. **Inflammatory skin diseases** are generally patchy sites of acute or chronic inflammation referred to as **dermatitis.** Dermatitis often includes associated symptoms of itching and some scaling of the epidermis. Certain viruses can lead to warts or rashes. Bacteria, foreign bodies, and plugged sebaceous glands are some of the causes that may lead to acne or other skin abscesses.

12

Neoplastic skin diseases (skin cancer) include basal cell carcinoma, squamous cell carcinoma, and malignant melanoma, which are the three most common types of cancer associated with the integument. Although other causes are possible, extensive exposure to sunlight is the most common etiology for each of these cancers.

PRINCIPLES OF EXAMINATION

Examination of a wound should include a thorough history and physical assessment of the cause, depth, and size of the wound and signs of infection. Some variations in actual examination procedures may be applicable to different etiologies (see later). The skin adjacent to or otherwise associated with the wound should also be examined for any alteration from normal function (e.g., sensation, temperature, hair growth, mobility, pliability) and appearance (e.g., texture and color [red for inflammation or bluish for cyanosis or poor perfusion]).

All ulcers, regardless of their etiology, should be examined for size and depth. The size of a wound can be charted by several methods, some of which are tracing diagrams of the wound, TBSA estimates (see discussion of burns), and photography. The depth of a wound can be measured by injecting known volumes of saline into the wound cavity (the amount of saline left over is subtracted from the total to give a volume). Depth may also be measured by use of a wound filler (such as dental alginate) that can be transferred to a volumeter to allow measurement of the depth of the wound via displacement of fluid from the volumeter. Depth can be further determined by observation of the exposed tissue. For example, a moist pink or red wound that is hypersensitive and on an even plane with adjacent, uninjured skin is probably a partial-thickness wound, whereas in deeper wounds subcutaneous adipose tissue or fascia can often be identified. In wounds that extend beyond defined subcutaneous tissue, muscle, tendon, ligament, bone, and other structures may be visible.

Besides assessing integrity of the integument, the PT should perform other tests and measures for a full evaluation of the patient. The patient's ability to communicate and comprehend, joint mobility, muscle performance, gait (if applicable), ventilation and circulation, and sensory tests (including assessment of pain) should be part of the physical therapy examination.

VASCULAR COMPROMISE

Arterial Wounds. Wounds caused by arterial insufficiency are commonly found on the lower part of the leg, including the feet and toes. Because of the poor circulation to the wound, minimal, if any, exudate is seen. The shape of these wounds is commonly irregular, and the wounds are often deep with a pale wound base. The diminished circulation contributes to poor wound healing. The pain associated with arterial wounds is severe and generally increases when the leg is elevated. Skin adjacent to these wounds is characterized by hair loss and pallor on elevation, is cool to the touch, and appears "thin" and shiny. Pulses associated with arterial wounds are weak or absent.

Venous Ulcers. Wounds caused by venous insufficiency are commonly found on the lower part of the leg. Exudate and edema are present, the shape of these wounds is commonly irregular, and the wounds are generally shallow with a red or pink wound base. Edema is a factor in poor wound healing. Some mild pain is associated with venous ulcers, and the pain can commonly be decreased when the leg is elevated. The skin adjacent to these wounds is characterized by inflammation, dilated veins, abnormal pigmentation, and induration (hardness) and may be dry or scaly. Pulses associated with venous ulcers are present.

Neuropathic Ulcers. Neuropathic ulcers are usually located on the plantar surface of the foot at pressure points or bony prominences. The wound may bleed easily unless the condition is coupled with arterial insufficiency. The shape of these wounds is commonly circular, and the wounds are often deep. Because of the sensory neuropathy that led to the wound, these ulcers are normally painless. The skin adjacent to the wounds is characterized by sensory deficit but might otherwise appear fairly normal.

Pressure Ulcers. Pressure ulcers may be located in diverse sites on the body but are generally found over bony prominences. Besides describing the location, the examiner should document the depth and size, which can vary. A well-accepted method for describing a pressure ulcer is to use a staging system provided by the U.S. Department of Health and Human Services.[34] Staging of the ulcer is based on wound characteristics, mainly depth. Table 12-2 outlines the criteria for staging pressure ulcers. Once an ulcer is staged, the assigned stage should not change as the wound changes. For example, a stage III ulcer that heals does not progress from a stage III to a stage II and then to a stage I ulcer (referred to as back-staging). Rather, healing of the wound is described in terms of changes in size, depth, and other characteristics and, when healed, the wound would be a healed stage III ulcer.

TRAUMA

Any traumatic wound of concern should be initially referred for primary medical intervention. This recommendation would hold true for wounds such as abrasions, lacerations, puncture wounds, avulsion injuries, degloving injuries, and burn injuries, regardless of the cause of the wound.

Burn injuries include skin damage from one or more of the following sources: flame, chemicals, scalding, radiation, and electrical current. The severity of the burn injury depends on several factors, including percent TBSA affected, location of the burn, depth of the wound, presence of associated trauma (e.g., fracture, nerve injury), and smoke inhalation. Figure 12-3 provides a method for calculating percent TBSA and documenting the location and depth of injury. The size of the wound, as reported in percent TBSA affected, and the location of the burns are important clues to sites of potential impairment and functional loss. Impairments may be acute when related to pain or wound contraction in superficial, partial-thickness, and full-thickness burns, whereas wound and scar contracture at a burn site can lead to chronic problems of decreased function and potential disability. The location of the burn may also have cosmetic implications for long-term socialization of a patient with burns. The depth of a wound can be determined by the presence of certain clinical findings.[35] A superficial burn injury is painful and erythematous (like a sunburn), with the

12

Table 12-2 Criteria for Staging and Pressure Ulcers	
Ulcer Stage	Description of the Ulcer
I	Nonblanchable erythema of intact skin, the heralding lesion of skin ulceration. In individuals with darker skin, discoloration of the skin, warmth, edema, induration, or hardness may also be indicators.
II	Partial-thickness loss involving the epidermis, dermis, or both. The ulcer is superficial and is clinically noticeable as an abrasion, blister, or shallow crater.
III	Full-thickness skin loss involving damage or necrosis of subcutaneous tissue, which may extend down to but not through underlying fascia. The ulcer is clinically manifested as a deep crater with or without undermining of adjacent tissue.
IV	Full-thickness skin loss with extensive destruction, tissue necrosis, or damage to muscle, bone, or supporting structures (such as tendon, joint capsule). Undermining and sinus tracts may also be associated with stage IV ulcers.

From Bergstrom N, Allman RM, Alvarez OM, et al: Treatment of Pressure Ulcers, Clinical Practice Guidelines NO 15. Rockville, MD, US Department of Health and Human Services, 1994.

possibility of minor localized swelling. Partial-thickness injuries are typically painful, red, and weepy. The skin is normally pliable. Blistering is also commonly associated with a partial-thickness burn. A full-thickness burn is generally not painful when palpated, may be tan or yellowish brown, and has a leathery, nonpliable texture.

Associated trauma can increase the severity of a burn injury because of the increased impairment the patient will experience beyond that caused by the burns. Documentation of any associated trauma is critical to the establishment of a comprehensive plan of care. Smoke inhalation (inhalation injury) may lead to cardiopulmonary impairment. In the plan of care the therapist may need to address impaired ventilation, gas exchange, aerobic capacity, and endurance related to inhalation injury.

DISEASE

A physician carries out the actual diagnosis and primary treatment of skin disease, but PTs and PTAs must be able to recognize the signs and symptoms of skin cancer so that they provide patients with an appropriate and prompt medical referral.[36] Key warning signs for skin cancer include a new skin growth, a sore that does not heal within 3 months, or a bump that is getting larger. Detection of melanoma is based on alterations in a growth on the skin or in a

Area	1 year	1–4 years	5–9 Years	10–14 years	15 years	Adult	Partial-thickness	Full-thickness	Total
Head	19	17	13	11	9	7			
Neck	2	2	2	2	2	2			
Ant. trunk	13	13	13	13	13	13			
Post. trunk	13	13	13	13	13	13			
Right buttock	2 1/2	2 1/2	2 1/2	2 1/2	2 1/2	2 1/2			
Left buttock	2 1/2	2 1/2	2 1/2	2 1/2	2 1/2	2 1/2			
Genitalia	1	1	1	1	1	1			
Right upper arm	4	4	4	4	4	4			
Left upper arm	4	4	4	4	4	4			
Right lower arm	3	3	3	3	3	3			
Left lower arm	3	3	3	3	3	3			
Right hand	2 1/2	2 1/2	2 1/2	2 1/2	2 1/2	2 1/2			
Left hand	2 1/2	2 1/2	2 1/2	2 1/2	2 1/2	2 1/2			
Right thigh	5 1/2	6 1/2	8	8 1/2	9	9 1/2			
Left thigh	5 1/2	6 1/2	8	8 1/2	9	9 1/2			
Right leg	5	5	5 1/2	6	6 1/2	7			
Left leg	5	5	5 1/2	6	6 1/2	7			
Right foot	3 1/2	3 1/2	3 1/2	3 1/2	3 1/2	3 1/2			
Left foot	3 1/2	3 1/2	3 1/2	3 1/2	3 1/2	3 1/2			
								Total	

Etiology of injury _____

Date of injury _____

Time of injury _____

Patient age _____

Patient sex _____

Patient weight _____

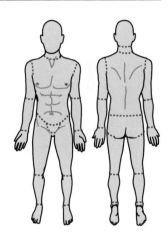

Figure 12-3 ■ Burn diagram used to calculate the size, location, and depth of a burn injury.

mole and may include changes in size, color, shape, elevation, surface appearance, or sensation.

SCAR TISSUE

As some wounds heal, scar tissue may form. Assessment of the scar tissue may be performed with the **Vancouver Burn Scar Scale**.[37] This scale rates characteristics of scars, including pigmentation, vascularity, pliability, and height (Table 12-3). A higher score on the Vancouver Burn Scar Scale correlates with more scarring. Scars are generally referred to as either hypertrophic scars or keloid scars. Both keloid scars and hypertrophic scars hypertrophy, but as keloid scars grow, they extend beyond the boundaries of the wound, whereas hypertrophic scars do not.[38] In addition to examination of the scar itself, the location of the scar should be assessed. Scars over or near joints may impede joint mobility, and scars in areas of cosmetic importance may have a detrimental effect on patient motivation and activity (Figure 12-4). Scar contraction, which can lead to contracture, is a major contributor to wound-related disability.

12

Table 12-3
Vancouver Burn Scar Scale

Score	Pigmentation	Vascularity	Pliability	Height
0	Normal pigmentation, close to the pigment over the rest of the body	Normal	Normal	Flat (normal)
1	Hypopigmentation	Pink	Flexible with minimal resistance	Raised <2 mm
2	Hyperpigmentation	Red	Gives way to pressure	Raised <5 mm
3		Purple	Firm, not easily moved	Raised >5 mm
4			Banding: raised tissue that blanches with stretching of the scar	
5			Contracture: permanent tightening that produces a deformity	

From Sullivan T, Smith J, Kermode J, et al: Rating the burn scar. J Burn Care Rehabil 1990;11:256-160.

PRINCIPLES OF EVALUATION, DIAGNOSIS, AND PROGNOSIS

Evaluation of a patient with a skin wound encompasses the extent of the condition, identification of related impairments, the level of associated loss of function, the patient's basic health condition, and social factors affecting care. The decisions made through an evaluation render a diagnosis about the meaning of a patient's signs and symptoms. The Guide to Physical Therapist Practice[39] provides groupings of signs and symptoms in "integumentary patterns" that can readily be associated with the various skin conditions presented in this chapter. The practice patterns presented in the Guide also provide diagnoses that can be used for patients with integumentary involvement.

The prognosis of a patient with integumentary involvement is related to the diagnosis and will be enhanced if the therapist ensures that the wound is stable, clean, healing, or healed. Some indication of the potential for scarring or the course of the scarring should be included in the prognosis because scarring clearly affects the time needed for treatment and follow-up. The prognosis of problems associated with wounds is influenced by the severity of the problems. For example, severe edema is associated with a poorer prognosis

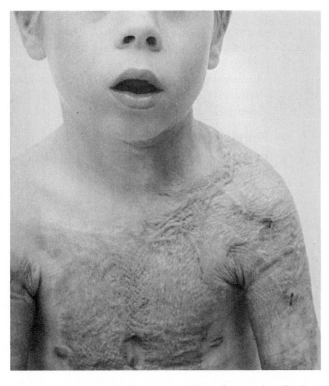

Figure 12-4 ■ Hypertrophic burn scar. (From Carrougher GJ: Burn Care and Therapy. St Louis, Mosby, 1998.)

than mild edema. In addition, the presence of any comorbidity or infection, the chronicity of the problem, and any number of other physical, psychological, or social factors will affect the prognosis.

PRINCIPLES OF DIRECT INTERVENTION

Proper attention by the PT and PTA to the integument ranges from preventing skin breakdown to promoting wound healing. Patients must also be educated about care of the wound, including management of the risks and signs of infection, wound care and dressing procedures, and management of scar tissue. Setting appropriate goals for interventions is imperative to minimize impairment and functional loss.

This section describes some basic elements of physical therapy intervention related to the integument. For details about integumentary management, the reader should refer to the Additional Resources at the end of the chapter and continue to peruse current literature on the topic.

PREVENTION

When patients are at risk for ulcers (e.g., because of decreased sensation, decreased vascularity, decreased mobility, poor nutrition, or incontinence), the preventive element of physical therapy care is important. Positioning, supports or cushions that reduce pressure, and self-inspection of the skin are important

12

elements of preventing ulcers secondary to decreased mobility, impaired sensation, or lack of circulation. Water-repellent lotions and absorbent products can be used to decrease the damaging effects of incontinence on the skin. Appropriate dressings and proper transfer techniques are important in preventing skin breakdown caused by shear and friction. When edema is associated with a wound, compression therapies such as intermittent compression pumps and compression garments may be beneficial.

WOUND MANAGEMENT

Depending on the depth of the wound and other complications, surgery such as grafting may be necessary to achieve wound closure. Many wounds, however, require short- or long-term conservative management with appropriate dressings and possibly topical agents. As noted in the Guide to Physical Therapist Practice,[39] the extent of physical therapy interventions is based on the depth of injury.

Conservative management of arterial wounds and neuropathic ulcers commonly consists of wound care, protection of the wound and surrounding tissue, and possibly bed rest. The wound should be cleansed when dressings are changed. Dressings that maintain or increase moisture at the wound site should be used because of the lack of exudate from the wound. Cushions or protective casting (total contact casting) may be useful in preventing further trauma to the wound as it heals. Bed rest may help to protect the wound, but it must be used with caution to avoid other impairments related to disuse.

Venous wounds should be managed by wound care and compression of the affected extremity.[40] Wound care should consist of cleansing the wound and applying a dressing. The dressing used depends on the amount of exudate at the wound site. The dressing of choice is usually a pliable semiabsorbent or gel-type dressing. If a dressing is to be worn during compression therapy, it should not be bulky. Compression of the extremity helps reduce swelling and venous hypertension in the limb. Activity such as ambulation, swimming, or cycling should be encouraged unless medically contraindicated.

Pressure ulcers require wound care and pressure relief. Much like venous ulcers, pressure ulcers should be cleansed and dressed in a way that provides a moist healing environment but still manages excess exudate. Pressure-relieving devices might include any of the following options. Seat cushions should decrease the likelihood of shear and pressure while also protecting against heat and moisture. Wheelchairs should be appropriately aligned to minimize the chance of pressure ulcer formation. Foam that is either premanufactured for certain anatomical areas or custom cut by the therapist can be used to help position patients in bed. Air mattresses and other pressure relief mattresses help to decrease the buildup of pressure in any one location on the body. Turning schedules should be established and followed. In a typical turning schedule the patient would be turned every 2 hours with equal time spent supine, prone, lying on the right side, and lying on the left side.

Treatment of burns is generally based on wound depth. Skin grafting is inevitable for full-thickness wounds of any consequential percent TBSA. Wounds of any depth should be carefully cleansed. After cleansing, superficial burns require only a moisturizer to help keep the skin moist, which may provide some pain relief. Partial-thickness burns are commonly covered with a topical agent, either an ointment such as Polysporin or a cream such as silver sulfadiazine. These wounds are then covered with nonadherent gauze and wrapped lightly with a gauze dressing. Full-thickness burns are characteristically treated with a topical silver sulfadiazine cream and wrapped in gauze dressing.

With any of these wounds, appropriate exercises and activities should be prescribed to decrease other impairments. Exercises should emphasize joint mobility, muscle performance, gait (if applicable), ventilation, and circulation.

SCAR MANAGEMENT

The major functional problem with scar tissue is the continuous contraction associated with it. Scar hypertrophy may not only contribute to loss of function, but also lead to cosmetic defects. Surgery to correct problems associated with scarring may be considered in an attempt to improve specific impairments or particular cosmetic deformities. Nonsurgical management of a scar is accomplished in a variety of ways. Positioning may be used to counter scar contraction by lengthening tissue for a maintained period.[24] Generally, anticontracture positions are positions of extension at each affected joint region, such as elbow extension with supination or a neutral ankle position with no flexion of the toes. Splints may be used as static positioning devices to hold a joint in a certain position.[41] Serial splinting may also be used to progressively increase joint range of motion.[42] Dynamic splints, which apply a gentle stretch to tissue, are used for mobilization or exercise purposes.[43] Some prefabricated splints are available, but most clinicians fabricate custom splints from malleable thermoplastic material. Passive stretching may be used to gently elongate contracting tissue. Active exercise (including ambulation) is used for the same purpose as passive stretching but provides a way to involve patients in their own rehabilitation.[44] With any stretching, passive or active, the patient should feel the tissue stretch and try to "push the stretch" as much as possible (Figure 12-5). Effective stretching does not require induction of pain in the affected tissue during the stretch or exercise.

Pressure garments are used to decrease hypertrophy of the scar (Figure 12-5). These supports also assist in conforming the scar to normal anatomical parameters. Typically, patients are prescribed pressure garments during the maturation phase of healing. The pressure garments can be custom ordered to fit a patient and can be made for any extremity, the face or head, the hands, the feet, and the torso.

PATIENT EDUCATION

The patient should be the most important member of the rehabilitation team. Those who will be assisting with care of the patient should also be included in all sessions preparing the patient for discharge. Obvious items that should be taught to the patient and other caregivers include skin care and wound management protocols, positioning techniques, exercise programs, and application and wearing of pressure garments (if needed). Demonstrating the technique and allowing the patient or caregiver to perform any of the protocols under observation should reinforce all these procedures. It is important to inform the

12

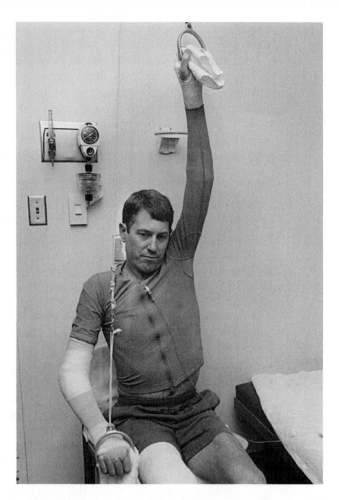

Figure 12-5 ■ Patient using overhead reciprocal pulleys to perform a self-stretch of scar tissue in the axillae and over the elbows. The patient is also wearing pressure garments to help control scar hypertrophy. (From Carrougher GJ: Burn Care and Therapy. St Louis, Mosby, 1998.)

patient about the reasons for the procedures being applied. If patients know what techniques or procedures they must perform, how to do them, and the reasons for the specific protocols assigned, they will be more apt to comply with their care.[45]

SUMMARY

This chapter outlined the many components of integumentary care. The anatomy of the skin and the phases of wound healing are important elements to understand when interventions are being considered. Common conditions of skin breakdown arise as a result of problems with local circulation, decreased sensation, long-standing pressure, and trauma. Understanding the implications of wound depth, size, and location is critical in developing treatments. Beyond direct management of the wound, interventions that stress prevention of further skin breakdown and decrease impairments related to other systems were discussed. Treatments that enhance wound healing and involve the patient directly as part of the rehabilitation team are most beneficial in generating optimum patient outcomes.

CASE STUDIES

CASE STUDY ONE

Mrs. George is a 53-year-old woman in whom venous insufficiency was diagnosed 5 years ago. She has managed it well until recently, when a small ulcer developed on the left lateral aspect of the lower part of her leg about 8 cm above her lateral malleolus. The ulcer is approximately 2 by 3 cm in size and is partial to deep partial thickness. A measurable amount of exudate is oozing from the wound. The limb is edematous (in comparison to the contralateral limb). Lower extremity pulses are palpable. The patient complains of mild pain at the wound site, but she is otherwise functionally independent in all activities.

Goals
Management goals include a reduction in risk factors for infection, reduced wound size, attainment of wound healing, and a reduction in edema. The patient should understand these goals and the desired outcomes from intervention.

Intervention
To decrease the risk for infection, the wound should be selectively debrided to remove nonviable tissue. Appropriate dressings should be applied, including (in this case) a semiabsorbent, nonbulky dressing that will maintain a moist wound environment but also absorb some of the exudate from the wound. Intermittent compression with an extremity lymphedema pump may be useful in decreasing edema. A graduated compression stocking should be fitted for the patient. She should be encouraged to ambulate and, if necessary, be prescribed a walking schedule. While seated, she should elevate the limb and perform ankle pumps. Standing for long periods should be discouraged. The patient should be educated and be able to demonstrate how to (1) perform dressing changes, (2) apply and operate the intermittent compression pump (one could be rented for home use), (3) apply and monitor the fit of the graduated compression stocking, and (4) describe the reasoning for the prescribed interventions and the importance of exercise and elevation in preventing further problems related to edema and venous stasis.

CASE STUDY TWO

Stan is 47 years old and was injured in a house fire. He incurred a 14% TBSA burn. Full-thickness injuries totaling 7% TBSA occurred on his right upper extremity and hand. The other 7% TBSA included the upper right portion of his chest and back. The patient is right hand dominant. He was previously healthy and suffered no associated injuries (i.e., smoke inhalation). Stan was employed as a worker in a warehouse and lives at home with his wife and three teenage children. Four days after his admission to the burn center, his right upper extremity and hand burns were skin-grafted.

12

Goals

Risk factors for infection need to be reduced to enhance partial-thickness wound healing and prepare full-thickness wounds for skin grafting. Joint mobility is to be maintained and soft tissue restriction (wound and scar contraction) reduced. The risk of impairment secondary to scar formation needs to be decreased. Independence in activities of daily living and the ability to perform tasks associated with Stan's work are goals to be regained. The patient should understand these goals and the desired outcomes from intervention.

Intervention

When dealing with such a burn, the patient must be treated before any surgery to alleviate and prevent increased impairment and disability. The patient must continue with postsurgical treatment to achieve the final desired outcomes of therapy intervention.

Presurgery

The wounds should be cleansed and dressed twice a day to reduce the risk of infection and promote healing of the partial-thickness wounds and to prepare the full-thickness wounds for skin grafting. Active range-of-motion exercises for the upper extremity and hand will enhance joint mobility and decrease the soft tissue restriction associated with wound contraction. Positioning of the upper extremity will also help prevent decreases in mobility and increases in soft tissue restriction. The patient should also be encouraged to participate in his personal care (e.g., brushing teeth, combing hair, and personal hygiene), which will aid in future independence in activities of daily living.

Postsurgery

Any remaining partial-thickness wounds should be cleansed and dressed twice a day to reduce the risk of infection and promote healing. Active range-of-motion exercises and positioning that began presurgically should be continued after surgery. Passive range of motion or stretching of the upper extremity might be helpful in overcoming any relentless contraction of the scar tissue forming at the sites of skin grafting. The patient should be required to manage his personal care independently. Strengthening exercises and exercises specific to preparation for return to work should also be included as the patient can tolerate them. The patient's upper extremity should be measured for and fitted with a scar control compression garment (specifically, an arm sleeve and a glove). Scar control will help maintain anatomical contours and decrease the risk of soft tissue restriction caused by scar formation.

The patient should be educated about and be able to demonstrate (1) assisting with dressing changes, (2) performing any of the specifically prescribed exercises, and (3) applying and monitoring the fit of the scar control compression garments. The patient should also be able to describe the rationale behind each of the interventions.

REFERENCES

1. Rankin JA: Biological mediators of acute inflammation. AACN Clin Issues 2004;15(1):3-17.
2. Park JE, Barbul A: Understanding the role of immune regulation in wound healing. Am J Surg 2004;187(5A):11S-16S.

3. Ford-Hutchinson AW, Bray MA, Doig MV, et al: Leukotriene B, a potent chemokinetic and aggregating substance released from polymorphonuclear leukocytes. Nature 1980;286:264-265.
4. Simpson DM, Ross R: The neutrophilic leukocyte in wound repair: A study with antineutrophil serum. J Clin Invest 1972;51:2009-2023.
5. Leibovich SJ, Ross R: The role of the macrophage in wound repair: A study with hydrocortisone and antimacrophage serum. Am J Pathol 1975;78:71-100.
6. Ward RS, Hayes-Lundy C, Reddy R, et al: Evaluation of topical therapeutic ultrasound to improve response to physical therapy and lessen scar contracture after burn injury. J Burn Care Rehabil 1994;15(1):74-79.
7. Fishel RS, Barbul A, Beschorner WE, et al: Lymphocyte participation in wound healing: Morphologic assessment using monoclonal antibodies. Ann Surg 1987;206:25-29.
8. Wahl SM, Wahl LM: Lymphokine modulation of connective tissue metabolism. Ann NY Acad Sci 1979;332:411-422.
9. Wahl SM, Wahl LM, McCarthy JB: Lymphocyte-mediated activation of fibroblast proliferation and collagen production. J Immunol 1978;121:942-946.
10. Peacock E: Wound Repair, ed 3. Philadelphia, Saunders, 1984.
11. Gogia P: Clinical Wound Management. Thorofare, NJ, Slack, 1995.
12. Hardy MA: The biology of scar formation. Phys Ther 1989;69(12):1014-1024.
13. Bell E, Ivarsson B, Merrill C: Production of a tissue-like structure by contraction of collagen lattices by human fibroblasts of different proliferative potential in vitro. Proc Natl Acad Sci USA 1979;76:1274-1278.
14. Eddy RJ, Petro JA, Tomasek JJ: Evidence for the nonmuscular nature of the "myofibroblast" of granulation tissue and hypertrophic scar: An immunofluorescence study. Am J Pathol 1988;130:252-260.
15. Gabbiani G, Ryan GB, Majne G: Presence of modified fibroblasts in granulation tissue and their possible role in wound contraction. Experientia 1971;27:549-550.
16. Gabbiani G, Hirschel BJ, Ryan GB, et al: Granulation tissue as a contractile organ: A study of structure and function. J Exp Med 1972;135:719-734.
17. Dunphy JE, Jackson DS: Practical applications of experimental studies in the care of primarily closed wounds. Am J Surg 1962;104:273-282.
18. Schumann D: The nature of wound healing. AORN 1982;35:1068-1077.
19. Rockwell WB, Cohen IK, Erlich HP: Keloids and hypertrophic scars: A comprehensive report. Plast Reconstr Surg 1989;84:827-837.
20. Ketchum L: Hypertrophic scars and keloids. Clin Plast Surg 1977;4:301-310.
21. Davies D: Scars, hypertrophic scars and keloids. BMJ 1985;290:1056-1058.
22. Deitch EA, Wheelahan TM, Rose MP, et al: Hypertrophic burn scars: Analysis of variables. J Trauma 1983;23:895-898.
23. Ketchum LD, Cohen IK, Masters FW: Hypertrophic scars and keloids. Plast Reconstr Surg 1974;53:140-154.
24. Rudolf R: Construction and the control of contraction. World J Surg 1980;4:279-287.
25. Paquette D, Falanga V: Leg ulcers. Clin Geriatr Med 2002;18(1):77.
26. Browse NL, Burnand KG: The cause of venous ulceration. Lancet 1982;2:243-245.
27. Coleridge Smith PD, Thomas P, Scurr JH, Dornandy JA: Causes of venous ulceration: A new hypothesis. BMJ 1988;296:1726-1727.
28. Daniel RK, Priest DL, Wheatley DC: Etiologic factors in pressure sores: An experimental model. Arch Phys Med Rehabil 1981;62:492-498.
29. Reuler JB, Cooney TG: The pressure sore: Pathophysiology and principles of management. Ann Intern Med 1981;94:661-666.
30. Husain T: An experimental study of some pressure effects on tissues, with reference to the bedsore problem. J Pathol Bacteriol 1953;66:347-358.
31. Lindon O, Greenway R, Piazza JM: Pressure distribution on the surface of the human body. Arch Phys Med Rehabil 1965;46:378-385.
32. Kosiak M: Etiology and pathology of ischemic ulcers. Arch Phys Med Rehabil 1981;62:492-498.
33. Allman RM, Goode PS, Patrick MM, et al: Pressure ulcer risk factors among hospitalized patients with activity limitations. JAMA 1995;273:865-870.
34. Bergstrom N, Allman RM, Alvarez OM, et al: Treatment of Pressure Ulcers, Clinical Practice Guideline No. 15. Rockville, MD, US Department of Health and Human Services, 1994.

12

35. Ward RS: The rehabilitation of burn patients. Crit Rev Phys Rehabil Med 1991;2(3):121-138.

36. Rhodes AR: Public education and cancer of the skin: What do people need to know about melanoma and nonmelanoma skin cancer? Cancer 1995;75(2 Suppl):613-636.

37. Sullivan T, Smith J, Kermode J, et al: Rating the burn scar. J Burn Care Rehabil 1990;11(3):256-260.

38. Rudolf R: Wide spread scars, hypertrophic scars and keloids. Clin Plast Surg 1987;14:253-260.

39. Guide to Physical Therapist Practice, revised ed 2. Alexandria, VA, American Physical Therapy Association, 2003.

40. Phillips TJ: Current approaches to venous ulcers and compression. Dermatol Surg 2001;27(7):611-621.

41. Waymack JP, Fidler J, Warden GD: Surgical correction of burn scar contractures of the foot in children. Burns 1988;14:156-160.

42. Hunter JM, Mackin EJ, Callahan AD (eds): Rehabilitation of the Hand, ed 4. St Louis, Mosby, 1995.

43. Duncan R: Basic principles of splinting the hand. Phys Ther 1989;69:1104-1116.

44. Schnebly WA, Ward RS, Warden GD, Saffle JR: A nonsplinting approach to the care of the thermally injured patient. J Burn Care Rehabil 1989;10(3):263-266.

45. Peloquin S: Linking purpose to procedure during interactions with patients. Am J Occup Ther 1988;42:775-781.

ADDITIONAL RESOURCES

Carrougher GJ: Burn Care and Therapy. St Louis, Mosby, 1998.
This nicely written textbook covers broad issues in burn care from both a nursing and a therapy perspective.

McCulloch JM, Kloth LC, Feedar JA: Wound Healing: Alternatives in Management. Philadelphia, FA Davis, 1995.
A very useful textbook that reviews wound healing and management of wounds.

Richard RL, Staley MJ: Burn Care and Rehabilitation: Principles and Practice. Philadelphia, FA Davis, 1994.
This excellent textbook provides the essential information one requires to understand and treat patients with burn injuries and selected serious skin diseases.

Sussman C, Bates-Jensen BM: Wound Care: A Collaborative Practice Manual for Physical Therapists and Nurses. Gaithersburg, MD, Aspen, 1998.
A well-written textbook that focuses on clinical examination and management of many common wounds.

1. Describe the three phases of wound healing and develop a rationale for physical therapy involvement in each phase.
2. List the variables that should be identified during your examination of a patient to determine the etiology and seriousness of the wound. How might these variables affect your intervention?
3. What characteristics differentiate a venous ulcer from an arterial ulcer, as well as these ulcers from a pressure ulcer?
4. Explain the differences involved in treating a superficial wound versus a deep wound.
5. How might an increased understanding of integumentary wounds and wound healing help you better understand injuries to tissues you cannot visualize (e.g., soft tissue injury, fracture, tissue necrosis)?
6. Why is it important for physical therapists to be aware of scar formation?

What path will we take? Let us not take one that others have made. . . . Instead, let us make our own path.
Ruth Wood, PT, FAPTA

13 Physical Therapy for Pediatric Conditions

Angela Easley Rosenberg and Stacey C. Dusing

KEY TERMS

anencephaly
cerebral palsy (CP)
clubfoot
cystic fibrosis (CF)
developmental coordination disorder (DCD)
developmental delay
developmental dysplasia of the hip (DDH)
developmental milestones
disablement process
Down syndrome
Duchenne muscular dystrophy (DMD)
dynamical systems theory
eclectic approach
enablement process
family assessment
fetal alcohol syndrome (FAS)
goal-directed movement approach
Individualized Education Plan (IEP)
Individualized Family Service Plan (IFSP)
juvenile rheumatoid arthritis (JRA)
meningocele
meningomyelocele
neural tube defect
neurodevelopmental treatment (NDT)
norm referenced
normal developmental theory
osteogenesis imperfecta (OI)
prenatal cocaine exposure
scoliosis
secondary condition
sensory integration (SI)

spina bifida
spina bifida occulta
spinal muscular atrophy (SMA)
standardized testing

OBJECTIVES ■

After reading this chapter, the reader will be able to:
- Describe the relationship between body structure, functional abilities, and activity limitations as presented by the World Health Organization
- Describe the impact of federal legislation on the delivery of physical therapy services to children
- Describe the general features of common pediatric conditions seen by a physical therapist or physical therapist assistant
- Describe aspects of the patient/client examination that are unique to pediatric clients
- Describe the general features of four physical therapy treatment approaches for pediatric clients

Children will be children, first and foremost. They are not merely scaled-down versions of adults; rather, they progress through unique age-related movement stages, or developmental milestones. Pediatric physical therapists observe these milestones to determine whether discrepancies exist between the child's chronological or developmental age or whether inefficient motor patterns are limiting the child's function. If so, evaluation and subsequent intervention may be appropriate. More important, pediatric physical therapists must evaluate each child's ability to meet the task-related challenges of that child's daily environment. This type of evaluation and intervention planning requires thoughtful, structured strategies that often involve a constellation of players, including the child's family, caregivers, teachers, and community professionals. This chapter describes the examination and intervention techniques used by pediatric physical therapists. It includes common conditions and two case studies to illustrate a variety of approaches for the management of pediatric clients.

The primary focus for pediatric therapists is to observe children as they portray their individual strengths and abilities and to promote a functional, optimal developmental process. By acquiring knowledge of normal development through observation of movement patterns and transitions, the therapist can more accurately detect abnormal or inefficient movements. The challenge is differentiating normal delays from those that signal potential developmental problems.[1] For example, observations of generations of children tell us that walking is initiated at approximately 10 to 13 months, yet some infants take their first steps as early as 8 months or as late as 18 months. This type of variation occurs at all stages of child development and requires pediatric therapists to examine and provide interventions to children on a constantly changing developmental base.[2] Pediatric therapists play a crucial role in determining the absence of movement components that may impede the accomplishment of **developmental milestones** or functional goals for a child. In addition to child development, pediatric practice requires the therapist to acquire specific knowledge in basic areas ranging from child psychology to motor learning. The cognitive strategies and learning methods of adults are generally functionally oriented toward work, leisure, or daily living activities, whereas children learn from a different point of view—play. The pediatric physical therapist is often found in what might be called compromising situations—hopping, rolling, tumbling—to engage and invite the child to participate in therapeutic activities.

Play is the medium most used to promote therapeutic activities for young children, whereas for adolescents, therapy goals may be structured around social situations.[3] The primary goal is to identify meaningful activities that correspond to the learning style of each pediatric client, given the age, culture, and most natural social and physical environments (Figure 13-1).

Children who have health problems that require specialty or subspecialty care are often referred to as "children with special health care needs."[4,5] Pediatric therapists may provide direct or consultative therapy to these children over long periods, depending on the child's changing needs. When caring for children with special needs, physical therapists collaborate closely with the family and other health professionals in designing a long-term, family-centered plan of care (Figure 13-2). This plan includes a full range of services—prevention, early identification, evaluation, diagnostics, treatment, habilitation, and rehabilitation.[6] Throughout service provision, emphasis is placed on recognizing each child as part of a family system, with unique cultural characteristics that must be considered when designing treatment goals.

GENERAL DESCRIPTION

If the physical therapist (PT) focuses solely on the child's motor strengths and needs while neglecting the cultural impact of family and community factors on that child, a successful treatment outcome is unlikely. The World Health Organization (WHO) has issued an International Classification of Functioning, Disability and Health (ICF) that describes the impact of a person's health

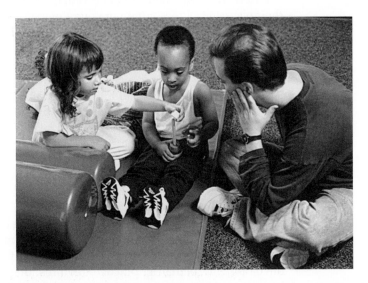

Figure 13-1 ■ Cooperative play provides an avenue for therapeutic activities. (Courtesy of Bruce Wang.)

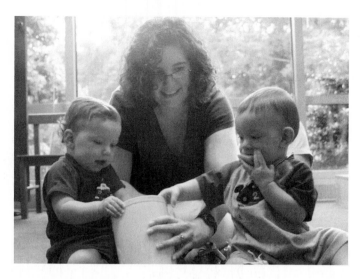

Figure 13-2 ■ A sibling incorporated into a therapy session to encourage participation and meet the family's goals. (Courtesy of Kathleen Hunter.)

condition on body functions and structures, daily activities, and social participation.[7] This model describes the process of *enablement* and *disablement* on several levels: body structures and functions, activities, and participation (Figure 13-3 and Table 13-1).[7]

Enablement processes and **disablement processes** represent the dynamic, interactive relationships a child has within different environmental contexts. This model shows that in the disease process, impaired body structures and functions (e.g., central nervous system abnormality) directly affect the child not only physically, but in several realms, all of which must be considered when a

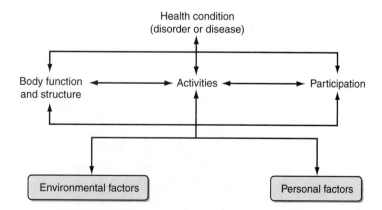

Figure 13-3 ■ Interaction between the components of the International Classification of Functioning, Disability, and Health. (Modified from International Classification of Functioning, Disability, and Health [ICF], Geneva, 2001, World Health Organization.)

Table 13-1
Classification of Disablement

Disablement Classification	Characteristics	Interaction Level
Impairment of body structures and body functions	Reflex development Joint motion Muscle length/strength Respiratory status Postural stability	Child
Activity limitations	Locomotion Communication Oral motor function Social/emotional	Child/daily environment
Participation restriction	Community recreation School participation Employment Access to facilities	Child/community and society

Modified from International Classification of Functioning, Disability, and Health (ICF). Geneva, 2001, World Health Organization.

plan of care is being designed. The child's activity limitations (e.g., inability to speak or walk) are influenced by the body's structure and function, as well as other factors, including the child's motivational level, environment, and course of rehabilitation. In turn, the child's activity limitations may have an impact on the family system (e.g., interaction style) and peer relationships. Participation restrictions, or the influence of social or environmental restrictions on child participation (e.g., access to schools, sports), is a result of the culture, society, and environment in which the child lives. (See Chapter 1 for further description of the ICF model.)

When the WHO model is used as a guide for care of a child, all these factors are considered important elements in the design of a plan of care. It is important to note that the WHO framework is consistent with the American Physical Therapy Association's Guide to Physical Therapist Practice[8] and the practice model adopted by the National Center for Medical Rehabilitation Research.[9] Throughout each of these frameworks, the physical therapist addresses body structure and function, activity limitations, and participation limitations as a result of disease or injury. Another important point is that the physical therapist can advance a child through an enabling process by addressing the body's structural integrity so that age-appropriate movement and interactive activities can occur. In a climate of radical health care reform and shifting venues for pediatric practice, a practitioner's understanding of the interdependence of all levels of the WHO model is germane to the evaluation process and success in achieving outcomes.

IMPACT OF FEDERAL LEGISLATION

The scope of pediatric specialization within the field of physical therapy is rapidly evolving as a result of a variety of factors that directly affect the care of children: public policy, family-centered care, and practice environments. These seemingly unrelated elements have become entwined through passage of federal legislation unique to the practice of pediatrics.

In 1975, Congress passed the Education of All Handicapped Children Act (EHCA), Public Law 94-142. This landmark legislation has continued to shape the evolution of pediatric practice for all professional disciplines.[10] The main premise of the EHCA was that all children from ages 6 to 21 years, regardless of disability, were entitled to free and appropriate public education. This premise set the basic framework for policy and standards, which were amended in 1986 with passage of Public Law 99-457 (Amendments to the EHCA) and again in 1991 and 2004 with reauthorizations as the Individuals with Disabilities Education Act (IDEA).[11,12] These amendments provide distinct policy for children from birth until 3 years and from 3 through 5 years of age.[13] Although the states must abide by a set of regulations for implementing services, each state can establish some of its own regulations, such as the inclusion of children who are "at risk" or transitioning from early intervention to school-based services.[12] Specific language in the amendments stipulates the concept of collaboration between parent and professional, as well as a family-centered focus throughout the process of pediatric examination, intervention, and care coordination. In addition, this legislation sets forth policy guidelines requiring that children be cared for in their "least restrictive" environment or in "natural" environments ranging from home to daycare centers as optimal sites for physical therapy intervention (Figure 13-4).[11,12,14]

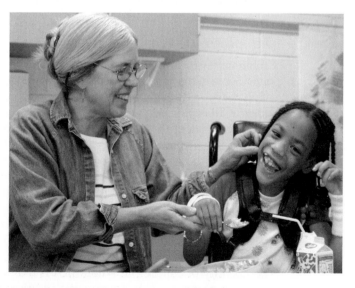

Figure 13-4 ■ Therapy at classroom—a natural environment. (Courtesy of Kathleen Hunter.)

The focus on the family system, family-centered care, individualized child and family plans, and natural environments is now commonplace in pediatric practice. This emphasis on family and community speaks to the evolving societal and cultural contexts in which pediatric physical therapists collaborate in the care of children with special needs.

COMMON CONDITIONS

The full range of pediatric diagnostic conditions is beyond the scope of this chapter. Children, like adults, have conditions that require expertise in all specialty areas. Many children are seen for acute, short-term orthopaedic needs, such as an adolescent who sprains an ankle while playing soccer. The majority of these pediatric clients are seen in physical therapy outpatient orthopaedics clinics or by sports physical therapy specialists.

Another subset of pediatric clients and the group most associated with pediatric practice are children with developmental delays and disabilities. A child with a **developmental delay** has not attained predictable movement patterns or behavior associated with children of a similar chronological age. During fetal development a multitude of factors have the potential to cause a developmental problem. Such factors as genetic and chromosomal anomalies, environmental toxins, or premature birth may cause impairment in the central or peripheral nervous system that results in immediate or eventual developmental delays. Affected children generally require some combination of short- and long-term therapies that continually shift with changes in the child's physical, cognitive, and emotional abilities.

The remainder of this section briefly describes selected orthopaedic and neuromuscular conditions of children. The etiology of many of these conditions remains unclear and may result from a combination of genetic and environmental factors. Later in the chapter, two of the conditions are described through case studies of children to provide the reader with snapshots of the many "faces" of pediatric practice.

ORTHOPAEDIC DISORDERS

Children may be born with or acquire problems with bones, muscles, fascia, and joints. Some of the more common disorders are discussed in the following sections.

Juvenile Rheumatoid Arthritis. One of many rheumatic diseases, **juvenile rheumatoid arthritis (JRA)** is characterized by inflammation of connective tissue manifested as a painful inflamed joint (arthritis). The cause of JRA is unknown, although genes associated with a variety of forms of JRA have been identified.[15] Similar to other autoimmune disorders, JRA appears to be the result of complex genetic and possibly environmental exposures.[16,17] JRA may be manifested in several distinct forms or subtypes, each with different characteristics. These subtypes vary in the number of joints affected, age at onset, male-to-female ratio, clinical findings, and prognosis. Signs and symptoms usually include joint pain, swelling, decreased motion, stiffness, and muscle atrophy. The majority of children in whom JRA is diagnosed lead active lives with the assistance of medications, therapeutic exercise, and specialized care programs. It is generally believed that an interdisciplinary team including parents, a pediatric rheumatologist, nurse, psychologist, physical therapist, and occupational therapist is best for total care coordination.

The primary role of the physical therapist is to assist in preventing deformity and improving the overall quality of life for the child. The primary focus is generally the child's musculoskeletal needs, with special emphasis on needs that affect function. Physical therapists also play a role in exercise prescription, since physical conditioning has been shown to increase functional abilities without exacerbating JRA.[18] Individualized goals are collaboratively planned to address posture, strength, mobility, and joint motion within the child's daily functional routine. Including the parent and child in decisions regarding education and instruction is vital because the home is where the majority of the child's goals will be reinforced.[19]

Clubfoot. The term **clubfoot** is derived from the position of the affected foot, which is turned inward and slanted upward. Because of this position, certain muscles become shortened and cause the foot to remain in a fixed position. Treatment includes progressive and prolonged casting or taping (or both), joint range of motion, and in some cases surgical correction.

Scoliosis. **Scoliosis** is characterized by a lateral curvature of the spine. The curve may vary in severity from mild to severe. Scoliosis may be idiopathic (of unknown origin), neuromuscular, or congenital (present at birth). Scoliosis is now detected more frequently because of school-based screening programs and is noted by asymmetry of the shoulders, breasts, and pelvis, among other factors. Treatment involves a wide range of external or internal fixations and, in select cases, electrical stimulation, depending on the degree of development of the curve. Exercise assists in reducing back pain and improving range of motion. For children with mobility limitations, positioning in appropriate seating systems is crucial to the prevention of scoliosis.

Developmental Dysplasia of the Hip. **Developmental dysplasia of the hip (DDH)** results from abnormal development of some of the structures surrounding the hip joint, such that the head of the femur can move into and out of the hip socket. The cause of DDH is unknown, but the disorder is thought to be related to a number of factors such as maternal hormonal changes during pregnancy, in utero positioning, large birth weight, multiple gestation pregnancy, birth trauma, or family history of DDH.[20] The incidence of DDH is unclear because debate exists over methods of screening and classification.[21-23] Treatment involves manual or surgical return of the femoral head to the hip socket and stabilization with splints or casts, depending on the degree of impairment and age of the child. Intensive postsurgical exercise protocols are required to regain full range of joint motion, muscle strength, and function. Children with spina bifida and certain forms of cerebral palsy (CP) are more prone to DDH and are monitored through regular physical examinations.

Osteogenesis Imperfecta. A common and severe bone disorder of genetic origin, **osteogenesis imperfecta (OI)** affects the formation of collagen during bone development, leading to frequent fractures during the fetal or newborn period.[24] The fetal form of OI is associated with high mortality, whereas the infantile form is less severe, with increased vulnerability to frequent fractures of the long bones in early childhood. Children with OI are identified through characteristic limb deformities, dental abnormalities, stunted growth, scoliosis, loose ligaments, and an unusually shaped skull. Treatment of fractures and prevention of deformity through positioning and joint range of motion are the major foci of intervention, as well as gentle exercise after postsurgical healing.[24,25]

NEUROMUSCULAR AND GENETIC DISORDERS

Neuromuscular disorders include all disorders that result in difficulty moving the body as a result of decreased control between the brain or central nervous system and the muscles of the body. The causes of these types of disorders are extremely variable and include trauma, genetic factors, premature birth, environmental factors, or a combination of several factors. Genetic factors include the inheritance of a trait, recessive or dominant, or a mutation that occurs during fetal development. A variety of risk factors affecting the health of either the mother or the fetus may present a risk to the newborn infant's health. Some of these factors include maternal health and nutrition (e.g., vitamin deficiency), radiation, drugs, infections, environmental toxins (e.g., lead), fetal hypoxia (lack of oxygen before or during labor), and birth trauma. Depending on the nature and timing of appearance of the risk factor during the pregnancy, the newborn may have a variety of developmental disabilities ranging from mild to severe. A complex interplay between genetics and the environment contributes to many neuromuscular disorders.

Duchenne Muscular Dystrophy. In **Duchenne muscular dystrophy (DMD)**, females do not manifest symptoms, but are carriers of the disease, whereas males do manifest symptoms. Boys with DMD usually develop normally until 6 to 9 years of age, when progressive pelvic muscle weakness and wasting become apparent and are combined with enlarged yet weak thigh muscles and tight heel cords. Associated complications include muscle contractures, spinal curvature (scoliosis), and wheelchair dependence by 10 to 12 years of age. Progressive weakness, pneumonia, and cardiac abnormalities reduce the life span of persons with DMD.[26] The use of nighttime ventilation may increase the life span for an individual with DMD to as much as 25 years.[26] Developmental effects of this type of muscular dystrophy may include mild mental retardation or learning disabilities, low muscle tone, and delays in attainment of motor milestones.[27] Activity limitations are closely associated with muscle strength and cognitive level.[28,29]

Spinal Muscular Atrophy. Symptoms of **spinal muscular atrophy (SMA)** include severe muscle weakness in infancy and progressive respiratory failure. Children with the infantile form of SMA have a decreased life span, whereas children with the juvenile form have a longer (but less than normal) life span and require aggressive physical therapy and orthopaedic management.[30]

Neural Tube Defects. A **neural tube defect** results from failure of the neural tube to close completely during the first month of gestational development. Although the etiology of the neural tube defect is unclear, some hypotheses suggest that this impairment may be a result of genetic expression in combination with factors in the fetal (maternal) environment.[31] Environmental factors such as organic solvents, ethanol, and valproic acid have been suggested, and maternal folate deficiency has been determined to exert a strong influence.[32-34] Studies have shown that daily folic acid supplementation (400 μg/day) can reduce the incidence of new cases of neural tube defects by at least 50%.[32] Recent advances in surgical techniques have led to attempts to close the neural tube in utero rather than delaying intervention until the infant has been born. Outcome studies regarding the benefit of this experimental procedure are under way.[35]

The following are several types of neural tube defects that differ in level of severity, depending on the degree and location of vertebral closure and spinal cord exposure.

SPINA BIFIDA. **Spina bifida** is the most common neural tube defect and involves orthopaedic malformations in its mild form and neurological malformations in its severe form (Figure 13-5).

SPINA BIFIDA OCCULTA. A common impairment of a vertebra (separation of the spinous process) that is not associated with disability, **spina bifida occulta** may be discovered only through diagnostic tests such as radiographic studies.

MENINGOCELE. A benign herniation of the meninges manifesting as a soft tissue cyst or lump that surrounds a normal spinal cord, **meningocele** does not cause any neurological deficits.

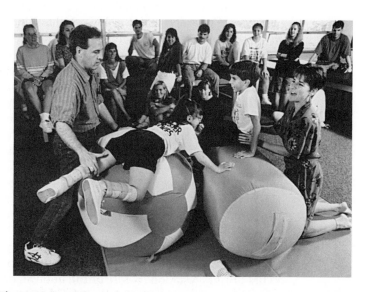

Figure 13-5 ■ Physical therapists promote interactive play to assist the movement patterns of two children with spina bifida. (Courtesy of Bruce Wang.)

MENINGOMYELOCELE. **Meningomyelocele** is an open lesion with minimal to no skin protection covering the deeper nerve roots. This condition is the most severe of the spinal closure defects, with the potential for leakage of spinal fluid and infection before surgical intervention and healing. Because this impairment is usually at the lower end of the spine, loss of motor function and sensation of the lower part of the body often results, including problems with bowel and bladder function.

ANENCEPHALY. **Anencephaly** is a form of neural tube defect that results from a lack of the neural tube closure at the base of the brain. This condition is not compatible with life and results in fetal death or death shortly after delivery.

Developmental Coordination Disorder. Children in whom **developmental coordination disorder (DCD)** is diagnosed may have a wide range of dysfunctions, including gross or fine motor coordination problems such as awkward running, frequent falling, slow reaction times, immature balance reactions, poor handwriting, and difficulty with activities of daily living such as dressing.[36-38] Children with DCD frequently have psychosocial problems in addition to their motor dysfunctions. The cause of DCD is unknown, but may be related to prenatal or perinatal insults to the central nervous system or damage to the neurotransmitter and receptor system.[38] DCD is more commonly diagnosed in children with attention deficit/hyperactivity disorder (ADHD) and learning disabilities than in children without these conditions. Treatment for DCD includes comprehensive management of all the child's areas of difficulty.[36]

Down Syndrome. **Down syndrome** is a congenital developmental disability caused by the presence of an extra copy of chromosome 21; it is also called trisomy 21. Routine prenatal care commonly includes screening for Down syndrome. New ultrasound techniques have increased the ability to prenatally diagnose Down syndrome in the first and second trimesters.[39] A child with Down syndrome is characterized by low muscle tone, a flat facial profile, upwardly slanted eyes, short stature, mental retardation, slowed growth and development, a small nose with a low nasal bridge, and congenital heart disease.[40-42] Associated complications may include instability of the first and second vertebrae, lax ligaments, seizures, leukemia, and premature senility.[43-47] The combination of these features is often manifested as deficiencies in balance, stability, and agility across many tasks and environmental contexts. Developmentally, a child with Down syndrome has decreased muscle tone, which improves with age. This abnormality is offset by loose ligaments that result in increased range of joint motion. The level of mental retardation varies, and the rate of developmental progress decreases with age.[47-49]

Cerebral Palsy. **Cerebral palsy (CP)** is a group of conditions, rather than a disease, and is caused by a nonprogressive lesion of the brain. Most often, CP occurs during gestation (before birth), at birth, or immediately after birth from interruption of oxygen to the brain of the fetus or newborn.[50,51] A variety of environmental toxins, maternal or infant infections, or early childhood trauma can cause this condition. The core problem with CP is an inability of the brain to control nerve and muscle activity. Manifestations of CP depend on the cause, timing (age of the fetus or child), and location and extent of the original impairment to the brain. Often, early signs of CP include poor sucking, irritability, stiff muscles (hypertonia), floppy muscles (hypotonia), or reduced movement quality.[52] Later manifestations may include delayed motor milestones, poor coordination, involuntary movements (dyskinesia), writhing movements (athetosis), poor visual tracking (ability of the eyes to follow a moving object), and language delay.[53] Approximately 60% to 70% of children with CP are mentally retarded.[54] Management emphasis is on attaining optimal growth and development. A variety of specialists may be involved in caring for a child with CP, including physical therapists, occupational therapists, and speech-language pathologists. In many cases, neurosurgical intervention, orthotic devices, adaptive equipment, strengthening programs, or pharmacological intervention is required to ameliorate or correct deformities (Figure 13-6).[55,56]

Fetal Alcohol Syndrome. The most severe condition in a continuum of alcohol-induced disabilities,[57,58] **fetal alcohol syndrome (FAS)** is related to a presumed history of significant maternal alcohol consumption during pregnancy.[57,59] Recent research suggests a genetic predisposition to fetal alcohol–related syndromes.[60] FAS is the leading known cause of mental retardation, even surpassing Down syndrome and spina bifida. Children are generally born at term (close to their due date), but are smaller than normal in weight and height. Children with FAS have distinct physical features that assist in identifying their condition. Complications are widespread and include an increased incidence of congenital heart defects, joint contractures, visual and auditory impairments, and hip dislocation.[61,62] A child with FAS may experience a range of developmental delays in the areas of language, fine motor control, eye-hand coordination, speech, IQ, and psychosocial behavior.[62-65]

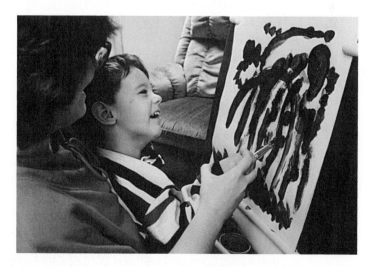

Figure 13-6 ■ All smiles when painting is a part of therapy for a child with cerebral palsy. (Courtesy of Bruce Wang.)

Prenatal Cocaine Exposure. **Prenatal cocaine exposure** refers to exposure to cocaine in utero from maternal cocaine use during pregnancy.[66,67] A number of studies conducted in the 1980s documented motor problems in children who were exposed to cocaine in utero,[68] but further studies[69,70] have been unable to support these findings when controlled for the environment where the child is raised, prematurity, and other risk factors.[71]

Cystic Fibrosis. The pulmonary disorder **cystic fibrosis (CF)** is the most common inherited chronic disease in white children. CF is characterized by the production of thick mucus with progressive lung damage, and children with CF require frequent hospitalization for acute respiratory attacks. A variety of medications and therapies can help to decrease the side effects of this disease, but no cure has been found. Genetic research has resulted in isolation of the defective gene for CF.[72] The life span of persons with CF has increased significantly in the past two decades. The median life expectancy is estimated to be 40 years of age.[73-75]

PRINCIPLES OF EXAMINATION

The process of examination and evaluation of children involves measures to determine whether a child needs physical therapy intervention, in addition to monitoring the child's progress after physical therapy has been initiated. If a child is suspected of having or is at risk for a developmental disability, an examination is conducted that involves the history, a systems review, screening, and tests and measures. After the examination the physical therapist makes an evaluation, using clinical judgment to synthesize the clinical and social information gathered during the examination. During the evaluation a prognosis is determined, as well as a plan of care, including the child's goals and objectives and any intervention strategies, if indicated.

Initial information about a child, the history, is generally obtained through a review of medical records and discussions with family members. For a child up to 5 years of age the discussion may take the form of a **family assessment.**[76] Family assessment is an essential part of the examination because the child will be treated in the context of that family system.[77] Family assessment may take the form of an interview, discussion, or standardized survey and is often initiated by the team member who will be the primary coordinator of care for the family. Regardless of the format, the purpose of family assessment is to obtain the family's insights regarding the child, including the family history, relationships, satisfactions, concerns, needs, and resources. The history has a direct impact on planning services for each child. As children get older, they may become more directly involved and state their own opinions and thoughts, thus providing vital information about their condition and areas of satisfaction or concern with their care coordination.

The administration of tests and measures, an initial and continuing part of any pediatric examination, primarily consists of two components: screening and assessment. Each component has a distinct purpose in determining a child's prognosis and ultimate plan of care (Table 13-2).[78-88]

Depending on the availability and type of diagnosis at the time of referral, screening may or may not be required as an initial measurement. Screening is

Table 13-2
Components of Tests and Measures in Pediatric Physical Therapy

Component	Description	Example
Screening	Short, inexpensive tests used to distinguish children with behavior different from that of other children of the same age; may indicate a need for further evaluation	Bayley Infant Neurodevelopmental Screener[78] Denver II Developmental Screening Test[79]
Assessment	Instruments used to gain a comprehensive profile of a child's physical, cognitive, social, emotional, communication, and adaptive abilities to assist in determining therapeutic service needs, as well as act as a guide for initial frequency and duration of service; assessment also involves the use of measures to determine the need for disability-related adapted equipment, as well as activity preferences addressed by the child and family	Bayley II Scales of Infant Development[80] Gross Motor Function Measure[81] Peabody Developmental Motor Scales, ed 2[82] School Function Assessment[83] Test of Infant Motor Performance[84,85] Bruininks-Oseretsky Test of Motor Proficiency[86] Pediatric Evaluation of Disability Inventory[87] Canadian Occupational Performance Measure[88]

usually indicated when a child is at risk for developmental delay or disability and is a quick way to determine whether the child is in need of further diagnostic services.

If a child has a definite diagnosis, screening is generally bypassed and a comprehensive assessment is recommended. Assessment measures are used to gain more in-depth information about the child's strengths and needs in all developmental domains. In the case of an orthopaedic condition, assessment may entail an examination of posture or movement, as well as special diagnostic tests such as radiographs. Assessment measures for a child with a developmental disability are generally obtained through **standardized testing**, which refers to a type of formal test in which the procedures remain the same when administered by different therapists and at variable test locations. A large variety and number of standardized measures are available for pediatric testing, and these measures are targeted according to the specific purpose of the assessment (Figure 13-7). Many standardized tests are also **norm referenced,** meaning that a large number of children have been assessed to create a comparison group for the assessment. Assessments that are norm referenced can be used to compare a child's functional abilities or activities to other children of the same age.

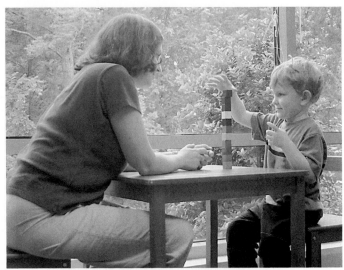

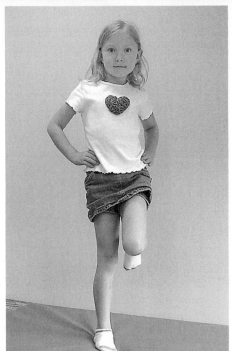

Figure 13-7 ■ Standardized testing. **A**, Assessment of eye-hand coordination and fine motor skills. **B**, Assessment of static balance. (Courtesy of Kathleen Hunter.)

In addition to choosing an assessment tool that meets the needs of the child being tested, it is imperative to review each measure for (1) validity, or the ability of the test to measure the content area or areas that it claims to measure (e.g., evaluation of mobility); (2) reliability, or the consistency of the test between separate administrations or examiners; and (3) appropriateness of the instrument for the specific disability or culture of the child being assessed. An equally important element of objective measurement is the information provided through observation of the child and reports by the child's caregivers in a variety of natural environments (home, daycare, school).

PRINCIPLES OF EVALUATION, DIAGNOSIS, AND PROGNOSIS

The results of tests and measures performed during the examination are used in the evaluation process to confirm, revise, or establish a diagnosis, prognosis, and plan of care. The evaluation can be vital for the child, family, and medical professionals. In many cases, the diagnosis and corresponding prognosis provide a mechanism by which physical therapists can determine treatment priorities and design the plan of care. With certain conditions that have defined physical manifestations, initial therapy can be planned to counteract negative physical outcomes, or **secondary conditions** of disability (e.g., muscle contractures). Diagnosis is also important for determining clinical conditions that contraindicate specific treatment regimens. Several positive outcomes are associated with establishing a clinical diagnosis, as are negative outcomes, many of which can have psychological and social ramifications (Box 13-1). For children and their families and friends the impact of childhood disablement is multifaceted, and all those who are touched by it continually experience the phases of grief and acceptance.

BOX 13-1   *Outcomes of Establishing a Diagnosis for a Pediatric Patient*

Positive Outcomes
- Gives the ability to establish a prognosis
- Validates the need for services and supports
- May indicate a need for genetic counseling
- Assists in possible prevention of secondary disabilities
- Knowledge may assist the family with coping mechanisms
- Aids research efforts targeted to specific conditions
- May assist in obtaining funding from government agencies for services

Negative Outcomes
- May lead to a negative stereotype (label)
- May disenfranchise the child from obtaining certain services
- May cause a state of depression or denial
- A false-positive diagnosis has negative immediate consequences for both the child and family
- A false-negative diagnosis will have long-term consequences for both the child and family
- May result in difficulty obtaining private insurance coverage

During the evaluation, individualized goals and objectives are developed from the information derived from the examination (family assessment, child observations, and standardized assessment measures). The SOAP note format is rarely used as a documentation method for pediatric patients, with the possible exception of specific hospital or rehabilitation settings (see Chapters 2 and 9 regarding the SOAP note). Instead, the necessary information is contained in an **Individualized Family Service Plan (IFSP)** or an **Individualized Education Plan (IEP)** developed for each child. These plans are reviewed on a regular basis as the framework for treatment and serve as a baseline by which progress is monitored.

As the name implies, the IFSP describes in detail the total plan of care for the child in the context of the family unit.[89-91] This type of plan, designed for children from birth to 3 years of age, is always determined in collaboration with the family, and therapeutic needs are intertwined with family needs and priorities. This strategy recognizes that the family unit must remain healthy to provide optimum care for the child. The IFSP might include such services as special babysitting assistance, transportation provisions, or specialized medical care at home. The IFSP also includes the different therapeutic services that the child will receive, the specific duration and frequency of these services, and location of the intervention.

On entry into the school system, physical therapy objectives shift to interface with an educational service delivery system and become part of the IEP. Through this model, therapists often interact with the family, educators, and other health team members to provide direct intervention in the classroom setting.[92-94] The physical therapist may work individually with the child, may work in a group setting, or may serve as a consultant to direct care providers. In the latter case the physical therapist instructs persons who directly care for the child. Instruction may include certain positioning or movement techniques to provide therapeutic benefit throughout the day. Regardless of the environment, treatment should be provided in a context in which activities can be targeted to achieve the manner or quality of movement desired.

Young children may be seen by a physical therapist at a variety of locations with different therapist-child ratios, depending on the particular objectives of therapy. Generally, the site of choice is the child's most natural environment, which may be the home, school, or a daycare setting. Therapists may choose to work with a child in a 1:1 ratio, in a group with other children, or with the parents. Often, some mixture of formats and environments provides treatment variety and the greatest benefit for the child.

It is important to remember that the initiation of therapy does not signal the end of examination. Examination is an ongoing process that begins with the history and continues throughout each therapy session. It includes assessment of each child's strengths and needs and evolves as the child, family, and therapist continue to determine appropriate therapeutic activities. Annual, biannual, or monthly reexamination is extremely important for monitoring the child's progress and redirecting intervention if necessary and is usually required by insurance companies. By applying the results of the examination and subsequent evaluation, the health care team and family work in a partnership to determine a well-coordinated plan of care for each child.

PRINCIPLES OF DIRECT INTERVENTION

Intervention in pediatric physical therapy involves helping each child gain abilities to assist in meeting the daily challenges of the most natural environments. As mentioned earlier, the initial task of the therapist, in collaboration with the family, is an examination of the child's individual strengths and needs. With this information a unique plan of care is developed that supports the child's strengths while facilitating skills in needed areas. Depending on the child's needs or diagnosis, intervention may involve a variety of approaches.

To initiate therapy with pediatric orthopaedic patients, PTs will find it useful to have specific knowledge in the area of pediatric orthopaedics (Box 13-2).[95] Orthopaedic examination and intervention vary according to the condition, but certain procedures are common to all orthopaedic clients, such as measurement of range of motion, muscle and sensory testing, gait assessment, and postural evaluation. (See Chapter 9 for a further description of these procedures.) Children may require specialized orthopaedic management for acute and long-term orthopaedic conditions, as well as for neuromuscular diseases. Intervention in both cases requires knowledge of the specific diagnoses, as well as of protocols for management if any exists. For example, specialized surgical procedures often require the therapist to know specific postoperative management protocols (e.g., positioning or weight bearing) in order to maintain the surgical correction. Often physical therapists are requested to fabricate splints or casts for a pediatric patient to assist in muscle lengthening, joint stabilization, or improved alignment (Figure 13-8).

In addition to orthopaedic techniques, physical therapists use a range of therapeutic techniques to enhance the rehabilitation process. A variety of neuromotor approaches are used to treat a child with neurological and orthopaedic disabilities. These approaches were primarily developed between 1950 and 1980 and were based on the theory, literature, and patient observations current at that time. These approaches have been and continue to be reviewed and adapted in light of current nervous system theories.[96,97] A primary task for both new and veteran pediatric physical therapists is to continue to research the effectiveness of each approach and assess the use of these approaches in a

BOX 13-2 *Knowledge Base for Pediatric Orthopaedic Assessment and Treatment*

- Normal pediatric biomechanical alignment
- Specific orthopaedic assessment procedures
- Presurgical evaluation of posture and movement
- Postoperative management of specialized surgical interventions
- Rationale and indications and contraindications for using manual therapy
- Use of casts and orthotics for correction or management of musculoskeletal malalignment
- Appropriate use of modalities and exercise protocols for children

From Pediatric Orthopedics. Alexandria, VA, American Physical Therapy Association, 1992.

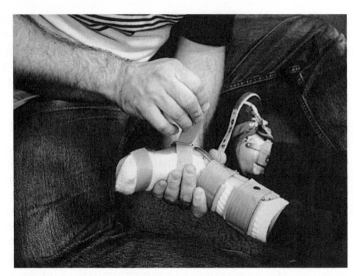

Figure 13-8 ■ Ankle-foot orthosis is used to assist the orthopaedic needs of a child. (Courtesy of Bruce Wang.)

variety of settings and their ability to facilitate the neuromotor changes they purport. It is also imperative that physical therapists evaluate the effectiveness of each approach in facilitating the child's achievement of targeted goals.

Most pediatric physical therapists continue to rely on an "eclectic," or multiple-method, approach when providing therapy. An **eclectic approach** includes some combination of therapeutic strategies used by the physical therapist that are thought to be helpful in the treatment of a given client.[98-100] Although the common use of eclectic practice has made it difficult to isolate and study the effectiveness of each specific approach, numerous published articles have discussed both the controversial nature and the effectiveness of a variety of neuromotor approaches.[101-112] Additional clinical research is necessary to achieve a sound basis of support for the continued use of many therapeutic approaches.

Regardless of the type of intervention, pediatric therapy should pave the way for a healthy, high-quality life for each child. Campbell outlined a checklist, or "defining strategy," for the evaluation of pediatric interventions.[113] The questions she poses can be used to evaluate intervention collaborations in the home, school, or other community venues. The answers to these questions provide a litmus test for successful pediatric intervention.

1. Does the intervention encourage the child to initiate a program of lifelong fitness activities, including proper nutrition, exercise, weight control, and stress management?
2. Does the intervention encourage the child to assume responsibility for personal health, including knowledge of the condition? Is the child encouraged to become personally involved in decisions on rehabilitation?
3. Does the intervention motivate the child and foster self-esteem?

4. Does the intervention promote meaningful pursuits that will foster the prevention of secondary conditions and thereby lead to lifelong musculoskeletal health and improved cardiovascular fitness?

A variety of approaches continue to be used to habilitate and rehabilitate pediatric clients. The following brief descriptions provide an objective overview of the more common neuromotor approaches in use.

DYNAMICAL SYSTEMS THEORY

In the **dynamical systems theory,** both the internal components of the patient and the external context of the task are equally important and contribute to functional movement.[114] This theory emphasizes the process of moving rather than the product of a movement. Cooperating systems included, but are not limited to, the musculoskeletal system, sensory system, cardiopulmonary system, and limbic system. The interactions of all the body's systems with the environment facilitate or inhibit movements. Therapists must work with the interplay of all systems rather than each system in isolation. To improve a child's ability to move independently, a therapist may modify the task or the environment (e.g., using an assistive device, adjusting surface texture) in addition to helping a child improve strength, endurance, and motor control.

NEURODEVELOPMENTAL TREATMENT APPROACH

The **neurodevelopmental treatment (NDT)** approach was originated by Berta and Karel Bobath in England almost 50 years ago to both analyze and treat neurological disorders of posture and movement.[115-117] Through the use of a motivating environment and the child's active participation, the therapist uses manual facilitation and inhibition techniques to present the child with a "normal" sensory experience and thereby encourage facilitation of a more functional motor response.[115,118,119] Continued active repetition of normal developmental skills is theorized to assist the child in establishing more coordinated, efficient movement patterns.[117-121] The primary emphasis of the NDT approach is on movement quality, and training of the parent or provider is stressed for the purpose of incorporating movement concepts into the child's functional daily routines. Pediatric therapists using this approach should realize that although some studies have demonstrated the efficacy of NDT,[120,122] other studies do not support its usefulness as a treatment approach.[123] Despite the controversy, NDT continues to be one of the most widely used and documented therapeutic approaches in the United States for the treatment of upper motor neuron lesions such as CP (Figure 13-9).[124,125]

SENSORY INTEGRATION THEORY

The **sensory integration (SI)** technique is based on the theory that poor integration of the use of sensory information (e.g., tactile or visual feedback) prevents the organization of resultant motor behavior (e.g., walking or jumping). This approach assesses the child's sensory systems through reports by the parent and child, clinical observations of limited tolerance for sensory experiences, and tests before initiation of therapy. The provision of controlled vestibular and

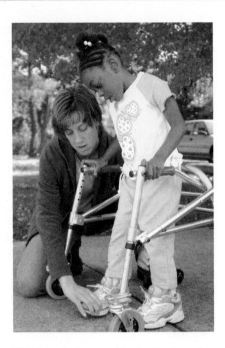

Figure 13-9 ■ Child ambulates with facilitation from the therapist. (Courtesy of Kathleen Hunter.)

somatosensory experiences within meaningful environments is believed to enable the child to integrate the sensory information and evoke a spontaneous functional response (Figure 13-10).[111,126-128]

NORMAL DEVELOPMENTAL THEORY

Therapy goals and objectives are designed to follow the progression of normal motor development (developmental milestones), as well as developmental theory (e.g., development proceeds in a proximal-to-distal direction). This **normal developmental theory** approach is based on a model of higher level cortical control that dictates the maturation process. The theory assumes that children with central nervous system damage will acquire motor skills in a fashion similar to that of children with normally developing nervous systems.[98] Many of the neuromotor therapies used today were originally based on this theoretical foundation.[129]

TASK-ORIENTED MOVEMENT MODEL

Based on the work of Gentile,[130] a **goal-directed movement approach** to intervention has been established by Sheperd[131] and by others[132] who were seeking to use environmental task conditions as an impetus for improved motor control and motor learning. In Gentile's paradigm, goal-directed movements include both the investigative and the adaptive behaviors resulting from a child's interactions with the environment. In observing such behavior, the pediatric physical therapist can orient therapy so that it focuses on the child's impairments, on task reorganization, and on environmental modifications that may

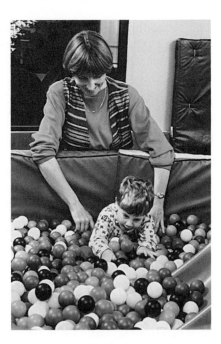

Figure 13-10 ■ Sensory integration can be fun. (Courtesy of Bruce Wang.)

improve child outcomes. Therapy is specific to the environment and task and is designed to promote a child's development of solutions to movement problems.

SUMMARY   Physical therapists who work with pediatric patients focus on child development, psychology, and learning. They may provide services to the patient for a long period, for a short time, or on a consultant basis. Intervention is family centered and usually incorporates activities adapted to play. Physical therapy is frequently rendered in the home or school setting as directed by federal entitlement programs.

Common conditions seen by pediatric physical therapists are generally classified as orthopaedic or neuromuscular disorders. Screening, examination, and assessment techniques are used to complete an evaluation and establish functional goals and objectives, which are incorporated into an IFSP or IEP. Intervention is often eclectic; that is, it combines components from a variety of approaches, including dynamic systems theory, neurodevelopmental treatment, sensory integration, normal developmental theory, and a task-oriented model. Early and continuing intervention programs for children are designed to incorporate a child's motivation and desire to play or participate in community-based recreation and leisure activities. Parents are active partners in assessing their child's individual interests and helping to design the optimal environment(s) that will support therapy goals while matching the child's interests. With careful observation and the use of environmental adaptations and assistive devices, community activities (e.g., soccer, art class) can be modified to embrace a child with special needs. Pediatric physical therapy is challenging and rewarding. Research, legislation, and new techniques create a changing practice environment to enhance the quality of care. The result is an exciting specialty in physical therapy.

CASE STUDIES

CASE STUDY ONE

Matthew is 3 years old and one of many preschoolers at Rosedale Preschool. He has Down syndrome.

Matthew attends preschool with other infants and toddlers. He plays with balls and puzzles and loves to swim. A formal evaluation revealed that Matthew has many strengths as well as needs in the gross and fine motor domains. Matthew is severely hypotonic (low muscle tone) and has difficulty running without falling. This problem was noted on the formal examination as well as in observations by Matthew's parents and preschool teacher. It was also noted that his automatic reactions to disturbances in balance (righting reactions and protective responses) were delayed, especially when moving into and out of various positions (transitions). Matthew was able to grasp objects in a manner appropriate for other 3-year-olds and enjoys drawing and playing with building blocks. He continues to exhibit needs in feeding skills because of the low muscle tone in muscles used for chewing and mouth closure. His medical history reveals that Matthew has a congenital heart problem, as well as several other features associated with Down syndrome.

Researchers have attempted to determine appropriate physical therapy interventions for children with Down syndrome.[133] Conclusions drawn from this research indicate that it appears most important to provide a child with Down syndrome opportunities to explore a variety of environments requiring different postural adjustments or movement patterns in response to changing task conditions. In accordance with this research, the therapist must observe the individual motor learning style of each child and respond by creating motivating and challenging learning situations.

In Matthew's case, the physical therapist will provide therapy in the school as designed in his IEP and collaborate with his preschool staff by instructing them to carry out physical therapy goals throughout his daily school routine. An inclusion program, such as the one at Rosedale Preschool, maintains a philosophy that children with a variety of developmental abilities should play and learn together in an atmosphere that fosters a sense of belonging and personal growth for all its members. This type of environment is naturally where a child as special as Matthew belongs.

Matthew's Individualized Education Plan

Because of Matthew's diagnosis of congenital heart disease, it is important that he avoid excessive exertion and fatigue. Activities that involve impact to the cervical vertebrae should also be avoided because of his vertebral instability. In designing a plan for Matthew, the therapist focuses on family goals and Matthew's current interests. Several pediatric assessment tools can assist in identifying and prioritizing Matthew's therapy goals. The Canadian Occupational Performance Measure is one measure designed specifically to identify and determine the importance of the child's and family's goals for therapy.[134] It is from this frame of reference that therapeutic goals and objectives will be designed. Specific objectives might involve achieving a task that is appropriate for Matthew's developmental abilities, as well as his functional level. Most objectives target a particular skill, the manner of performance or assistance, and the criterion to be met (Box 13-3).

The same skill can also be scaled[112] so that Matthew will always achieve different measures of success and his individual progress can be monitored over time (Box 13-4). Initial therapeutic goals are vital for assessing his response to intervention, as well as for maintaining treatment consistency. Through the ongoing assessment process, Matthew's progress will be monitored with alterations made to his care plan if warranted.

Intervention. Physical therapy intervention may first involve assisting Matthew in developing a relationship with his environment. Matthew may initially move too quickly or slowly, take steps that are too large or uneven, or resist the challenge to ambulate altogether. During an activity the therapist may use NDT techniques such as guided handling to assist with movement. Another strategy may involve Matthew's active participation through the use of cognitive and verbal reinforcement during a motivating recreational activity to reinforce learning. As mentioned previously, some combination of techniques may best accomplish the task (see the section Principles of Direct Intervention). If each of Matthew's goals can be

---

BOX 13-3   *Example of a Goal and Criterion for Matthew*

Goal: Matthew will run across a level (hard) mat surface without falling when prompted with his favorite toy.
Criterion: Three to four times during four play sessions.

BOX 13-4   *Goal Attainment Scaling*

−2 Matthew will walk across a level mat surface without falling when prompted with his favorite toy.
−1 Matthew will run across a level mat surface with one stop to regain his balance (hands down on mat) when prompted with his favorite toy.
 0 Matthew will run across a level mat surface without falling when prompted with his favorite toy.
+1 Matthew will run across a level mat angled 10 degrees with one stop to regain his balance (hands down on mat) when prompted with his favorite toy.
+2 Matthew will run across a level mat raised by a 10-degree angle without a stop or fall when prompted with his favorite toy.

designed according to his motivations (e.g., eating, play, recreation), the inclusion of therapeutic approaches and techniques becomes more functional and likely to meet with success.

CASE STUDY TWO

Emmie began her life in the neonatal intensive care unit of Eastern Shore Memorial Hospital. Her first experiences were the sounds of the slow beeps and hums of the infant monitors. Her first visions were obstructed by glass, and her human touch was limited to persons performing routine checks of her medical status. Unlike other newborn infants who experience the sounds of home and the arms of friends or siblings, Emmie will have to wait until she has surgery, because she was born with spina bifida (meningomyelocele). Children with spina bifida have no choice but to begin their lives in the hospital environment. Although diligent efforts have improved the comfort and familiarity of hospital neonatal intensive care and pediatric units, they continue to be a threatening, imposing environment for families.

Management

The general goals of physical therapy management for Emmie and other children with spina bifida are (1) to prevent her body structure from causing participation limitations that are a potential consequence of activity limitations (e.g., "can't crawl"), and (2) to improve the quality of life for her and her family by preventing activity limitations from limiting her participation in daily activities and social events (e.g., "can't go to the school dance").[135] Accomplishing these goals requires a collaborative approach involving the child, the family, and the health care team. Physical therapy examination should be comprehensive and take into account the observations and examinations of other health care team and family members. Evaluation and continued follow-up (monitoring) should include the following specific objectives:

- General multidomain screening and evaluation of developmental level
- Neurological examination, including monitoring for signs of increased intra-cranial pressure
- Orthopaedic examination for joint range and mobility, kyphosis, scoliosis, or dislocations
- Examination of bowel and bladder function
- Examination of skin integrity
- Activities of daily living
- Examination of mobility
- Promotion of recreational activities

Emmie's Individualized Family Service Plan

Activities are generally centered on the goals and objectives indicated in the child's individualized plan. For a child of Emmie's age the format would probably be an IFSP. A child with spina bifida often has a range of cognitive delays and delayed skills in the psychosocial area. Consideration of these abilities, as well as physical and environmental factors, is essential when designing a plan of care. During the first few years of life, Emmie will develop a sense of her autonomy and self-esteem, so physical therapy will focus on her ability to explore her environment.

Depending on each child's abilities, the physical therapist will explore options to accomplish mobility goals. Many children with spina bifida use orthoses or braces to assist in locomotion. Therapy goals may also focus on other functional activities, such as position transitions, muscle strengthening, and self-care activities. Assistive technology devices such as an adapted computer keyboard will be especially useful in creating a more accessible environment for Emmie as she enters school.[136] As Emmie reaches adolescence, she will probably choose to use a wheelchair that allows greater speed and efficiency for daily living. The team should encourage Emmie to explore a variety of recreational activities that are motivating and will improve general fitness and quality of life. She may continue to be seen on a periodic basis through the hospital's outpatient clinic or opt for private outpatient care. Therapy will continue only on an "as-needed" basis to assist with problems that arise during transitional developmental phases.

REFERENCES

1. Cherry DB: Pediatric physical therapy: Philosophy, science and techniques. Pediatr Phys Ther 1991;3(2):70-76.
2. Bottos M, Dalla Barba B, Stefani D, et al: Locomotor strategies preceding independent walking: Prospective study of neurological and language development in 424 cases. Dev Med Child Neurol 1989;31:25-34.
3. Linder TW: Transdisciplinary Play-Based Assessment: A Functional Approach to Working with Young Children. Baltimore, Brookes, 1990.
4. Surgeon General's Report: Children with Special Health Care Needs. Rockville, MD, US Department of Health and Human Services, Public Health Service, 1987.
5. McPherson M, Arango P, Fox H, et al: A new definition of children with special health care needs. Pediatrics 1998;102:137-140.
6. National Maternal & Child Health Resource Center: Community-Based Service Systems for Children with Special Health Care Needs and Their Families. Washington, DC, US Department of Health and Human Services, 1988.
7. International Classification of Functioning, Disability and Health. Geneva, World Health Organization, 2001.
8. Guide to Physical Therapist Practice, revised ed 2. Alexandria, VA, American Physical Therapy Association, 2003.
9. National Advisory Board of Medical Rehabilitation Research: Research Plan for the National Center for Medical Rehabilitation. Bethesda, MD, National Institute of Child Health and Human Development, National Institutes of Health, 1993.
10. Education of All Handicapped Children Act of 1975. Public Law 94-142, 20 USC 1401, 1975.
11. Individuals With Disabilities Education Act Amendments of 1991. Public Law 102-119, 105 STAT.587, 1991.
12. Individuals with Disabilities Education Improvement Act of 2004. Public Law 108-443, STAT. 2647, 2004.
13. Fischer J: Physical therapy in education environments: Moving through time with reflections and visions. Pediatr Phys Ther 1994;6(3):144-147.
14. Strain P: Least restrictive environments for preschool children with handicaps: What we know, what we should be doing. J Early Intervent 1990;14:291-296.
15. Miterski B, Drynda S, Boschow G, et al: Complex genetic predisposition in adult and juvenile rheumatoid arthritis. BMC Genet 2004;5:2.
16. Thompson SD, Moroldo MB, Guyer L, et al: A genome-wide scan for juvenile rheumatoid arthritis in affected sibpair families provides evidence of linkage. Arthritis Rheum 2004;50(9):2920-2930.
17. Prahalad S: Genetics of juvenile idiopathic arthritis: An update. Curr Opin Rheumatol 2004; 16:588-594.
18. Klepper SE: Effects of an eight-week physical conditioning program on disease signs and symptoms in children with chronic arthritis. Arthritis Care Res 1999;12:52-60.

19. Scull S: Juvenile rheumatoid arthritis. *In:* Tecklin JS (ed): Pediatric Physical Therapy. Philadelphia, Lippincott, 1998.

20. Omeroglu H, Koparal S: The role of clinical examination and risk factors in the diagnosis of developmental dysplasia of the hip: A prospective study in 188 referred young infants. Arch Orthop Trauma Surg 2001;121:7-11.

21. Patel H: Preventive health care, 2001 update: Screening and management of developmental dysplasia of the hip in newborns. CMAJ 2001;164:1669-1677.

22. Bialik V, Bialik GM, Blazer S, et al: Developmental dysplasia of the hip: A new approach to incidence. Pediatrics 1999;103:93-99.

23. Goldberg MJ: Early detection of developmental hip dysplasia: Synopsis of the AAP Clinical Practice Guideline. Pediatr Rev 2001;22:131-134.

24. Zeitlin L, Fassier F, Glorieux FH: Modern approach to children with osteogenesis imperfecta. J Pediatr Orthop B 2003;12:77-87.

25. Binder H: Rehabilitation of infants with osteogenesis imperfecta. Connect Tissue Res 1995;31:S37-S39.

26. Eagle M, Baudouin SV, Chandler C, et al: Survival in Duchenne muscular dystrophy: Improvements in life expectancy since 1967 and the impact of home nocturnal ventilation. Neuromuscul Disord 2002;12:926-929.

27. Hyser CL, Mendell JR: Recent advances in Duchenne and Becker muscular dystrophy. Neurol Clin 1988;6:429-453.

28. Nair KP, Vasanth A, Gourie-Devi M, et al: Disabilities in children with Duchenne muscular dystrophy: A profile. J Rehabil Med 2001;33:147-149.

29. Uchikawa K, Liu M, Hanayama K, et al: Functional status and muscle strength in people with Duchenne muscular dystrophy living in the community. J Rehabil Med 2004;36:124-129.

30. Chung BH, Wong VC, Ip P: Spinal muscular atrophy: Survival pattern and functional status. Pediatrics 2004;114:e548-e553.

31. Mitchell LE, Adzick NS, Melchionne J, et al: Spina bifida. Lancet 2004;364:1885-1895.

32. Shaw GM, Lammer EJ, Zhu H, et al: Maternal periconceptional vitamin use, genetic variation of infant reduced folate carrier (A80G), and risk of spina bifida. Am J Med Genet 2002; 108:1-6.

33. Cragan JD, Roberts HE, Edmonds LD, et al: Surveillance for anencephaly and spina bifida and the impact of prenatal diagnosis—United States, 1985-1994. MMWR CDC Surveill Summ 1995;44:1-13.

34. Blatter BM, Roeleveld N, Bermejo E, et al: Spina bifida and parental occupation: Results from three malformation monitoring programs in Europe. Eur J Epidemiol 2000;16:343-351.

35. Bruner JP, Tulipan N, Reed G, et al: Intrauterine repair of spina bifida: Preoperative predictors of shunt-dependent hydrocephalus. Am J Obstet Gynecol 2004;190:1305-1312.

36. Dewey D, Kaplan BJ, Crawford SG, Wilson BN: Developmental coordination disorder: Associated problems in attention, learning, and psychosocial adjustment. Hum Mov Sci 2002;21:905-918.

37. Dewey D, Wilson BN: Developmental coordination disorder: What is it? Phys Occup Ther Pediatr 2001;20:5-27.

38. Barnhart RC, Davenport MJ, Epps SB, Nordquist VM: Developmental coordination disorder. Phys Ther 2003;83:722-731.

39. Filkins K, Koos BJ: Ultrasound and fetal diagnosis. Curr Opin Obstet Gynecol 2005;17:185-195.

40. Batshaw M, Perret Y, Shapiro B: Normal and abnormal development. *In:* Batshaw M, Perret Y (eds): Children with Disabilities: A Medical Primer, ed 4. Baltimore, Brookes, 1997.

41. Roche AF: The cranium in mongolism. Acta Neurol 1966;42:62-78.

42. Spicer RL: Cardiovascular disease in Down syndrome. Pediatr Clin North Am 1984;31:1331-1343.

43. American Academy of Pediatrics, Committee on Sports Medicine: Atlantoaxial instability in Down syndrome. Pediatrics 1984;74:152-154.

44. Agha MM, Williams JI, Marrett L, et al: Congenital abnormalities and childhood cancer. Cancer 2005;103:1939-1948.

45. Menendez M: Down syndrome, Alzheimer's disease and seizures. Brain Dev 2005;27:246-252.

46. Barden HS: Growth and development of selected hard tissues in Down syndrome: A review. Hum Biol 1983;55:539-576.

47. Pueschel SM: Clinical aspects of Down syndrome from infancy to adulthood. Am J Med Genet Suppl 1990;7:52-56.

48. Cooley WC, Graham JM Jr: Common syndromes and management issues for primary care physicians: Down's syndrome: An update and review for the primary pediatrician. Clin Pediatr (Phila) 1991;30:233-253.

49. Galley R: Medical management of the adult patient with Down syndrome. JAAPA 2005;18:45-46, 48, 51-52.

50. Scher MS, Belfar H, Martin J, Painter MJ: Destructive brain lesions of presumed fetal onset: Antepartum causes of cerebral palsy. Pediatrics 1991;88:898-906.

51. Murase M, Ishida A: Early hypocarbia of preterm infants: Its relationship to periventricular leukomalacia and cerebral palsy, and its perinatal risk factors. Acta Paediatr 2005;94:85-91.

52. Einspieler C, Prechtl HF: Prechtl's assessment of general movements: A diagnostic tool for the functional assessment of the young nervous system. Ment Retard Dev Disabil Res Rev 2005;11:61-67.

53. Allen MC, Capute AJ: Neonatal neurodevelopmental examination as a predictor of neuromotor outcome in premature infants. Pediatrics 1989;83:498-506.

54. Blackman JA: Medical Aspects of Developmental Disabilities in Children Birth to Three, ed 2. Rockville, MD, Aspen, 1990.

55. Styer-Acevedo J: Physical therapy for the child with cerebral palsy. *In:* Tecklin JS (ed): Pediatric Physical Therapy. Philadelphia, Lippincott, 1994.

56. Morton JF, Brownlee M, McFadyen AK: The effects of progressive resistance training for children with cerebral palsy. Clin Rehabil 2005;19:283-289.

57. Kvigne VL, Leonardson GR, Neff-Smith M, et al: Characteristics of children who have full or incomplete fetal alcohol syndrome. J Pediatr 2004;145:635-640.

58. National Institute on Alcohol Abuse and Alcoholism (NIAA): Sixth Special Report to the U.S. Congress on Alcohol and Health. Washington, DC, US Department of Health and Human Services, 1987.

59. Stratton K, Howe C, Battaglia F (eds): Fetal Alcohol Syndrome: Diagnosis, Epidemiology, Prevention, and Treatment. Washington, DC, National Academy Press, 1996.

60. Warren KR, Li TK: Genetic polymorphisms: Impact on the risk of fetal alcohol spectrum disorders. Birth Defects Res A Clin Mol Teratol 2005;73(4):195-203.

61. Graham JM Jr, Hanson JW, Darby BL, et al: Independent dysmorphology evaluations at birth and 4 years of age for children exposed to varying amounts of alcohol in utero. Pediatrics 1988;81:772-778.

62. Streissguth A: Fetal Alcohol Syndrome: A Guide for Families and Communities. Baltimore, Brookes, 1997.

63. Streissguth AP, Barr HM, Sampson PD, et al: Attention, distraction and reaction time at age 7 years and prenatal alcohol exposure. Neurobehav Toxicol Teratol 1986;8:717-725.

64. Larkby C, Day N: The effects of prenatal alcohol exposure. Alcohol Health Res World 1997;21:192-198.

65. Faden VB, Graubard BI: Maternal substance use during pregnancy and developmental outcome at age three. J Subst Abuse 2000;12:329-340.

66. Chasnoff IJ, Burns KA, Burns WJ: Cocaine use in pregnancy: Perinatal morbidity and mortality. Neurotoxicol Teratol 1987;9:291-293.

67. Schneider JW, Griffith DR, Chasnoff IJ: Infants exposed to cocaine in utero: Implications for developmental assessment and intervention. Infants Young Children 1989;2(1):25-36.

68. Newald J: Cocaine infants: A new arrival at hospitals' step? Hospitals 1986;60:96.

69. Doberczak TM, Shanzer S, Senie RT, Kandall SR: Neonatal neurologic and electroencephalographic effects of intrauterine cocaine exposure. J Pediatr 1988;113:354-358.

70. Schneider JW, Chasnoff IJ: Cocaine abuse during pregnancy: Its effects on infant motor development: A clinical perspective. Topics Acute Care Trauma Rehabil 1987;2:59-69.

71. Blanchard Y: Neurobehavioral and neuromotor long-term sequelae of prenatal exposure to cocaine and other drugs: An unresolved issue. Pediatr Phys Ther 1999;11:140-146.

72. Rommens JM, Iannuzzi MC, Kerem B, et al: Identification of the cystic fibrosis gene: Chromosome walking and jumping. Science 1989;245:1059-1065.

73. Jaffe A, Bush A: Cystic fibrosis: Review of the decade. Monaldi Arch Chest Dis 2001;56:240-247.

74. Frank DA, Augustyn M, Knight WG, et al: Growth, development, and behavior in early childhood following prenatal cocaine exposure: A systematic review. JAMA 2001;285:1613-1625.

75. Messinger DS, Bauer CR, Das A, et al: The maternal lifestyle study: Cognitive, motor, and behavioral outcomes of cocaine-exposed and opiate-exposed infants through three years of age. Pediatrics 2004;113:1677-1685.

76. Bailey D, Simeonsson R: Family Assessment in Early Intervention: Rationale and Model for Family Assessment in Early Intervention. Columbus, OH, Merrill, 1988.

77. Foster M, Phillips W: Family systems theory as a framework for problem solving in pediatric physical therapy. Pediatr Phys Ther 1992;4(2):70-73.

78. Aylward G: Bayley Infant Neurodevelopmental Screener (BINS). San Antonio, TX, Psychological Corporation, 1995.

79. Frankenburg WK: Denver Developmental Screening Test Manual. Denver, LADOCA Project & Publishing Foundation,1973.

80. Bayley N: Bayley Scales of Infant Development. San Antonio, TX, Psychological Corporation, 1993.

81. Russell D, Rosenbaum P, Cadman D, et al: The gross motor function measure: A means to evaluate the effects of physical therapy. Dev Med Child Neurol 1989;31:341-352.

82. Folio RM, Fewell RR: Peabody Developmental Motor Scales: Examiner's Manual, ed 2. Austin, TX, Pro-Ed, 2000.

83. Coster W, Deeney T, Haltiwanger J, Haley S: School Function Assessment. Austin, TX, Pro-Ed, 1998.

84. Campbell SK, Hedeker D: Validity of the Test of Infant Motor Performance for discriminating among infants with varying risk for poor motor outcome. J Pediatr 2001;139:546-551.

85. Campbell SK, Kolobe TH, Wright BD, Linacre JM: Validity of the Test of Infant Motor Performance for prediction of 6-, 9- and 12-month scores on the Alberta Infant Motor Scale. Dev Med Child Neurol 2002;44:263-272.

86. Bruininks-Oseretsky Test of Motor Proficiency. Circle Pines, MN, AGS, 2005.

87. Haley SM, Coster WJ, Ludlow LH, et al: Pediatric Evaluation of Disability Inventory (PEDI): Development, Standardization and Administration Manual. Boston, New England Medical Center Hospitals and PEDI Research Group,1992.

88. Law M, Baptiste S, McColl M, et al: The Canadian Occupational Performance Measure: An outcome measure for occupational therapy. Can J Occup Ther 1990;57(2):82-87.

89. Bailey DB Jr, Hebbeler K, Scarborough A, et al: First experiences with early intervention: A national perspective. Pediatrics 2004;113:887-896.

90. American Academy of Pediatrics, Committee on Children with Disabilities: The pediatrician's role in development and implementation of an Individual Education Plan (IEP) and/or an Individual Family Service Plan (IFSP). Pediatrics 1999;104:124-127.

91. McGonigel MJ, Garland CW: The individualized family service plan and the early intervention team: Team and family issues and recommended practices. Infants Young Children 1988;1(1):10-21.

92. Giangreco M: Delivery of therapeutic services in special education programs for learners with severe handicaps. Phys Occup Ther Pediatr 1986;6(2):5-15.

93. Krehbiel R, Munsick-Bruno G, Lowe JR: NICU infants born at developmental risk and the Individualized Family Service Plan/Process (IFSP). Child Health Care 1991;20:26-33.

94. Henry B: The role of physical therapists in development of individualized educational plans. Totline 1986;12:13-15.

95. Pediatric Orthopedics. Alexandria, VA, American Physical Therapy Association, 1992.

96. Montgomery P: Neurodevelopmental treatment and sensory integrative theory. *In:* Lister MJ (ed): Contemporary Management and Motor Control Problems: Proceedings from the II Step Conference. Alexandria, VA, Foundation for Physical Therapy, 1991.

97. Umphred D: Merging neurophysiologic approaches with contemporary theories. *In:* Lister MJ (ed): Contemporary Management of Motor Control Problems: Proceedings from the II Step Conference. Alexandria, VA, Foundation for Physical Therapy, 1991.

98. Campbell PH: Posture and movement. *In:* Tingey C (ed): Implementing Early Intervention. Baltimore, Brookes, 1989.

99. Fetters L, Kluzik J: The effects of neurodevelopmental treatment versus practice on the reaching of children with spastic cerebral palsy. Phys Ther 1996;76:346-358.

100. O'Flaherty S: International perspectives on paediatric rehabilitation—Australia. Pediatr Rehabil 2004;7:267-270.

101. Cotton E: Improvement in motor function with the use of conductive education. Dev Med Child Neurol 1974;16:637-643.

102. DeGangi GA, Royeen CB: Current practice among NeuroDevelopmental Treatment Association members. Am J Occup Ther 1994;48:803-809.

103. Bartlett DJ, Palisano RJ: Physical therapists' perceptions of factors influencing the acquisition of motor abilities of children with cerebral palsy: Implications for clinical reasoning. Phys Ther 2002;82:237-248.

104. Kaminker MK, Chiarello LA, O'Neil ME, Dichter CG: Decision making for physical therapy service delivery in schools: A nationwide survey of pediatric physical therapists. Phys Ther 2004;84:919-933.

105. Golden GS: Controversial therapies in developmental disabilities. *In:* Gottlieb MI, Williams JE: Developmental Behavioral Disorders: Selected Topics, Vol 3. New York, Plenum, 1990.

106. Golden GS: Nonstandard therapies in the developmental disabilities. Am J Dis Child 1980;134:487-491.

107. Goodgold-Edwards SA: Principles for guiding action during motor learning: A critical evaluation of neurodevelopmental treatment. Phys Ther Pract 1993;2(4):30-39.

108. Harris S: Early intervention: Does developmental therapy make a difference? Topics Early Child Special Educ 1988;7:20-32.

109. Harris SR, Atwater SW, Crowe TK: Accepted and controversial neuromotor therapies for infants at high risk for cerebral palsy. J Perinatol 1988;8:3-13.

110. Ottenbacher KJ, Biocca Z, DeCremer G, et al: Quantitative analysis of the effectiveness of pediatric therapy: Emphasis on the neurodevelopmental treatment approach. Phys Ther 1986;66:1095-1101.

111. Ottenbacher K: Sensory integration therapy: Affect or effect. Am J Occup Ther 1982;36:571-578.

112. Palisano RJ, Haley SM, Brown DA: Goal attainment scaling as a measure of change in infants with motor delays. Phys Ther 1992;72:432-437.

113. Campbell S: Physical therapy programs that last a lifetime. Phys Occup Ther Pediatr 1997;17(1):115.

114. Kamm K, Thelen E, Jensen JL: A dynamical systems approach to motor development. Phys Ther 1990;70:763-775.

115. Bobath K, Bobath B: The neuro-developmental treatment. *In:* Scrutton D (ed): Management of Motor Disorders in Children with Cerebral Palsy. Philadelphia, Lippincott, 1984.

116. Bobath B: A neuro-developmental treatment of cerebral palsy. Physiotherapy 1963;49:242-244.

117. Bobath K: A Neurophysiological Basis for the Treatment of Cerebral Palsy. Philadelphia, Lippincott, 1980.

118. Bly A: Historical and current view of the basis of NDT. Pediatr Phys Ther 1991;3:131-135.

119. Bobath K, Bobath B: The facilitation of normal postural reactions and movements in the treatment of cerebral palsy. Physiotherapy 1964;50:246-262.

120. Tsorlakis N, Evaggelinou C, Grouios G, Tsorbatzoudis C: Effect of intensive neuro-developmental treatment in gross motor function of children with cerebral palsy. Dev Med Child Neurol 2004;46:740-745.

121. Cammisa K, Calabrese D, Myers M, et al: NDT theory has been updated. Am J Occup Ther 1995;49:176.

122. Girolami GL, Campbell SK: Efficacy of a neuro-developmental treatment program to improve motor control in infants born prematurely. Pediatr Phys Ther 1994;6(4):175-184.

123. Palisano R: Research on the effectiveness of neurodevelopmental treatment. Pediatr Phys Ther 1991;3(3):143-148.

124. Conner F, Williamson G, Sieff JA: Programming for the Infants and Toddlers with Neuromotor and Other Developmental Disabilities. New York, Teachers College Press, 1978.

125. Finnie N: Handling Your Young Cerebral Palsied Child at Home. New York, Dutton, 1975.

126. Ayres AJ: Sensory Integration and Learning Disorders. Los Angeles, Western Psychological Services, 1972.

127. Olson LJ, Moulton HJ: Use of weighted vests in pediatric occupational therapy practice. Phys Occup Ther Pediatr 2004;24:45-60.

128. Fisher AG, Bundy AC: Sensory integration theory. Med Sport Sci 1992;36:16.
129. Campbell PH, Finn D: Programming to influence acquisition of motor abilities in infants and young children. Pediatr Phys Ther 1991;3(4):200-205.
130. Gentile AM: Skill acquisition: Action, movement, and neuromotor processes. *In:* Carr JA, Shepherd R (eds): Movement Science: Foundations for Physical Therapy in Rehabilitation. Rockville, MD, Aspen, 1987.
131. Shepherd RB: Training motor control and optimizing motor learning. *In:* Shepherd RB (ed): Physiotherapy in Paediatrics, ed 3. Oxford, Butterworth-Heinemann, 1995.
132. Shumway-Cook A, Woollacott M: Motor Control: Theory and Practical Applications. Baltimore, Williams & Wilkins, 1995.
133. Shea AM: Motor attainments in Down's syndrome. *In:* Lister MJ (ed): Contemporary Management of Motor Control Problems: Proceedings of the II Step Conference. Alexandria, VA, Foundation for Physical Therapy, 1991.
134. Law M, Narrah J, Pollock N, et al: Family-centered functional therapy for children with cerebral palsy: An emerging practice model. Phys Occup Ther Pediatr 1998;18(1):83-102.
135. Hirst M: Patterns of impairment and disability related to social handicap in young people with cerebral palsy and spina bifida. J Biosoc Sci 1989;21:1-12.
136. Langone J, Malone MD, Kinsley T: Technology solutions for young children with developmental concerns. Infants Young Children 1999;11(4):65-78.

It is always the season for the old to learn.

Aeschylus, 500 BC

14 Physical Therapy for the Older Adult

Jennifer E. Collins

KEY TERMS

activities of daily living (ADLs)
adaptive equipment
assistive device
dynamic balance
frail elderly
Functional Reach Test
hypokinesis
instrumental activities of daily living
    (IADLs)
osteoarthritis
osteoporosis
presbycusis
rheumatoid arthritis
static balance
well elderly

OBJECTIVES ■■■■■■■

After reading this chapter, the reader will be able to:
- Identify three specific reasons that a physical therapist would modify an intervention for an older person
- Differentiate between static and dynamic balance
- Describe the primary role for the physical therapist in each of the common conditions discussed in this chapter
- Explain why an interdisciplinary approach is important when developing a plan of care for an older person

Senior citizen, older American, elder, aged. What kind of individual comes to mind when you see or hear these words? Is it a white-haired gentleman struggling to move a walker through long hallways? Is it a silver-haired woman swimming laps at the community pool? Both of them should come to mind, as well as countless other descriptions of appearance, abilities, and challenges. In health care, professionals tend to think first of the multiple medical problems many older people have. But physical therapists (PTs) and physical therapist assistants (PTAs) may be as likely to intervene with an 85-year-old athlete as with a 70-year-old person who has had a stroke. So as the words senior, elderly, and older person are used for this population group, consider the wide variation of functional abilities that may be present. While keeping this individual variation in mind, also recognize the commonality that we are all part of the aging population.

GENERAL DESCRIPTION

DEMOGRAPHICS

For many decades PTs have provided services to individuals with conditions common to people over the age of 65. Only in the last decade, however, have PTs and PTAs worked with older persons in such large (and growing!) numbers. Current trends in health care and life expectancy have rapidly increased the numbers of older adults requiring some type of physical therapy services, whether rehabilitative or preventive. For example, according to U.S. census data, in July 2004, there were 36.3 million people over the age of 65 in the United States, or 12% of the population. This is expected to increase 147% between 2000 and 2050, while the remainder of the population is expected to increase by only 49%.[1] For an individual born in 1997 the life expectancy is 76.5 years, the longest life expectancy ever experienced in the United States.[2]

As people live longer, they tend to display more physical or medical conditions that require a PT's assistance in maintaining or regaining skills necessary for maximum function in their daily activities. While each individual requiring physical therapy benefits from specific, unique interventions, the goals for most people include skills in independently performing such activities as bathing, cooking, dressing, and shopping. These are described as **activities of daily living (ADLs).** More complex activities necessary for community living are called **instrumental activities of daily living (IADLs).**

ADLs and IADLs are skills that allow an older person to be less dependent on caregivers. For instance, shopping is a difficult skill for many older adults with physical impairments. If therapists assist older adults in improving balance and provide an appropriate assistive device, more individuals may be able to complete shopping trips with less assistance.

Figure 14-1 presents data on ADLs and IADLs of persons 70 years of age and over who are not institutionalized.[3] The data indicate that nearly 47% of these individuals have difficulty in performing one or more of the activities. The percentage increases with age and is higher for women in all categories. This information confirms that PTs have an important role in improving functional performance.

Although individual differences exist, the aging process includes changes that are common in older persons. Sometimes professionals find it useful to differentiate between "well elderly" and "frail elderly," since people in each group have needs quite distinct from those of people in the other group. **Well elderly** refers to people 65 years and over who are not experiencing physical limitations or who have age-related changes that are not significant enough to affect function. The 86-year-old woman in Figure 14-2 is a good example of a person described as one of the "well elderly." Although she has minor medical problems, these do not significantly affect her daily activities. The primary goal of physical therapy for someone like her is to maintain good physical function and prevent conditions that might limit her ability to continue at this level. In

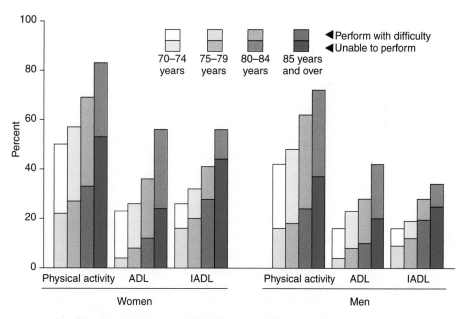

Figure 14-1 ■ Percentage of persons 70 years and older who have difficulty performing one or more physical activities, activities of daily living (ADLs), and instrumental activities of daily living (IADLs), by age and sex: United States, 1995. (From Health, United States, 1999, with Health and Aging Chartbook. Hyattsville, MD, National Center for Health Statistics, 1999.)

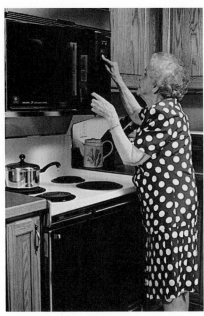

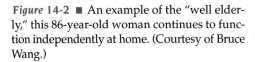

Figure 14-2 ■ An example of the "well elderly," this 86-year-old woman continues to function independently at home. (Courtesy of Bruce Wang.)

contrast, the term **frail elderly** is used to describe people over 65 with conditions that significantly impair their daily function or that require frequent medical intervention. For these people PTs offer strategies to regain mobility skills or to modify the environment to maximize the individual's function.

SETTINGS

Because the abilities and disabilities of older adults are diverse, so are the environments in which these individuals live. PTs and PTAs may work with older individuals in a wide variety of settings. People with acute medical conditions such as pneumonia, cardiovascular dysfunction, or hip fractures are treated in hospitals. Older people with conditions such as cerebrovascular accident (CVA; stroke), Parkinson's disease, or amputation may be seen for physical therapy in rehabilitation centers once they are medically stable. A variety of long-term care centers (skilled nursing facilities, extended care facilities, and others) provide services to older people who are not acutely ill but require nursing care or assistance with functional activities. PTs and PTAs in long-term care settings generally provide two types of services. Rehabilitative services improve skills so that people may return to their homes or will be less dependent on caregivers in the long-term care facility. Functional maintenance programs, often implemented by facility staff under the supervision of PTs, assist older adults to maintain the skills they currently possess and prevent further limitations or disability.

Many older people with functional limitations are healthy enough to live at home independently or have family members who are able to care for them. Depending on the medical condition of the individual and availability of appropriate transportation, older people living at home who require physical therapy may receive those services at an adult daycare facility, in an outpatient clinic, or through a home health care agency.

Healthy older people who want to maintain or improve their optimum physical status may attend exercise classes at senior centers or those sponsored by such groups as the Arthritis Foundation. Traditional or aquatic exercise programs may be conducted, supervised, or developed by PTs. These exercise programs may be aimed at general fitness and health promotion or at the prevention of conditions responsive to exercise, such as osteoporosis or poor balance.

ROLES FOR PHYSICAL THERAPISTS WITH OLDER ADULTS

It is easy to envision the PT as a clinician who provides hands-on services (direct intervention) to older adults. In each of the settings described above, however, PTs are also educators. With valuable knowledge of the physiological aging process, PTs are the ideal professionals to educate patients, family members, and other professionals about preventing and minimizing impairments, functional limitations, and disability. Armed with facts, older people will be better able to exercise appropriately and maintain or regain skills. For example, the woman in Figure 14-3 is being taught how to use her arms to more easily get up from a reclined position. The PT is in an excellent position to teach older persons that strength and endurance can be increased with properly designed programs.

PTs may act as consultants to individuals and programs. PTs are effective advocates for older people in developing appropriate activity programs and in ensuring accessibility to all environments. For an individual, the PT provides information necessary to acquire appropriate adaptive equipment or assistive devices that improve safety and convenience. **Adaptive equipment** allows an individual to perform a functional task with increased ease or independence. An example is a grab bar secured to the wall in the bathroom near the shower or toilet so the individual can safety attend to ADLs without assistance from a

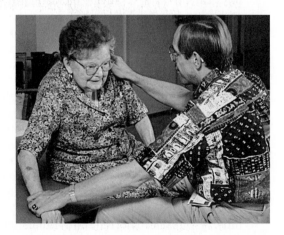

Figure 14-3 ■ Instruction is a major component of physical therapy. The woman in the photo is being taught how to use her arms to sit up from a reclined position. (Courtesy of Bruce Wang.)

caretaker. An **assistive device** provides the individual with assistance during periods of mobility. For example, a cane may assist an individual in climbing stairs safely. As a program consultant, the PT makes recommendations for group activities to maintain strength and endurance. The PT acts as a resource for other staff members to determine how to incorporate goals related to mobility into other components of the day program.

Other roles PTs may assume relating to the older adult are those of manager and researcher. PTs are prepared to assume such roles as managers of rehabilitation services or case managers. In these positions the educational background of PTs in managing resources and leadership, combined with their knowledge about issues of aging, allows them to take on additional responsibilities to serve clients. Research related to such topics as the aging process, prevention of disability related to aging, and effective intervention for older adults is a priority in the health care field. Discipline-specific studies of the cost effectiveness of particular interventions are essential in determining reimbursement policies for health care for older individuals. PTs are also essential team members in interdisciplinary studies that expand the knowledge of all health care professionals related to aging.

AGING-RELATED CHANGES

PTs and PTAs must be familiar with the changes that occur in "normal" aging and be able to distinguish them from pathological changes. Age-related changes, which vary with each individual, are considered when conducting examinations, formulating evaluations that include a prognosis, designing programs, and setting goals for people over 65 years of age. Although there are biological changes associated with aging, many changes once thought to be an inevitable part of aging are now considered to be related to the reduced activity and sedentary lifestyle of many elders. The PT, with the health care team, has an important role in evaluating older adults to determine what impairments and limitations can be addressed or what disabilities can be minimized through physical therapy. Changes that are not amenable to improvement may be addressed through adaptation, accommodation, or compensation.

The physical changes observed in older adults that affect the musculoskeletal system (bones, muscles, and connective tissues) often result in poor posture and decreased strength and flexibility. Decreased strength is often related to **hypokinesis** (decreased activity or movement) and the decreased muscle mass typically seen in older people. Muscle mass is reduced because of a decrease in the number of muscle fibers.[4] The reduction in fibers is related to loss of motor neurons (nerves innervating muscles) and active motor units (single motor neuron and all muscle fibers it innervates).[5]

Changes in flexibility with age are related to both hypokinesis and biological changes in connective tissue. Connective tissue tends to become less hydrated and stiffer in older persons. If they move less and become more sedentary, the muscles are not required to lengthen as often and actually become shorter over time. As muscles shorten, individuals tend to assume more flexed positions, potentially leading to postural changes.

Bone also undergoes changes with age. In studies of vertebral bodies, bone mass was shown to decrease by 35% to 40% between the ages of 20 and

80 years.[6] This finding suggests that bone is weaker in older people. This change may eventually advance to osteoporosis (see Common Conditions).

The central nervous system shows a reduction in conduction velocity associated with age.[4] The reduction affects the ability of the nerve to transmit impulses. This change tends to make movement responses slower in older persons and may explain the reduced ability to respond rapidly to loss of balance or slowed gait pattern often seen in later life.

Several of the sensory systems display changes that significantly affect mobility, specifically in the ability to move safely in the environment. The visual system is important in providing the older person with accurate information regarding the environment. The lens becomes less elastic, and the muscles around the lens decrease in their ability to accommodate rapidly from seeing far to near distance.[7] Visual acuity is also reduced. These changes make lighting and contrasting colors important in offering the older person cues about objects or surfaces that might interfere with safe mobility.

Older people display a group of characteristics called **presbycusis** ("old people's hearing"). This term refers to decreased ability to perceive higher pitches and to distinguish between similar sounds.[8] Auditory acuity is also reduced. These changes must be considered when instructions are given or an older person is taught about physical therapy.

The tactile system is another sensory system whose changes may affect mobility. The tactile system provides important information regarding the texture and changes in the walking surface. Age-related changes reduce the amount of tactile information the individual receives regarding the environment. If an older person does not receive accurate information regarding the surface underfoot, ambulation may become altered or a loss of balance may occur.

Age-related changes in the cardiovascular system are complicated by the characteristic cardiovascular diseases of old age. For example, 64% of people between the ages of 65 and 74 have hypertension (high blood pressure).[9] It appears, however, that overall cardiac performance at rest is not altered by age in healthy people, although cardiac response to stress does differ. This is demonstrated by a decrease in maximum cardiopulmonary function and work capacity.[10] Increased stiffness in the chest wall affects the respiratory system, which further reduces the effectiveness of cardiopulmonary function. These changes should be considered carefully in the design of exercise programs for individuals over 65 years of age.

Balance is a skill essential for safe and independent daily function. Limitation in balance and an increase in the risk for falling are common problems in older adults. Falls have been reported to occur in more than 35% of people over the age of 75.[11] Static balance and dynamic balance are the result of a complex interaction of the systems subject to age-related changes mentioned above. If any of these systems undergoes change, balance may be affected as well. A fall from a loss of balance could expose the elder to a multitude of subsequent impairments, such as fracture or other trauma, pneumonia, decubitus ulcers, and loss of strength or range of motion. The psychosocial impact on the individual can also be disabling. Fear of falling and loss of confidence may cause the individual to become isolated or more sedentary. If the fall is serious enough to cause injury, it is common for the elder to lose the ability to safely live independently.

For many years one of the most common myths of aging was that cognitive function always significantly decreases with advanced age. In fact, people seemed to assume that dementia was inevitable. It is now known that deterioration of cognitive function characterized as dementia is related to Alzheimer's disease or some other pathological condition, not to aging itself. Reports indicate that 10% of the general population over 65 years of age, and 20% of people over 85, display dementia.[12] Health professionals serving older people are aware of how to recognize dementia and how to interact with people with dementia; however, the characteristics of dementia are not displayed universally among people over 65 or even those over 85.

Significant cognitive changes that do fall in the category of normal aging are in memory and conceptualization (tasks requiring abstract thinking).[13] Specifically, the manner in which new information is stored (encoded) in the memory is altered. This leads to difficulty in retrieving newer information. Studies show that training in memory techniques, such as list organization, can improve recall in older persons.[14]

Psychosocial changes may affect people in older population groups. These vary widely based on the individual, family, environment, and presence of other changes or actual disease. What is important for the PT to remember is that psychosocial issues are crucial to the success of any rehabilitation program. Social considerations such as adjustment to retirement, loss of lifetime roles (worker, parent, homeowner, athlete, etc.), living environment, and presence or absence of health insurance have tremendous impact on the elder's life. Older persons may be required to adjust to the loss of spouses, friends, and siblings. Psychiatric disorders such as depression, dysthymia (disorder of mood), and anxiety are more common among homebound older people than those who are able to be out in the community.[15] The PT or PTA has a responsibility to bring signs of psychological problems to the attention of other members of the health care team.

COMMON CONDITIONS

Many impairments that are more prevalent in older people can benefit from physical therapy intervention. Individuals with the following common conditions are frequently seen by PTs and PTAs. Problems for older adults that are neurological in nature, such as Parkinson's disease and cerebrovascular accident (CVA), are discussed in Chapter 10.

Therapists should be aware of the impact of medical conditions on the older person's ability to recover from functional limitations. A retrospective analysis of a group of more than 1000 people over 65 showed that an older person who has two or more medical conditions is less likely to recover function in such tasks as dressing or carrying 10 pounds. Diabetes mellitus, stroke, depression, and hip fracture had the greatest effect on recovery.[16]

ARTHRITIS

By far the most common problem for older people is one of the joint diseases described as arthritis. In 1990, 38 million people in the United States were affected by arthritis.[17] There are two primary types of arthritis. **Osteoarthritis** most commonly affects the hands, spine, knees, and hips and occurs when the cartilage deteriorates after many years of use. This disease causes pain on movement. It is important for the person with osteoarthritis to maintain at least a moderate activity level while protecting the joints. PTs and PTAs can teach older adults appropriate exercise routines to maintain flexibility without excessively stressing the joints.

In contrast to osteoarthritis, **rheumatoid arthritis,** a disease of the immune system, is a chronic inflammation of the joints. It is more common among women than men, and the peak incidence is between 40 and 60 years of age.[18] It is characterized by enlarged joints that are often reddened and warm to the touch. The affected joints are stiff and painful, usually more so in the morning or after extended periods of inactivity. This disease process leads to limited range of motion, joint deformity, and eventually, progressive joint destruction. Typical physical therapy goals for the person with arthritis are pain relief, increased joint movement, assistive devices to facilitate independent function, and rehabilitation when joint surgery is required.

Pain relief may be provided by heat modalities such as hot packs or paraffin baths. The PT may teach the individual positioning principles for pain relief when in resting postures. Active range-of-motion exercises assist the individual in maintaining movement and flexibility necessary for function. Assistive devices such as canes or walkers may reduce pain in the affected joints during ambulation.

Total joint replacements of the hip and knee are common surgeries for older adults, undertaken to decrease the pain associated with arthritis and to improve function. When joint replacements are performed for a person with arthritis, the PT is involved with the patient or client before surgery as well as during the rehabilitation process. Before surgery the PT teaches the older person strengthening and flexibility exercises so the patient will go into surgery in the optimal condition. The therapist also teaches the individual important guidelines to follow after surgery, orders assistive devices, and reinforces the importance of exercise and rehabilitation after surgery. After joint replacements the PT provides interventions for regaining muscle strength, joint motion, and ADLs.

OSTEOPOROSIS

Osteoporosis is an extremely common disease in older people. Osteoporosis is characterized by decreased mineralization of the bones, which results from decreased production of new bone cells and an increased resorption of bone. The condition is measured by dual-energy x-ray absorptiometry, and the results are described according to bone mass density (BMD).[19] Osteoporosis is more common in women than men. In an analysis of data from a national survey, 56% of women over 50 years of age had reduced bone density, and 16% of these had osteoporosis. Among women over 80 years of age, 87% had reduced BMD.[19] Other factors that predispose people to osteoporosis are postmenopausal state, family history, lack of physical activity, smoking, diet, and certain medications.[18] The most important problem related to osteoporosis is bone fracture, which affects especially the wrist and hip in the older population.

The PT's primary role in osteoporosis is prevention. This is discussed in the next section, which addresses hip fracture.

HIP FRACTURE

The combination of osteoporosis and accidental falls has made hip fracture one of the most important health care issues for older people. People 65 years and older sustain 86% of the hip fractures in the United States. More than 300,000 hospitalizations for these fractures occur annually, with a mortality rate of nearly 25%.[20] As larger proportions of the population enter the over-65 age group, these numbers are likely to increase. Hip fracture is considered by many to be a major public health problem. A study conducted in Boston illustrates the significant impact that hip fracture has on the functional skills an elderly person may hope to regain after surgery to repair the hip. Only 33% of the people in that study had regained their prefracture status in five basic ADLs 1 year after the fracture.[21] Another study showed that 2 months after hospital discharge about 40% had regained ADLs but only 18% had returned to previous levels of IADLs.[22]

PTs are essential in the rehabilitation of patients after hip fracture. Transfer skills, ambulation, and use of assistive devices are taught in the hospital. Often patients are not discharged until they demonstrate safe transfers and ambulation. These skills are continued at a rehabilitation center, skilled nursing facility, or the person's home (Figure 14-4). As these basic skills are attained, PTs teach the person to regain additional functional skills, such as showering or transfers to and from automobiles, within the setting where the individual will be living.

PTs play an important role in preventing both osteoporosis and hip fractures. The most beneficial programs are directed at maintaining activity level, maintaining weight-bearing abilities and flexibility, strengthening, and education regarding a safe physical environment. Prevention of falls requires input from

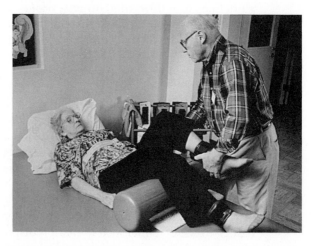

Figure 14-4 ■ After instruction by the physical therapist, a volunteer provides assistance in an exercise program to regain hip and knee strength after surgery to repair a hip fracture. (Courtesy of Bruce Wang.)

the entire health care team.[23] Falls may be related to any of several medical conditions, musculoskeletal or neurological changes, side effects of medication, cognitive status, the environment, or any combination of these factors. The health care team needs to be alert to these issues and teach the older person and family members the importance of prevention. Routine opportunities for weight bearing and walking are important as prevention strategies (Figure 14-5).

DIABETES

Diabetes mellitus affects 10% to 20% of Americans over the age of 60 years.[24] Diabetes is a chronic disorder with effects on many body systems. It is a disease of insufficient insulin action, affecting the efficient transport of glucose into muscle, adipose, and liver cells. Glucose is not transported into these cells, but accumulates in the blood. Some of the common complications of diabetes include renal failure, neurological lesions (termed diabetic neuropathies), neuropathic skin ulcerations, atherosclerotic vascular disease (which makes heart attack and stroke more common in people with diabetes), and retinopathies (which may lead to blindness). Many of these complications lead to specific problems for which physical therapy may benefit the person with diabetes. For instance, common physical therapy interventions for foot ulcers are hydrotherapy, debridement, other wound care techniques, and the provision of adaptive footwear. When not responsive to treatment, foot ulcers may lead to the development of gangrene and often amputation. The rehabilitation process after an amputation requires physical therapy for care of the residual limb, prosthetic training, and gait training, resulting in return to independent ambulation.

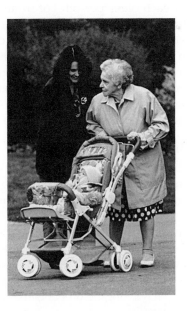

Figure 14-5 ■ The home care physical therapist uses another family member (child) as a meaningful approach to increasing the strength and endurance of an older individual. (Courtesy of Bruce Wang.)

For people with non-insulin-dependent diabetes, management of the disease through diet and exercise is important. PTs play an important role in developing exercise programs that consider the problems associated with diabetes.

PRINCIPLES OF EXAMINATION

Physical therapy for an older adult begins with examination and evaluation. The PT's examination is one component of a team evaluation. It is necessary for professionals from a variety of disciplines to critically examine the older person. If they all effectively share their findings, each will be better able to serve the individual.

As was pointed out earlier, older people constantly undergo a wide variety of changes after receiving services from a myriad of providers. Only if all these changes are considered and all providers are aware of the others' interventions will the health care be of optimum benefit. Many settings, however, do not have every health care discipline available to their clients. In these situations the PT should be able to make observations about the individual that include not only musculoskeletal, neurological, cardiovascular, and integumentary status, but also basic information regarding cognitive status, social situation, and communication abilities. Table 14-1 lists the components of a physical therapy examination with examples of possible sources of data and information.[25] Only a sampling of tests and measures are listed, and the array of tests and measures selected will vary substantially from one individual to the next. The Guide for Physical Therapist Practice contains a comprehensive list of tests and measures for use in examination.

Examination and evaluation should be specifically oriented to the skills and capabilities needed for maximum independence. These capabilities will differ for each older person. For example, a 70-year-old who has been inactive and sedentary since retirement at age 55 will have very different needs for rehabilitation from those of a 78-year-old who walks 2 miles every day and continues to work 4 hours a day as a volunteer in a recreation program. In each case the health care team considers how the individual functioned before the condition requiring therapy. A thorough examination includes information related to the person's typical daily function and what the person hopes to accomplish after the intervention.

HISTORY

The information described above is obtained through interviews with the patient and family as part of the process of obtaining the patient/client history. This is the first part of the examination. When interviewing the older person, the PT seeks information about how he or she views the current problem. A person's perceptions of the seriousness of the problem and expectations of therapy are important to consider when the plan of care and the interventions are being developed. Information from the person regarding any culturally based beliefs about illness, disability, and health is also important. An older person may have long-held beliefs that the PT should consider.

Interviewing the older person will also give the PT general impressions of cognitive function to determine whether a more formal examination of cognition is necessary. The individual should be able to give the PT information about

Table 14-1
Physical Therapy Examination for an Older Person

Components of Examination	Sources of Information
History	Patient/client interview Family interview Caregiver interview Medical chart Referral information

System review	Limited examination of:
	    Cardiopulmonary status
	    Integumentary status
	    Musculoskeletal status
	    Neuromuscular status
	    Communication ability
	    Affect
	    Cognition

Tests and measures*	Aerobic capacity and endurance Human body measurements Arousal Assistive devices, orthoses, prostheses ADLs/IADLs Gait and balance Joint integrity and mobility, ROM Motor function Muscle performance Neuromotor status Pain Posture Sensation Ventilation and respiration

ADLs, Activities of daily living; *IADLs*, instrumental ADLs; *ROM*, range of motion.
Data from Guide to Physical Therapist Practice, revised ed 2. Alexandria, VA, American Physical Therapy Association, 2003.
*This entry is a sampling of possible tests and measures and should not be considered comprehensive.

family support, typical activity level, occupation or former occupation, and the living environment.

Input from family members and other caregivers is an important component of the history. This information is essential in determining the amount of assistance a person may need from other sources. In some circumstances caregivers can verify or clarify information for the practitioner. In Figure 14-6 both the client and her spouse are providing essential information to the PTs. A thorough

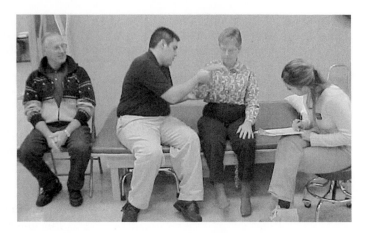

Figure 14-6 ■ The spouse (on the far left) is able to provide additional important information for the physical therapist during the history portion of the examination.

chart review is also important for a complete history. Objective information is gained from reports, records, and patient charts, including such information as the medical diagnosis, dates of hospitalization, lab reports, and other documented facts about the present illness or complaint, as well as past problems that could influence the plan of care for the current problem.

SYSTEMS REVIEW

The examination continues with a systems review, which entails a brief examination of the individual's systems to provide the PT with information regarding the older adult's general health. Data from other health care providers may provide pertinent information for the systems review. The information from the brief examination helps the PT to select the most appropriate tests and measures for the individual.

TESTS AND MEASURES

The examination of an older person proceeds much like the PT's examination of any individual, except that the PT is especially alert to the common problems of this age group. The PT may adapt some examination procedures to be more appropriate to the older individual. Tasks that are requested of the individual are explained as they relate to function. For example, the older adult may resist an examination activity such as creeping or kneeling on the floor. The person may be afraid of the positions or feel foolish. If, however, the PT explains that the activity is necessary to determine whether the person could get up from the floor if a fall occurred, he or she may be more willing to cooperate. This explanation provides a meaningful context for the request.

In examining the musculoskeletal system of the older person, the PT keeps in mind the potential for age-related changes described earlier. The therapist examines strength in terms of what activities the individual wants or needs to be able to perform. In other words, strength is examined in terms of function. Norms for range of motion in people over 65 years have not been established, nor are any norms universally accepted. Based on the person's activity level, some deficits may be expected. The therapist determines, with the older person, how much limitation of movement at the joints is acceptable. Posture of the older adult is examined in the same way as for other patients. The PT determines whether the observed posture is due to actual structural changes or whether it is a result of habit or functional issues. If the changes are not structural, education and exercise may significantly improve abnormal postural findings.

The neurological examination of the older person is similar to that of any individual. Some responses may be slow as described earlier, but it is a matter of determining what impact, if any, this has on the person's quality of life. The neurological examination includes specific sensory testing, such as two-point discrimination, proprioception, and visual and auditory testing performed by other members of the health care team. Sensory deficits may significantly affect functional tasks such as balance. As was noted earlier, balance is a complex interaction of cognitive, visual, perceptual, and motor skills. The PT needs to examine each of these systems individually to determine which may be contributing to a balance problem.

Both static (while standing still) and dynamic (while moving) balance should be examined. Tests and measures for examining **static balance** include such tests as observing the person standing with eyes open and eyes closed, timing of standing on one foot, and degree of postural sway. A specific balance test that can predict the likelihood of falling is the **Functional Reach Test**.[26] In this test a simple measure of how far the person can reach in front of the body gives an indication of the likelihood of falls.

Dynamic balance is assessed in a number of ways. Gait and functional mobility are important aspects of dynamic balance. The PT may measure how long it takes the older person to walk a set distance, using a measure such as the Timed Up and Go (TUG).[27] Other tests include the Berg Balance Scale, the Performance Oriented Mobility Assessment (POMA), and the Dynamic Gait Index.[28-30] The Gait Abnormality Rating Scale (GARS) looks at several components of gait and relates them to balance.[31] These are just a few of many tools available to assess balance. The PT selects an appropriate tool based on such factors as the individual's ability to follow directions, the person's living situation, and the specific features of the test. Gait examination should always include the use of any required assistive device and a description or consideration of the type of footwear the person uses. The type of sole or the weight of the shoe will affect the way the person ambulates. In Figure 14-7 the PT is performing an initial gait examination of a man approximately a month after hospital discharge following a stroke. The quadruped cane is needed at this time to assist with dynamic balance.

Information regarding balance and potential for falling is useful to the entire interdisciplinary team working with the older person. Another balance measure that may reveal information useful to the team is a self-efficacy measure, such as the Falls Efficacy Scale (FES).[32] This type of test focuses on the individual's confidence regarding balance and provides useful information for program

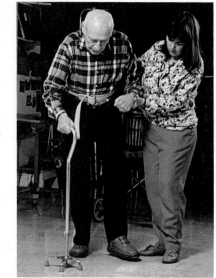

Figure 14-7 ■ Gait assessment using a quadruped cane after a stroke. (Courtesy of Bruce
Wang.)

planning. The team will be able to develop strategies in fall prevention that
range from exercise and environmental modification to teaching fall prevention
skills to the older person.

Standard tests of cardiopulmonary function are used for older persons.
Older people receiving physical therapy often fatigue easily and have reduced
endurance. PTs examine and evaluate these individuals to determine if exercise
programs should be modified. Measurements of cardiopulmonary function help
the PT to determine whether goals to increase endurance are realistic and
appropriate (see also Chapter 11).

An important part of the examination of the older person is to determine
whether he or she is experiencing pain related to movement. A description of
pain location, intensity, and circumstances that elicit or alleviate the pain is
needed. It should be noted whether the pain is acute or chronic and whether it
increases or decreases from one session to the next. Since pain is perceived
differently from one individual to the next, it is important to assess how much
discomfort the person is willing to tolerate to maintain independent function.

One simple means of measuring pain is on a Visual Analog Rating Scale
(VAS).[33] The individual indicates the amount of pain being experienced along
a 10-cm scale (see Figure 9-2). If an objective pain index such as this is used,
decreasing pain from one measurable point to another on the scale may be an
appropriate goal for an older adult. Another approach is to set a goal for a
specific functional task to be performed within a tolerable level of pain.

The tests and measures just described relate to specific impairments or functional limitations. It is also important for the PT to examine the older adult's
overall function. For many years PTs have used checklists to indicate whether
a patient or client can perform particular tasks. More recently, several standardized measures have been developed. Standardized measures allow health care
professionals to compare a person's scores as the individual moves from one

setting to another. They can also measure change at specific time intervals. Measures generally fall under the categories of self-report or performance measures. Examples of standardized self-report measures are the Functional Status Questionnaire (FSQ)[34] and the Functional Status Index (FSI),[35] in which the older person or the caregiver reports the person's ability to perform functional activities. In performance tests such as the Physical Performance Test (PPT), the therapist observes the older person performing tasks and scores the performance according to the instructions for the tool.[36]

Information about the environment in which the older person lives is essential. Whether the individual is in a nursing home, at a relative's house, or living alone, several aspects of the environment must be considered. The physical layout of the living area, the access to and from the residence, and the access from the home to outside services are important. Ideally, the PT should visit the residence rather than rely on reports from others.

The PT investigates access to and from the residence based on the individual's specific abilities and limitations. The following items are important in determining how much assistance the older person will require to be as independent in the living environment as possible:

- Ground surfaces—gravel, pavement, grass, sidewalks
- Curbs and curb cuts
- Ramps or steps outside of home
- Stairways within the home
- Presence or absence of handrails
- Size of door openings
- Door handles, latches
- Furnishings and floor coverings
- Arrangement of kitchen and bathroom fixtures
- Distance between rooms used most often

In addition to the above, a thorough examination should include such items as lighting, doorways, floor plans, furniture, and adequate space for adaptive equipment. Since the clinician has so many items to consider, a checklist with space for individual notation is most efficient for this assessment.

An environmental examination is equally important whether the older person is in a private home or a long-term care facility. According to federal regulations, long-term care facilities receiving federal reimbursement (such as Medicare or Medicaid) are obligated to ensure that residents are as free from the use of restraints as is practical. Such items as seat belts in wheelchairs, chest or hand straps in beds, and bedrails are to be used as infrequently as possible. PTs in these settings are obligated to assess mobility skills and safety and make recommendations to the interdisciplinary team regarding the need, if any, for these devices. The team must attempt to modify the physical environment to meet individual needs for safety before considering restraints. Only when other options have been exhausted should the team recommend the use of such supports.

As described earlier, few cognitive changes are solely the result of aging in a healthy older person. However, many of the conditions common in the elderly have the potential for development of dementia. For this reason the PT should either obtain information from other health care professionals or make observations during the physical therapy evaluation regarding cognitive function. The older person's cognitive abilities have great influence on how the PT provides instructions, the number of repetitions required when demonstrating, and how much practice is required when teaching a new skill. A standard, quick cognitive assessment tool, such as the Mini-Mental Status Exam, can easily be used by PTs without extensive training.[37]

As with all patients, the PT must obtain psychosocial information as part of the complete evaluation of the older person. The person's success in adjusting to the present disability is important information that will help the therapist determine the individual's level of motivation and whether special strategies are necessary to increase that level. An older person may become depressed, viewing a problem such as stroke or heart attack as "the beginning of the end." The therapist benefits from knowing the significant people in the patient's life—spouse, family, friends, or caregivers.

It is also extremely important to know the setting to which the person will return, so that available social support can be determined. Social workers or case managers are able to provide the PT with pertinent details regarding each patient's specific health insurance coverage and financial status so that the impact on rehabilitation services can be considered. The health care team plans and prioritizes intervention for each individual, based not only on the findings of the examination, evaluation, and prognosis, but also on social supports.

PRINCIPLES OF EVALUATION, DIAGNOSIS, AND PROGNOSIS

Once information about the patient or client is obtained, the next step in providing physical therapy intervention for the older adult is to evaluate the findings of the examination. From the evaluation the PT then determines a diagnosis that directs the course of rehabilitation. The diagnosis is a label or classification assigned to the cluster of findings related to a particular individual. It is important to remember that older adults frequently have multiple medical diagnoses. The PT considers these medical conditions, impairments, and functional limitations and evaluates how they affect the individual's ability to function. The physical therapy diagnosis reflects the result of the evaluation process and determines appropriate interventions.

Similarly, all the variables must be weighed to arrive at a prognosis that will direct the planning and goal-setting process for the older adult. Two 80-year-old individuals with identical medical conditions will not necessarily have the same prognosis or subsequent plans for physical therapy. Social supports, environmental factors, internal factors such as cognitive level, and other variables all contribute to determination of a prognosis.

PRINCIPLES OF DIRECT INTERVENTION

The individual's diagnosis and prognosis form the basis of the plan for physical therapy intervention. Physical therapy for any patient focuses on the problems identified from the evaluation. Care for the older person, however, requires emphasis on certain aspects of intervention, including (1) direct intervention techniques with the expectation of improved function, (2) instruction, (3) modification of accepted intervention techniques as necessary for the effects of aging, (4) recommendations for environmental modification, (5) training in the use of appropriate adaptive equipment, (6) teaching of health promotion, wellness, and prevention, (7) communication with other members of the health care team, and (8) setting.

DIRECT INTERVENTION

The first consideration in establishing goals for direct intervention with the older person is to set meaningful goals that address daily function. In other words, a goal to have the person reach full or normal shoulder flexion (arm up over head to 180 degrees) may not be meaningful if the person does not have the need to reach straight up overhead. If the highest cupboards in the house require only partial flexion and the person does not put any clothing on over the head, perhaps valuable time for direct intervention should be spent on other activities. However, if this older adult continues to work part time and must reach overhead to do so, full shoulder flexion is important.

To set meaningful and functional goals, the therapist involves the older person throughout the process. This may require some encouragement from the professional, especially if the person believes that the role of the health care professional is to issue direction and wait for patient compliance. Many older people feel that determining treatment is not the patient's role. In this case the professional encourages the older adult to be more involved in decision making regarding care.

The interdisciplinary approach mentioned throughout this chapter is important when setting goals. The individual may have multiple medical and rehabilitative needs. The team, including the patient and family, examines all those needs and prioritizes which should be addressed initially and which are more long term.

INSTRUCTION

Effective instruction of the older person encompasses both general and specific information. General, factual information about the effects of aging on the various body systems gives the older person a good background and model from which to judge changes the individual is experiencing. This information helps the older person appreciate the importance of achieving or maintaining an active lifestyle to prevent changes that are linked to inactivity. More specific information pertaining to the particular problem the older adult is experiencing is also important. A basic understanding of the disablement process, including the relationships among pathology, impairments, function, and disability, may help the older person understand why the PT is selecting particular interventions. Such topics as the typical course of the disorder, expected type and length of treatment, expectations for the home program, and impact on function should be clearly outlined for the individual and family members.

Education plays a role in motivating older adults, but other techniques can increase motivation as well. Often, older people enjoy therapy if social interaction is built into the process. Establishing a group of people with similar abilities for exercise may be beneficial and fun. Designing intervention in such a way that the person is competing, either with results of the last session or with peers, may also increase motivation to perform.

For some individuals motivation is not an issue. These people may be highly motivated but not confident of their ability to carry out a program on their own while the therapist is working with another person or when they perform the program at home. Lists of activities, diagrams, charts with spaces to check off, or a notebook may be valuable in assisting such a person to take control of the routine.

MODIFICATION

Intervention for older adults focuses on improving daily function. Programs should incorporate movement patterns that normally occur during the person's routine. For example, treatment for balance problems is most beneficial if it includes such activities as balance during transitional movements (up and down from chairs, in and out of bed) and on uneven surfaces. On the other hand, one-legged standing is probably not meaningful for most older persons. In most cases direct intervention does not need modification based solely on aging factors. Healthy older persons can increase strength, range of motion, endurance, and overall performance using traditional approaches. For example, 86- to 96-year-old nursing home residents who participated in exercise (resistance training) programs were able to increase quadriceps strength.[4] In Figure 14-8 the woman is engaged in resistive exercise to increase strength in hip and knee musculature. Modification may be necessary, however, in the presence of certain medical conditions. Cardiovascular and cardiopulmonary conditions, arthritis, and diabetes are common in older individuals and may necessitate modifications of accepted approaches. The PT and PTA working with elderly persons should be alert to these and prepared to modify programs accordingly.

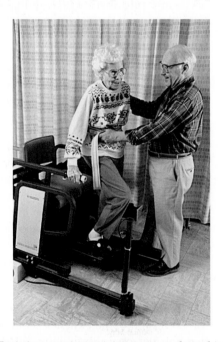

Figure 14-8 ■ Resistive exercises to increase strength, in this case in the hip and knee musculature, are effective in the elderly. (Courtesy of Bruce Wang.)

Some medications taken by older individuals also necessitate the modification of intervention. Certain medications affect the ability to perform physical activity. Older people commonly take multiple medications, both prescribed and over the counter. The PT should be aware of the medications taken by the individual, possible drug interactions, and side effects. For example, dizziness is a side effect of many drugs. A PT who is working with someone on getting out of bed, getting up from the floor, or performing more advanced balance activities must be alert to any signs of dizziness. If the person is taking medication that increases dizziness, the PT must take greater safety precautions while performing these activities. For information related to medical conditions and medications, the PT should remain in close contact with the physician and other team members.

ENVIRONMENTAL MODIFICATION AND ADAPTIVE EQUIPMENT

When providing services to an older person, the PT considers the need for environmental modification and adaptive equipment. Simple changes in the environment (improved lighting, removal of throw rugs, or furniture rearrangement) may make the individual safer and better able to function in the living environment. Appropriate adaptive equipment and training in its use may enable the older person to be more independent. Training in adaptive equipment should include demonstration and repeated opportunities to practice.

TEACHING OF HEALTH PROMOTION, WELLNESS, AND PREVENTION

An important component of any physical therapy plan of care is to provide the client with information about how to maintain or improve his or her health and prevent further problems that could limit physical function. Elders should be taught the benefits of exercise, regardless of age. Prevention of falls is also important to teach elders. Strategies to improve balance or to modify the environment to be safer are examples of teaching to prevent falls and fractures.

COMMUNICATION WITH MEMBERS OF THE HEALTH CARE TEAM

Communication with other members of the team is important for good physical therapy intervention. Team members provide information that assists the therapist in selecting the most appropriate strategies. Team members also reinforce the goals of other disciplines and share successful approaches to advance the individual's progress.

SETTING

A final consideration in determining the most appropriate intervention for an older person relates to the setting. In a physical therapy department within a health care facility, multiple pieces of equipment are available for use in improving strength and mobility or decreasing pain. The PT may have to be creative, however, to ensure that enhanced performance on objective tests in this setting will translate into improvement in daily function in a more home-like environment. Physical therapy provided in the home setting provides the

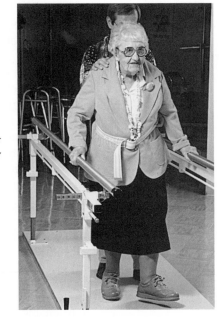

Figure 14-9 ■ Gait training is enhanced by using parallel bars in a clinical setting. (Courtesy of Bruce Wang.)

opposite challenge. There will be many opportunities in a home to improve functional skills, but it may be difficult to increase strength or endurance over long distance. The therapist must keep these advantages and limitations in mind when planning programs for intervention. In Figure 14-9 parallel bars are used to assist a woman in gait training. When she is ready to return to a home environment, another device, such as a walker, may be necessary to increase the distance she is able to walk.

SUMMARY

As the baby boomers grow older, the proportion of the U.S. population over 65 years of age, and especially over 85, will continue to grow. PTs and PTAs serve older adults in every type of setting, not solely in long-term care facilities. Certainly, some therapists will choose to specialize in working with people over 65 years, but almost all therapists and assistants will have contact with patients in this age group at some point. To provide high-quality services to the older population, PTs should recognize the similarities and differences between the older person and any other individual in need of physical therapy. The therapist should be ready to modify interventions as needed to address documented age-related changes. He or she should be able to educate the older person requiring services and all significant others in methods that will enhance the person's function. Finally, the therapist must be able to communicate and cooperate with the older individuals, the family, and team members to develop a meaningful and successful plan for intervention.

ACKNOWLEDGMENT

The author wishes to acknowledge the staff and members of The Friendly Home and the clients, staff, and faculty at Nazareth College Physical Therapy Clinic, both of Rochester, New York, for their assistance.

CASE STUDY

CASE STUDY ONE

This example is provided with the intent of demonstrating the complex medical, cognitive, psychosocial, and ethical issues facing the health care practitioner who works with older people and their families.

Margaret Evans is an 81-year-old woman who has been hospitalized for 7 days following a total hip replacement. She has the multiple diagnoses of rheumatoid arthritis, osteoporosis, and hypertension. She is also hearing impaired. The arthritis causes almost constant pain in her hips, knees, and hands. The surgery was performed to relieve pain in her right hip, which was the side with more severe pain. Mrs. Evans lives alone in the home where she has resided for 40 years. Payment on her home mortgage was completed 6 years ago. Her husband is deceased, her son lives 250 miles away, and her daughter lives with her family about 10 miles away. Mrs. Evans has a limited income (Social Security), and her medical coverage is Medicare.

Mrs. Evans is considered medically ready for discharge from the hospital. She has been receiving physical therapy once a day, consisting of (1) range of motion to all extremities, focusing on hip and knee musculature; (2) transfer training (moving from wheelchair to toilet, bed to standing, etc.); and (3) gait training with a walker. The PT made a home visit and noted that (1) there are four steps into the house, (2) the bedroom Mrs. Evans uses is upstairs (13 steps), (3) there are many throw rugs on the hardwood floors, (4) both bathrooms have tubs with showers, and (5) the laundry facilities are in the basement.

Mrs. Evans wants to go home as soon as possible. She has never been away from her home more than 3 days and has been very lonely for her neighbors while in the hospital. She sometimes awakes at night disoriented and confused about where she is. Her daughter, who works full time, is concerned about her mother's safety at home and is not sure whether her mother is ready to go home alone. She has also stated that she wants to be sure her mother has every opportunity for full rehabilitation and is advocating for daily physical therapy.

The team, including Mrs. Evans and her daughter, meets to discuss a discharge plan. A short-term placement is proposed. In this plan, Mrs. Evans would be discharged to a skilled nursing facility where daily physical therapy could be provided. Mrs. Evans is opposed to that move, although her daughter tries to convince her that it is a good proposal. The social worker suggests discharge to home and asks the team what other support services are necessary to ensure her success at home. The PT indicates that Mrs. Evans should learn to navigate stairs safely with crutches, obtain adaptive equipment such as a bathing chair and a raised toilet seat, and modify the home environment to be successful at home. Moving her bedroom to the first floor is another possibility to improve safety. Physical therapy services could be provided two to three times weekly through a home health care agency. The social worker suggests that a home health aide would be appropriate to assist Mrs. Evans with personal care, housework, and laundry.

Mrs. Evans is pleased, but her daughter is still concerned for her safety. The rehabilitation nurse suggests an emergency call button for Mrs. Evans to obtain assistance if she falls or experiences any other urgent situation. A bedroom will be set up for her on the first floor so she can avoid excessive stair climbing. The team agrees to the plan, and the social worker will monitor the services on a weekly basis.

REFERENCES

1. Longley R: Census offers statistics on older Americans. US Gov Info Resources, Apr 25, 2005.
2. National Vital Statistics Report—Preliminary Data, Vol. 47, No. 4. Hyattsville, MD, National Center for Health Statistics, 1997.
3. Health, United States, 1999, with Health and Aging Chartbook. Hyattsville, MD, National Center for Health Statistics, 1999.
4. Fiatarone MA, Marks EC, Ryan ND, et al: High intensity strength training on nonagenerians: Effects on skeletal muscle. JAMA 1990;263:3029-3034.
5. Doherty TJ, Vandervoort AA, Taylor AW, et al: Effects of motor unit losses on strength in older men and women. Appl Physiol 1993;74(2):868-881.
6. Mosekilde L: Normal age-related changes in bone mass, structure, and strength—consequences of the remodeling process. Dan Med Bull 1993;40(1):65-83.
7. Lewis CB: Aging: The Health Care Challenge, ed 3. Philadelphia, FA Davis, 1996.
8. Schaknecht HF: Pathology of the Ear. Philadelphia, Lea & Febiger, 1993.
9. Subcommittee on Definition and Prevalence of the 1984 Joint National Committee: Hypertension prevalence and the status of awareness, treatment, and control in the United States. Hypertension 1985;7:457-468.
10. Schneider EL, Rowe JW (eds): Handbook of the Biology of Aging. New York, Academic Press, 1990.
11. Tinnetti ME, Speechly M, Ginter SF: Risk factors for falls among elderly persons living in the community. N Engl J Med 1985;319:1701-1707.
12. Evans DA, Funkenstein HH, Albert MS, et al: Prevalence of Alzheimer's disease in a community population of older persons. JAMA 1989;262:2551-2556.
13. Salthouse TA: Age related changes in basic cognitive processes. In Storundt M, VandeBos G (eds): The Adult Years: Continuity and Change. Washington, DC, American Psychiatric Association, 1989.
14. Norris MP, West RL: Activity memory and aging: The role of motor retrieval and strategic processing. Psych Aging 1993;8(1):81-86.
15. Bruce ML, McNamara R: Psychiatric status among the homebound elderly: An epidemiological perspective. Am Geriatr Soc 1992;40:561-566.
16. Miller R, Zhang Y, Silliman RA, et al: Effect of medical conditions on improvement in self-reported and observed functional performance of elders. J Am Geriatr Soc 2004;52(2):217-223.
17. Schumacher HR: Primer on the Rheumatic Diseases. Atlanta, Arthritis Foundation, 1988.
18. Centers for Disease Control and Prevention: Prevalence of Arthritis—United States, 1997. MMWR Morb Mortal Wkly Rep 2001;50:334-336.
19. Osteoporosis. National Health and Nutrition Examination Survey (NHANES). Available at http://www.cdc.gov/nchs/nhanes.htm. Accessed June 16, 2005.
20. Hip Fracture Outcomes in People Age 50 and Over—Background Paper (OTA-BP-H-120). US Congress, Office of Technology Assessment. Washington, DC, US Government Printing Office, 1994.
21. Jette AM, Harris BA, Cleary PD, et al: Functional recovery after hip fracture. Arch Phys Med Rehabil 1987;68:735-740.
22. Magaziner J, Simonsick EM, Kashner TM, et al: Predictors of functional recovery one year following hospital discharge for hip fracture: A prospective study. J Gerontol 1990;45(3):M101-M107.
23. Kalchthaler J, Bascon R, Quintos V: Falls in the institutionalized elderly. J Am Geriatr Soc 1978;26:424.
24. Lipson LG: Diabetes in the elderly: Diagnosis, pathogenesis, and therapy. Am J Med 1986;80 (suppl 5A):10-21.
25. Guide to Physical Therapist Practice, revised ed 2. Alexandria, VA, American Physical Therapy Association, 2003.
26. Duncan PW, Weiner DK, Chandler J, et al: Clinical measure of balance. Gerontology 1990; 45(6):M192-M197.

27. Podsiadlo D, Richardson S: The Timed "Up & Go": A test of basic functional mobility for frail elderly persons. J Am Geriatr Soc 1991;39:142-148.
28. Berg KO, Wood-Dauphinee SL, Williams JI, Maki B: Measuring balance in the elderly: Validation of an instrument. Can J Public Health 1992;83(suppl 2);S7-S11.
29. Tinnetti M: Performance oriented assessment of mobility problems in elderly patients. J Am Geriatr Soc 1986;34(2):119-126.
30. Shumway-Cook A, Woolacott MH: Motor Control: Theory and Practical Applications. Baltimore, Williams & Wilkins, 1995.
31. Wolfson L, Whipple R, Amerman P, et al: Gait assessment in the elderly: A gait abnormality rating scale and its relation to falls. J Gerontol 1990;45(1):M12-M19.
32. Tinetti ME, Richman D, Powell L: Falls efficacy as a measure of fear of falling. J Gerontol 1990;45(6):P239-P243.
33. Scott J, Huskisson EC: Graphic representation of pain. Pain 1976;2:175-184.
34. Jette AM, Davies AR, Cleary PD, et al: The Functional Status Questionnaire, J Gen Intern Med 1986;1:143-149.
35. Jette AM: The Functional Status Index: Reliability and validity of a self-report functional disability measure. J Rheumatol 1987;14:15-19.
36. Reuben DB, Sui AL: An objective measure of physical function of elderly outpatients: The Physical Performance Test. J Am Geriatr Soc 1990;38:1105-1112.
37. Folstein MF, Folstein SE, McHugh PR: "Mini Mental State": A practical method for grading the cognitive state of patients for the clinician. J Psych Res 1975;12:189-198.

Glossary

A Normative Model of Physical Therapist Assistant Education Approved by the House of Delegates, this document is a guide for physical therapist assistant education programs to ensure that the academic program meets the quality and comprehensiveness established by the members of the profession.

A Normative Model of Physical Therapist Professional Education Approved by the House of Delegates, this document is a guide for physical therapist education programs to ensure that the academic program meets the quality and comprehensiveness established by the members of the profession.

access Ability for an individual to obtain health care services when needed.

accessory motion Ability of the joint surfaces to glide, roll, and spin on each other.

active assisted range of motion Joint movement in which the patient may be assisted either manually or mechanically through an arc of movement.

active free range of motion Joint movement in which the patient does not receive any support or resistance through an arc of movement.

active member Former membership category in the APTA for the physical therapist.

active range of motion (AROM) Ability of the patient to voluntarily move a limb through an arc of movement.

active resisted exercise Joint movement in which an external force resists the movement.

activities of daily living (ADLs) Activities in which individuals participate daily to meet their basic needs. Examples include bathing, dressing, using the toilet, and eating.

adaptive equipment Pieces of equipment that allow individuals to perform functional tasks with increased ease or independence.

aerobics training Exercise program that uses oxygen as the major energy source.

affective domain The domain of learning that deals with attitudes, values, and character development and that influences all other professional skills.

Affiliate Assembly Past component of the APTA that represented and was composed of physical therapist assistants; precursor to National Assembly.

affiliate member Former membership category in the APTA for the physical therapist assistant.

Affiliate Special Interest Group Past component of the APTA that served the interests of the physical therapist assistant; precursor to Affiliate Assembly.

akinesia Poverty of movements.

alliance Collaboration of several health care facilities and practices.

ambulatory center Any facility in which health care is provided on an outpatient basis; the patient is able to walk into the facility, receive care, and walk out of the facility the same day.

American Board of Physical Therapy Specialties (ABPTS) Unit created by the House of Delegates to provide a formal mechanism for recognizing physical therapists with advanced knowledge, skills, and experience in a special area of practice.

American Physical Therapy Association (APTA) National organization that represents and promotes the profession of physical therapy.

American Physiotherapy Association (APA) Organization (formerly called American Women's Physical Therapeutic Association) responsible for maintaining high standards and educational programs for physiotherapists; precursor to APTA.

American Women's Physical Therapeutic Association First national organization representing "physical therapeutics." Established in 1921 to maintain high standards and provide a mechanism to share information.

amyotrophic lateral sclerosis (ALS) Also known as Lou Gehrig's disease; rapidly progressive neurological disorder associated with a degeneration of the motor nerve cells.

anencephaly A form of neural tube defect that results from a lack of the neural tube closure at the base of the brain. It is not compatible with life and results in fetal death or death shortly after delivery.

angina Condition in which chest pain occurs from ischemia.

angiography Technique in which radiopaque material is injected into the blood vessels to better visualize and identify problems such as occlusion (blockage) of blood vessels, aneurysms, and vascular malformations.

angioplasty   Process of mechanically dilating a blood vessel.

annual conference and exposition   Yearly (usually June) meeting of the APTA, held in accordance with the bylaws, and including an extensive program of educational presentations, meetings, and activities.

aquatic physical therapy   Therapeutic use of water for rehabilitation or prevention of injury.

arterial insufficiency   Deficiency or occlusion of blood flow through an artery.

arteriosclerosis   Hardening of the arteries.

assembly   Component of APTA whose purpose is to provide a means by which members of the same class may meet, confer, and promote the interest of the respective membership class.

assessment   Measurement or assigned value by which physical therapists make a clinical judgment.

assistive device   Device that provides individuals with assistance to perform tasks or during periods of mobility. Examples include canes, walkers, and adapted keyboards.

autonomous practice   Services provided by physical therapists using independent, professional judgment within their scope of practice.

Bad Ragaz method   Aquatic therapy technique using proprioceptive neuromuscular facilitation techniques while the patient is suspended by rings in the water.

Balanced Budget Act of 1997 (BBA)   Federal legislation, passed by Congress and signed by President Clinton, that cut health care expenditures for Medicare and other government-sponsored programs to achieve a balanced budget.

beginning professional behaviors   Professional behaviors that develop during the didactic (academic) portion of the physical therapy curriculum.

beneficiary   Individual who is covered by a health insurance policy; as a result of this coverage, the person can receive health care benefits.

blood gas analysis   Assessment of blood (usually arterial) to determine the concentrations of oxygen and carbon dioxide.

Board of Directors (BOD)   APTA unit consisting of six APTA officers and nine directors, whose duty is to carry out the mandates and policies established by the HOD.

bradykinesia   Slowness of movements.

Brunnstrom's approach   Neurological technique based on the natural sequence of recovery following stroke.

bursitis   Inflammation of bursae, fluid-filled sacs located throughout the body that decrease the friction between two structures.

capitation   Method of payment (reimbursement) in some health maintenance organizations (HMOs). The HMO pays the health care provider a fixed dollar amount per member per month (PMPM) in advance (before services are delivered).

cardiac catheterization   Passage of a catheter (a flexible tube) into an artery in the arm or leg, then along the artery to reach the heart and measure pressure, inject dye, or take a tissue sample.

cardiac muscle dysfunction   Various pathological conditions associated with heart failure.

cardiac pacemaker   Electronic device that produces a pulse to control heart depolarization.

career ladder   Employer's structure, creating levels within a specific field or position to enable promotion of employees in that category.

case management   Process used to monitor and coordinate treatment delivered to patients usually requiring costly and extensive services.

case-mix   Method used to measure the mix of cases (patients) being treated by a health care provider and the scope of resources needed to serve this combination of patients.

Centers for Medicare and Medicaid Services (CMS)   Government agency within the Department of Health and Human Services responsible for directing the Medicare and Medicaid programs.

cerebral palsy (CP)   Group of conditions caused by a nonprogressive lesion on the brain. Most often CP has its origin during gestation (before birth), at birth, or immediately after birth, owing to an interruption of oxygen to the brain of the fetus or newborn.

certification   Process by which a state legally regulates the use of a professional title without creating a separate scope of practice. State law will not permit use of the title unless state standards are met. This differs from the private certification offered by private organizations for meeting the standards of that organization.

chapter   Organizational unit of the APTA that is defined by specific legally constituted boundaries such as a state, territory, or commonwealth of the United States or the District of Columbia. Membership is automatic and is based on location of residence or employment, education, or greatest active participation.

chronic inflammation   Low-grade, protracted inflammatory process.

chronic obstructive pulmonary disease (COPD)   Group of disorders that produce certain specific physical symptoms, including chronic productive cough, excessive mucus production, changes in the sound produced when air passes through the bronchial tubes, and shortness of breath (dyspnea).

civil law   Law of a jurisdiction concerned with private rights and remedies; the administration of justice involving the violation of private duties owed by individuals.

claims   Bills submitted by health care providers to health insurance and managed care companies for payment (reimbursement). Sometimes these claims are denied (not paid).

client   Individual who seeks the services of a physical therapist to maintain health, or a business that hires a physical therapist as a consultant.

closed kinetic chain exercise Exercise incorporating several muscle groups through the use of several joints with the end segment fixed.

clubfoot Disorder in which the foot is turned inward and slanted upward.

Code of Ethics Principles set forth for the physical therapy profession by the APTA for maintaining and promoting ethical practice.

coinsurance Cost-sharing obligation required by a health insurance policy. The subscriber assumes a percentage of the costs incurred.

collagen Supportive, strong, and fibrous connective tissue protein that is found in the dermis, tendon, cartilage, fascia, ligament, and bone.

Combined Sections Meeting Early February meeting of APTA sections' members to provide an opportunity for sharing information.

Commission on Accreditation in Physical Therapy Education (CAPTE) Unit responsible for evaluating and accrediting professional (entry level) physical therapist and physical therapist assistant education programs.

common law Law created by court decision rather than by legislative action.

components Organizational units within the APTA currently limited to chapters, sections, and assemblies as established by APTA bylaws.

computed (axial) tomography (CAT or CT) Computer synthesis of x-rays transmitted through a specific plane of the body.

conducting airways Passageways and tubes that allow air to pass into or out of the lungs.

congestive heart failure (CHF) Condition in which the heart muscle is compromised to the point that it cannot move blood volume effectively.

consumer-driven health plans Range of health insurance plans designed to allow different degrees of employer and employee responsibility. A common design allows for catastrophic (high severity–low incidence; high deductible) coverage combined with a health care spending account.

continuous quality improvement/total quality management (CQI/TQM) Method of examining and improving processes using data management tools.

continuum of care Health care provided within a system that meets all levels of need (e.g., from acute care, to inpatient medical rehabilitation or inpatient subacute rehabilitation, to home care, to outpatient care).

contract Agreement between two or more persons that creates a legal obligation to do, or not do, a particular thing.

copayment Fixed amount of money stipulated in the health insurance plan paid to the health care provider by a beneficiary at the time of service.

criminal law Administration of justice, through the enforcement of the criminal code of a state or of the United States; involves violations of duties owed to society at large.

coronary artery bypass grafting (CABG) Grafting (attaching) a small artery or a leg vein to a point beyond the blockage or plaque. This bypasses the blockage, reestablishing blood flow to the heart.

coronary heart disease (CHD) Arteriosclerosis, or a hardening of the arteries, affecting the coronary vessels.

covered services Services covered by a health insurance plan.

critical pathways Guidelines for patient hospital care using "milestones" to monitor progress; based on consensus, including only those aspects of care provided to affect patient outcomes.

cross-training Training health care professionals in treatment skills from a variety of professions to provide a multi-disciplinary team in a patient-focused care (PFC) model.

cryotherapy Application of cold agents to cause decreases in blood flow and metabolism, which result in a decrease in swelling and pain.

cultural continuum Theoretical model that describes six stages of culturally related behaviors, including cultural destructiveness, incapacity, blindness, precompetency, competency, and proficiency.

culture of medicine Beliefs, attitudes, and behaviors unique to the practice of medicine. Biomedical Western medicine operates primarily through low-context assumptions. These assumptions may conflict with those of practitioners, patients, and families who operate from more high-context assumptions.

Current Procedural Terminology (CPT) codes Standardized list of five-digit codes assigned to medical services and procedures.

customer satisfaction Satisfaction of the consumer receiving health care with the care and how it was provided.

cystic fibrosis (CF) Most common inherited chronic pulmonary disease among white children, characterized by the production of thick mucus with progressive lung damage.

deductible Amount of money that must be paid by the insured before a health insurer will assume any liability for covered services.

dermatitis Inflammation of the skin indicated by any one or all of the following: redness, rash, itching, irritation, and possible skin lesions.

dermis Portion of the skin directly under the dermis; it is made up of fibrous connective tissue and supports sweat glands, sebaceous glands, nerves and nerve endings, blood and lymph vessels, hair follicles, and their allied smooth muscle.

developing professional behaviors Professional behaviors that develop during the first half of each clinical internship of an education program.

developmental coordination disorder (DCD) Motor condition in children with a wide range of dysfunctions, including gross or fine motor coordination problems such as awkward running, frequent falling, slow reaction times, immature balance reactions, poor handwriting, and difficulty with activities of daily living such as dressing.

developmental delay Failure to attain predictable movement patterns or behaviors associated with children of a similar chronological age.

developmental dysplasia of the hip (DDH) Dislocation resulting from the abnormal development of some of the structures surrounding the hip joint, allowing the head of the femur to move in and out of the hip socket; cause is unknown.

developmental milestone Movement pattern that appears at a certain stage of growth and development.

diagnosis Final interpretation of findings based on examinations; in physical therapy the diagnosis must be made in accordance with a policy adopted by the APTA House of Delegates.

diagnostic related groups (DRGs) Classification scheme developed by the federal government as a means to establish uniform reimbursement for a variety of diagnostic conditions.

direct access Availability of the physical therapist to anyone seeking physical therapy services without stipulation of a referral by another health care provider.

disability Inability to perform a task in a particular context or environment.

disablement model Conceptual approach to health care based on the functional abilities of the patient/client that result from a medical condition. As applied to physical therapy, includes impairment, functional limitation, and disability.

disablement process Examination process that focuses on the individual's impairments, functional limitations, disability, and resultant restrictions in activities.

discharge Termination of services when goals have been achieved.

discontinuation Termination of services as determined by the patient/client or physical therapist (in the latter case when the patient/client is unable to continue or can no longer improve).

district Most local organizational unit in the structure of the APTA. Membership is automatic and may be based on location of residence or employment, as provided in the bylaws of the APTA.

doctor of physical therapy (DPT) Professional (entry level) degree in physical therapy at the clinical doctorate level.

Down syndrome Congenital developmental disability caused by a defect of chromosome 21; sometimes called trisomy 21.

Duchenne muscular dystrophy (DMD) Progressive pelvic muscle weakness and wasting in the male child, combined with enlarged, yet weak, thigh muscles and tight heel cords.

durable medical equipment Medical equipment prescribed by a medical provider for a patient's extended use.

dynamic balance Balance maintained with the body in motion.

dynamical systems theory Treatment approach in children that incorporates all of the body's systems with the environment to facilitate or inhibit movements. It emphasizes the process of moving rather than the product of a movement.

dysfunction Any functional disability.

dyspnea Shortness of breath.

echocardiography Technique using high-frequency ultrasound to assess the size of the heart chambers, the thickness of the chamber walls, and the motion of the chamber walls and heart valves.

eclectic approach Combination of therapeutic approaches used by the physical therapist and thought to be useful for treatment of a given client.

electrical stimulation Application of electricity at specified locations to stimulate nerves, muscles, and other soft tissues to reduce pain and swelling, to increase strength and range of motion, and to facilitate wound healing.

electrocardiogram (ECG) Readout produced by placing electrodes on the anterior chest wall to record depolarization or contraction of the heart muscle; assesses the heart's rate and rhythm.

electroencephalography (EEG) Technique for recording the electrical potential/activity in the brain by placing electrodes on the scalp.

electromyography (EMG) Technique for recording the electrical activity in the muscle during a state of rest and during voluntary contraction.

embolus Clot formed by a substance detached from elsewhere.

employer-sponsored health insurance Health insurance offered to employees by employers; offered as a benefit of employment.

enablement process Examination process that focuses on the individual's structural body and concurrent abilities while addressing age-appropriate movement patterns and activities.

entitlement Right or privilege.

entry level professional behaviors Professional behaviors that develop during the second half of each clinical internship of an education program.

epidermis Outer layer of the skin.

ergonomics Relationship between the worker, tasks, and work environment.

evaluation Judgment based on an examination.

Evaluative Criteria for Accreditation of Education Programs for the Preparation of Physical Therapists Standards and criteria approved by the House of Delegates to ensure quality and consistency in physical therapy education programs.

Evaluative Criteria for Accreditation of Education Programs for the Preparation of Physical Therapist Assistants Standards and criteria approved by the House of Delegates to ensure quality and consistency in physical therapist assistant education programs.

evidence-based practice Interventions used in physical therapy based on research that demonstrates the reliability and validity of the procedures.

examination Process of gathering information about the past and current status of the patient/client.

exercise stress testing Noninvasive method of determining how the cardiovascular and pulmonary systems respond to controlled increases in activity; most frequently used to diagnose or assess suspected or established cardiovascular disease.

expiration Breathing out.

expressive aphasia Impaired ability to express oneself.

family assessment Family interview, survey, or discussion used to obtain the family's insights regarding a patient, especially a child; includes family history, relationships, concerns, needs, and resources.

Federation of State Boards of Physical Therapy (FSBPT) National organization through which member state boards work together to promote and protect the health, welfare, and safety of the American public by identifying and promoting desirable and reasonable uniformity in physical therapy regulatory standards and practices.

fee-for-services (FFS) A method of health care reimbursement in which a health care provider bills the health insurer a fee for each service provided.

fee schedule A listing of health care services in which a specific amount of money is associated with each service.

fetal alcohol syndrome (FAS) Most severe condition in a continuum of alcohol-induced disabilities related to high levels of maternal alcohol consumption during pregnancy.

flexibility Ability to move a limb segment through a range of motion.

flexibility exercise Exercise performed over time, using stress, to change the length and elasticity of soft tissue such as muscle; usually performed for postural or ROM enhancement.

fluidotherapy Use of a self-contained unit filled with sawdust-type particles heated to the desired temperature and circulated by air pressure around the involved body part.

Foundation for Physical Therapy Organization, separate from the APTA, that promotes and provides financial support for scientific research, clinical research, and health services research in physical therapy.

fracture Break in a bone.

frail elderly People over 65 with conditions that significantly impair their daily function.

functional capacity evaluation Examination of a worker's physical abilities to perform required tasks.

functional exercise Exercise that mimics functional movements and activities. Functional movements incorporate strength, flexibility, balance, and coordination.

functional limitation Decreased ability of a person to perform a task, without regard to the context or environment.

Functional Reach Test Specific balance test that can predict the likelihood of falling.

gatekeeper Health care provider who provides the consumer with access to the health care system. Historically, this has been the primary care physician.

generic abilities Behaviors essential for physical therapy professionals that are not explicitly part of the profession's core of knowledge and technical skills but are required for success in the profession.

goal-directed movement approach Treatment approach that emphasizes the importance of both task and environmental features as a primary impetus for movement.

goals Measurable, functional objectives that are linked to a problem identified in a patient evaluation.

goniometer Instrument used to measure and document ROM.

goniometry Methods to measure and document ROM.

ground substance Supportive, amorphous gel-like substance secreted by fibroblasts; fills space between connective tissue fibers and cells.

Guide to Physical Therapist Practice Extensive description of the roles and scope of practice of a physical therapist. Describes tests and measures and procedural interventions for patients and clients for musculoskeletal, neuromuscular, cardiovascular and pulmonary, and integumentary conditions.

Halliwick method Aquatic therapy technique using a preswim stroke instruction and musculoskeletal rehabilitation.

health insurance Financial protection against health care costs arising from disease or injury.

health maintenance organization (HMO) Prepaid health insurance that may provide all health care services needed within one facility.

heart failure Decrease in the pumping capability of the heart muscle.

high-context assumptions Assumptions found in cultures in which the group is more important than the individual. Communication is indirect; meaning is based on implicit cues. Nonverbal aspects such as posture, eye contact, and gesture are considered.

history Description of the past and current health status of the patient/client.

hot pack Pouch filled with silica gel and soaked in thermostatically controlled water.

House of Delegates (HOD) Highest policymaking body of the APTA, consisting of voting chapter delegates and nonvoting section and assembly delegates and members of the Board of Directors.

hydrotherapy Use of the therapeutic effects of water by immersing the body part or entire body into a tank of water.

hypermobile joint Joint with excessive motion.

hypertonia High tone.

hypertrophic scar Excess of collagen deposited at the site of a healing or healed wound that is noticeably different from the normal skin; scar remains within the boundaries of the original wound.

hypokinesis State of decreased activity or movement.

hypomobile joint Joint with less motion than is considered functional.

hypotonia Low tone.

impairment Loss or abnormality in a function at the cellular, tissue, organ, or system level.

indemnity Health insurance plan that defines maximum amounts that will be paid for covered services.

independent practice association (IPA) model Organized form of prepaid medical practice in which participating providers remain in their own (independent) practice settings yet negotiate contracts with health insurers as a group (organization).

Individualized Education Plan (IEP) Model using collaboration of therapists, family, educators, and other health care team members to provide direct intervention in the classroom setting.

Individualized Family Service Plan (IFSP) Detailed total plan of care for the child in the context of the family unit.

inflammatory phase Phase of wound healing encompassing vascular reactions that decrease blood loss and initiate vessel repair, and cellular responses that moderate blood loss, fight infection, and provide nutrition and oxygen to initiate and sustain tissue repair.

inflammatory skin diseases Diseases of the skin whose etiologies invoke an inflammatory response (etiologies for these diseases commonly include immune reactions and contact irritants or allergens).

infringement Situation occurring in health care, in which one health care provider performs the skills and techniques of another health care provider.

inspiration Contraction of the muscles of respiration, resulting in an increase in the space contained within the thoracic cavity. This expansion causes the air pressure to drop inside the lungs, resulting in movement of air into the lungs.

instrumental activities of daily living (IADLs) Activities that individuals must perform to function in the community. Examples include shopping, driving, and paying bills.

insured Individual covered by a health insurance plan.

insurer Organization that offers health insurance plans.

integument Skin.

internal dialogue Communication within an individual ("silent talking" to oneself) that may affect nonverbal communication with other people.

intervention Procedure conducted with the patient/client to achieve the desired outcomes.

ischemia Insufficient oxygenation of tissues owing to a blocked blood vessel.

joint mobilization and manipulation Technique used when a patient's dysfunction is the result of joint stiffness or hypomobility (loss of motion); applies to a joint specific passive movements, either oscillatory (rapid, repeated movements) or sustained.

juvenile rheumatoid arthritis (JRA) One of the many rheumatic diseases characterized by an inflammation of the connective tissue that manifests as a painful inflamed joint (arthritis); begins in childhood.

keloid scar Excess of collagen deposited at the site of a healing or healed wound that is noticeably different from the normal skin; scar commonly extends beyond the boundaries of the original wound.

LAMP document Document created by the Section on Health Policy and Administration of the American Physical Therapy Association that describes behaviors for the development of Leadership, Administration, Management, and Professionalism in Physical Therapy (LAMP).

law Formal rule having binding legal force laid down, ordained, or established by a governing body.

licensure Process by which the state grants permission to practice a profession to an individual who has met state standards and grants legal recognition to a particular scope of practice.

low-context assumptions Assumptions found in cultures in which the individual is considered more important than the group. Communication is direct; meaning is based on explicit verbal cues. Communication is less dependent on cues or nuances and is influenced by what the speaker is saying.

lumbar puncture (LP) Injection of a hypodermic needle into the lumbar subarachnoid space.

magnetic resonance imaging (MRI) Creation of a computer image by placing the body part in a magnetic field.

malpractice Failure to do (or avoid doing) something that a reasonably prudent member of the profession would have done (or would not have done), with subsequent injury to a patient/client.

managed care Arrangement in which an insurance company contracts with health care providers to provide health care to the consumers who subscribe to the insurance plan.

managed care organization (MCO) Health insurer that offers managed care plans.

manual muscle testing (MMT) Test allowing the therapist to assign a specific grade to a muscle, based on whether the patient can hold the limb against gravity, how much manual resistance can be tolerated, and whether there is full range of motion at a joint.

massage Systematic use of various manual strokes designed to produce certain physiological, mechanical, and psychological effects.

matching One method of developing rapport. It may include mirroring the body language or using similar verbal pacing, tonality, intent, or speed of communication of the person with whom one is communicating.

maturation phase Phase of wound healing that includes collagen synthesis and lysis, as well as reorientation of the collagen fibers that remain at the wound site; this phase may also be referred to as the remodeling phase.

Medicaid Reimbursement system established at the state level to provide health care for those with limited financial means.

Medicare Reimbursement system established at the federal level for individuals over 65 years of age.

Medicare Advantage (Medicare Part C) Medicare program developed under the 1997 Balanced Budget Act that offers more flexibility for beneficiaries. Persons eligible for Medicare Parts A and B are also eligible for this program.

Medicare Fee Schedule Physician fee schedule (payments) allowed by Medicare to those who provide services to Medicare beneficiaries.

Medicare Modernization Act (MMA) Legislation (Medicare Prescription Drug Improvement and Modernization Act of 2003) that provides a prescription drug benefit, more choices, and better benefits to Medicare beneficiaries.

Medicare Part A—Hospital Insurance Hospital insurance covered under Medicare. This program helps to pay for care in hospitals as an inpatient, critical access hospitals (small facilities that give limited outpatient and inpatient services to people in rural areas), skilled nursing facilities, hospice care, and some home health care. Most people get Part A automatically when they turn age 65. They do not have to pay a monthly premium for Part A because they or a spouse paid Medicare taxes while they were working.

Medicare Part B—Supplementary Medical Insurance Medical insurance covered under Medicare. This program helps to pay for doctors' services, outpatient hospital care, and some other medical services that Part A does not cover, such as the services of physical and occupational therapists, and some home health care. Part B helps to pay for these covered services and supplies when they are medically necessary. Enrollment in part B is voluntary, and individuals pay a Medicare Part B premium ($88.50 per month in 2006).

meningocele Benign herniation of the meninges presenting as a soft tissue cyst or lump that surrounds a normal spinal cord and produces no neurological deficits.

meningomyelocele Open congenital spinal cord lesion with minimal to no skin protection covering the deeper nerve roots.

Minimum Data Set (MDS) A specified collection of data that is documented and used to measure the amount of care provided to a patient at a skilled nursing facility

motor control Ability to manipulate movement and non-movement of the body's musculoskeletal components.

motor development Age-related processes of change in motor behavior.

motor learning Body's mechanism for acquiring or learning voluntary motor control.

multiple sclerosis (MS) Disease in which patches of demyelination occur in the nervous system, leading to disturbances in conduction of messages along the nerves.

muscle endurance Ability to produce and sustain tension over a prolonged period of time.

muscular strength Maximal amount of tension an individual can produce in one repetition.

myocardial infarction Heart attack resulting from blockage by an embolus (clot) of one of the coronary arteries.

myofascial release Manual stretching of the layers of the body's fascia (connective tissue that surrounds muscle and other soft tissues in the body).

National Assembly of Physical Therapist Assistants (National Assembly) Former Component of the APTA that consisted of all affiliate (physical therapist assistant) and life affiliate (retired) members. Included officers and regional directors who represented the interests of its members.

National Foundation for Infantile Paralysis ("the Foundation") Foundation established in 1938 in response to repeated polio epidemics. Established to provide research, education, and patient services.

negligence Failure to do something that a reasonably prudent person would do, or behavior that would normally not be done under similar circumstances.

neoplastic skin diseases Cancers affecting the skin.

nerve conduction velocity (NCV) study Study that records the rate at which electrical signals are transmitted along peripheral nerves.

nerve entrapment Pressure on a nerve.

neural tube defect Condition in which the neural tube fails to close completely during the first month of gestational development.

neurodevelopmental treatment (NDT) Approach to both analyze and treat neurological disorders of posture and movement. Through the use of a motivating environment and a patient's active participation, manual facilitation and inhibition techniques are employed by the therapist to present the patient with a "normal" sensory experience, thereby encouraging facilitation of a more functional motor response.

neuropathic (neurotropic) ulcer Skin lesion caused by a decreased cutaneous sensation that disallows protective responses such as weight transfer; these ulcers are commonly associated with diabetes mellitus.

norm referenced Type of assessment based on a large number of participants to create a comparison group for the assessment. In children norm referenced assessments can be used to compare a child's functional abilities or activities with those of other children of the same age.

normal developmental theory Model asserting that therapy goals and objectives are designed to follow the progression of normal motor development. Assumes that children with central nervous system damage will acquire motor skills in a similar fashion to children with normally developing nervous systems.

objective examination Quantitative or qualitative measurements that are taken by the physical therapist or physical therapist assistant or by use of a mechanical device.

obstructive lung disease Pathological abnormality in airflow through the bronchial tubes.

open enrollment Specific period of time each year in which a health insurer must accept all who apply for health insurance coverage.

open kinetic chain exercise Exercise in which the end limb segment is free.

osteoarthritis Condition characterized by degeneration of cartilage as a result of many years of use. Hands, spine, knees, and hips are most commonly affected.

osteogenesis imperfecta (OI) Common and severe bone impairment of genetic origin. Affects the formation of collagen during bone development, resulting in frequent fractures during the fetal or newborn period.

osteoporosis Decreased mineralization of the bones caused by a decreased production of new bone cells and an increased resorption of bone.

paraffin treatment Use of a mixture of melted paraffin wax and mineral oil maintained at a specific temperature to promote relaxation and pain relief and allow greater comfort during range-of-motion exercises.

paraplegia Spinal cord damage and resultant loss of sensory or motor function affecting the lower trunk and legs.

Parkinson's disease Progressive condition, also referred to as paralysis agitans and idiopathic parkinsonism, characterized by a classic triad of symptoms: tremor, rigidity, and bradykinesia/akinesia.

passive range of motion (PROM) Amount of movement at a joint that is obtained by the therapist's moving the segment without assistance from the patient.

pathology/pathophysiology Interruption of normal processes, usually at the cellular level, exhibited as abnormal signs or symptoms.

patient Individual who has a disorder that requires interventions to improve function.

patient-focused care (PFC) Patient care model in which all departments in a hospital are decentralized and professional staff are assigned to work on multidisciplinary teams; usually involves cross-training of health care professionals.

perception Ability to integrate various simultaneous sensory inputs and to respond appropriately.

per diem Method of health care reimbursement; a set payment per day.

pharmaceutical formularies Usually a list of generic drugs and their indications for use.

physiatrist Title given to physicians who specialize in physical medicine.

physical therapist (PT) Professional who works to evaluate, treat, and/or prevent physical disability, movement dysfunction, and pain resulting from injury, disability, disease, or other health-related conditions.

physical therapist assistant (PTA) Health care provider who assists the PT in the provision of physical therapy and has graduated from an accredited physical therapist assistant associate degree program.

physical professional therapist education All academic programs that prepare students for *entry* into the field of physical therapy, regardless of the degree.

physical therapy Assessment, evaluation, treatment, and prevention of physical disability, movement dysfunctions, and pain resulting from injury, disease, disability, or other health-related conditions.

physical therapy aide Support personnel who perform designated tasks that do not require the clinical decision making of the physical therapist or the clinical problem solving of the physical therapist assistant.

physician-owned physical therapy service (POPTS) Physical therapy service owned or invested in by a physician.

physiotherapist Synonym for physical therapist, commonly used outside the United States.

physiotherapy Synonym for physical therapy, commonly used outside the United States; used by the first national organization, American Women's Physical Therapeutic Association.

plan of care Goals, interventions (including duration and frequency), desired outcomes, and criteria for discharge.

point-of-service (POS) Health insurance plan in which subscribers can select the type of health care at the time of need; allows more subscriber choice, usually at a higher cost.

policy Plan or course of action designed to influence and determine decisions. APTA further defines this as "a decision which obligates actions or subsequent decisions on similar matters."

post–entry level professional behaviors Professional behaviors that develop once the physical therapist is working in the profession of physical therapy.

postprofessional education Advanced education of a licensed physical therapist, at the certificate, master's, or doctorate level.

postural drainage Use of gravity through appropriate positioning and chest wall percussion to promote removal of excessive secretions from the tracheo-bronchial tree.

practice act State's official statement or document of definition and regulation of a specific profession, setting down guidelines for those practicing the profession within its jurisdiction.

preferred provider organization (PPO) Organization formed by hospitals and other health care providers that provides health care services to purchasers, usually at discounted rates.

premium Money owed to the health insurance company upfront to guarantee future health insurance coverage.

prenatal cocaine exposure Fetal exposure to cocaine in utero owing to maternal cocaine use during pregnancy. Infants often show clinical signs of exposure after birth such as hyperirritability, poor feeding patterns, high respiratory and heart rates, increased tremulousness, and irregular sleeping patterns.

presbycusis Decreased ability to perceive higher pitches and to distinguish between similar sounds.

pressure ulcer Skin lesion caused by ischemia of the integument secondary to pressure; these ulcers are generally located at bony prominences.

prevention Services designed to avoid the occurrence of pain and dysfunction or to limit or reduce those that exist.

primary care Level of health care delivered by a member of the health care system who is responsible for the majority of the health care needs of the individual.

primary care provider (PCP) Generalist physician who provides primary care; commonly a family practice, internal medicine, or general pediatric physician.

profession Career or means of employment demonstrating five characteristics: commitment to field, a representative organization, knowledge in a specific area, social service, and recognized autonomy.

professional misconduct Violation of the state statutes and/or regulations that define competent professional practice by those professionals regulated by the state.

prognosis Prediction of the level of improvement and time necessary to reach that level.

proliferative phase Phase of wound healing that involves increased activity of fibroblasts, instigation of aggressive wound contraction, and epithelialization.

proprioception One's awareness of position and movement.

proprioceptive neuromuscular facilitation (PNF) Technique used to enhance movement and motor control, emphasizing proprioceptive (joint and position sense) stimuli but also using tactile, visual, and auditory stimuli.

proprioceptors Receptors found in the skin and joints that respond to such stimuli as pressure, stretch, and position.

prospective payment system (PPS) Establishment of a reimbursement rate to be paid in advance of the delivery of care. It is often based on the diagnosis and level of care needed.

provider contracting The process used by managed care companies to negotiate contracts (formal, legal relationships) with providers for the future provision of health care services.

provider network (panel) Formal affiliations of health care providers with third party payers.

PTA Caucus A body consisting of one physical therapist assistant representative from each chapter of the American Physical Therapy Association. It meets annually just before the House of Delegates and provides input to the latter through five delegates from the Caucus.

pulmonary function test Assessment of the effectiveness of the respiratory musculature and the integrity of the airways and lung tissues to help classify the lung disease pattern as obstructive or restrictive.

quadriplegia Spinal cord damage resulting in loss of sensory or motor function affecting all limbs.

range of motion (ROM) Movement at a joint.

range-of-motion exercise Exercise for mobility of a joint. Falls into two categories: active or passive. Active ROM exercise involves voluntary movement of a limb through an arc of movement; passive ROM exercise involves the *therapist's* moving the limb without patient assistance.

rapport—cultural, verbal, and behavioral Communication that is characterized by mutual collaboration and respect but does not necessarily indicate agreement. It occurs at the cultural (style of greeting and form of dress), verbal (verbal pacing, tonality, speed), and behavioral levels (body language and gestures).

receptive aphasia Diminished ability to receive and interpret verbal or written communication.

reconstruction aide Aide (exclusively a woman) responsible for providing physical reconstruction to persons injured in war; forerunners of the profession and practice of physical therapy in the United States.

registration Process by which the state tracks regulated professionals by requiring updated listing of names, addresses, and qualifications. This generally does not involve a review of whether standards of practice are met.

regulation Administrative or departmental rules issued to carry out the intent of the law.

reimbursement The process of payment for the provision of health care services. Typically health care providers are reimbursed by third party payers who insure patients.

Representative Body of the National Assembly (RBNA) Former deliberative body for the physical therapist assistant with representatives from each chapter. Replaced by the PTA Caucus.

resisted exercise Form of active movement in which some form of resistance is provided to increase muscular strength and endurance.

resisted test Test that allows the therapist to determine the general strength of a muscle group and assess whether any pain is produced with the muscle contraction.

resource-based relative value scale (RBRVS) Medicare payment rules for physician services established as part of the Omnibus Reconciliation Act of 1989.

resource utilization groups (RUGs) The Balanced Budget Act (1997) changed Medicare reimbursement for skilled nursing facilities (SNFs) from cost-based to a prospective payment system (PPS). Under the PPS, SNFs are required to assign residents to 1 of 44 resource utilization groups that are calculated based on a clinical assessment tool.

respiration Process of exchanging oxygen and carbon dioxide between the air a person breathes and the cells of the body.

restrictive lung disease Pathological reduction of the volume of air in the lungs.

retrospective reimbursement Payment made to providers after health care services have been rendered.

rheumatoid arthritis Chronic inflammation of the joints, of unknown etiology.

rigidity Disturbance of muscle tone; manifests as a resistance when the limbs are passively moved.

risk Probability of a financial loss.

risk management Process by which coordinated efforts are made by an organization to identify, assess, and minimize the risk of harm and loss to the organization, employees, and clients.

Rood's approach Neurological treatment using a variety of sensory stimuli to influence motor behavior.

scar contraction Dynamic movement of the edges of a scar (wound boundaries) toward each other.

scar contracture Permanent or relatively permanent lack of mobility of the scar tissue that results in functional and/or cosmetic impairment.

scoliosis Lateral curvature of the spine; may be idiopathic (of unknown origin), neuromuscular, or congenital (present at birth).

screening Procedure to determine if there is a need for further services of a physical therapist or other health care professional.

secondary care Services provided by individuals on a referral basis.

secondary condition Condition that is potentially preventable and is a direct or indirect consequence of inadequate attention to (or inadequate amelioration of) an impairment or disability.

section National level of organizational unit of the APTA for members of all classes to promote similar interests. Membership is voluntary.

self-assessment Ability to critically examine and evaluate one's own cognitive, affective, and psychomotor behaviors in the professional setting.

sensation Ability to receive sensory input from within and outside the body and transmit it through the peripheral nerves and tracts in the spinal cord to the brain, where it is received and interpreted.

sensory integration (SI) Technique based on the theory that poor integration and use of sensory input (feedback) prevent subsequent motor planning (output). Providing controlled vestibular and somatosensory experiences enables the child to integrate the sensory information to evoke a spontaneous, functional response.

short-wave diathermy Use of electromagnetic energy to produce deep therapeutic heating effects.

SOAP note Documentation format taken from the Problem-Oriented Medical Record System; its components are (1) Subjective (what the patient/family member describes), (2) Objective (what the physical therapist observes/measures), (3) Assessment (clinical judgment based on evaluation; includes goals), and (4) Plan (of care).

soft tissue mobilization One of a variety of "hands-on" techniques designed to improve movement and decrease pain.

special interest group (SIG) One of many groups existing at multiple levels of the APTA to enable members at all levels to organize into smaller specialty areas.

special tests Tests designed for examination of specific joints to indicate the presence or absence of a particular problem.

spina bifida Congenital incomplete closure of a vertebra.

spina bifida occulta Congenital incomplete closure of a vertebra (separation of the spinous process) that is not associated with disability.

spinal cord injury (SCI) Damage to the spinal cord that results in neurological dysfunction.

spinal muscular atrophy (SMA) Genetic disorder characterized by severe muscle weakness in infancy and progressive respiratory failure.

spirometer Instrument measuring the various volumes and airflow rates, which are then compared to a normal scale.

sprain Overstretching of a joint ligament accompanied by a tearing of the fibers, causing pain and instability of the joint.

staff model (of HMO) A managed care organizational (MCO) model in which the health care providers are employed by the MCO.

standardized testing Type of formal test in which the evaluation procedures remain the same when administered by different therapists and at variable test locations.

Standards of Ethical Conduct for the Physical Therapist Assistant Principles set forth by the APTA for maintaining and promoting high standards of professional conduct among affiliate member physical therapist assistants.

Standards of Practice for Physical Therapy Document approved by the House of Delegates of the APTA that identifies conditions and performances essential for the provision of high-quality physical therapy.

State Children's Health Insurance Program (SCHIP) Program under the Centers for Medicare and Medicaid Services administered by the states for uninsured children. Matching funds are provided by the federal government to help states expand health care coverage.

static balance Balance maintained while standing still.

statute Formal written enactment by the legislative department of government.

strain Tearing of muscle fibers, caused by a sudden contraction of a muscle or excessive stretch to the muscle.

strength Amount of force produced during a voluntary muscular contraction.

stroke or cerebrovascular accident (CVA) Neurological problem arising from disruption of blood flow in the brain.

Student Assembly Component of the APTA whose members are physical therapist and physical therapist assistant students; provides a forum in which physical therapist and physical therapist assistant students can better understand their roles.

subjective examination Interview of the patient about the extent and nature of an injury; a qualitative measurement based on the patient's perception of the problem.

subscriber Individual who makes an advance payment for something; specifically, an employee who pays a health insurance premium through his or her employer to purchase a health insurance policy.

systems review Brief examination to provide information about the general health of the patient/client, including the physiological, anatomical, and cognitive status.

target heart rate (THR) Appropriate heart rate to be maintained during the peak period in aerobic training; calculated as a percentage of the individual's maximum heart rate.

tendinitis Inflammation of a tendon, a structure that is located at the ends of muscles and attaches muscle to bone.

tendinopathy Disorder of a tendon.

tendinosis Degeneration of a tendon from overuse.

tertiary care Service provided by specialists, who are commonly employed in facilities that focus on particular health conditions.

tests and measures Specific procedures selected and performed to quantify the physical and functional status of the patient/client.

thermal agent Agent used to modify the temperature of surrounding tissue, resulting in a change in the amount of blood flow to the injured area.

third party administrator/payer Organization that pays (or insures) health and medical expenses on behalf of beneficiaries.

tone Tension exerted and/or maintained by muscles at rest and during movement.

tort Civil injury for which the injured party can seek legal relief from the courts.

total body surface area (TBSA) Represents the extent of the surface of the body covered by skin. The percent TBSA used to describe the size of a skin injury (routinely used to estimate the size of a burn injury).

training zone Individual's ideal range of minimum and maximum heart rates (see target heart rate) that must be achieved for that individual to produce an aerobic training effect.

traumatic brain injury (TBI) Damage to the brain caused by physical means and resulting in neurological dysfunction.

tremor Alternating contractions of opposing muscle groups.

Trialliance Organization that consists of the APTA, the American Occupational Therapy Association, and the American Speech-Language and Hearing Association and meets to discuss issues of mutual concern.

ultrasound Therapeutic application of high-frequency sound waves that penetrate through tissue and cause an increase in the tissue temperature to promote healing and reduce pain.

usual, customary, and reasonable (UCR) Range of fees allowable for physician reimbursement based on typical charges that fall within a reasonable cost of service.

utilization Use of services.

utilization review (UR) An evaluation of the need, correctness, and efficiency of the health care services and procedures.

Vancouver Burn Scar Scale Clinical method for assessing scar tissue. The characteristics of scar that are examined include pigmentation, vascularity, pliability, and height.

venous insufficiency Deficiency or occlusion of blood flow through a vein.

ventilation Process of inspiration and expiration; results in an exchange of oxygen and carbon dioxide between the air found in the lungs and the pulmonary circulation.

vertigo Sensation of spinning or whirling that occurs as a result of a disturbance in balance.

vicarious liability Principle by which one individual may be held indirectly liable legally for the acts of another; for example, the liability of an employer for the acts of an employee during the performance of job responsibilities.

Vision 2020 A statement (and sentence in abridged version) adopted by the American Physical Therapy Association House of Delegates in 2000 that establishes expectations for the practice of physical therapy in the year 2020. It addresses six components: autonomous practice, direct access, practitioner of choice, doctor of physical therapy, evidence-based practice, and professionalism.

well elderly   People 65 years and over who are not experiencing physical limitations or who have age-related changes that are not significant enough to affect function.

whirlpool   Tank of water used in hydrotherapy for immersing a body part or the entire body.

work-conditioning program   Intervention for an individual with a work-related injury, focusing mostly on physical dysfunctions (e.g., strength, range of motion, and cardiovascular endurance).

work-hardening program   Intervention for an individual with a work-related injury, broad in scope to include behavioral and vocational management (e.g., counseling) as well as physical dysfunctions.

World Confederation of Physical Therapy (WCPT)   International organization that represents physical therapy on a global level and consists of physical therapy organizations in member nations.

Index